Minimally Invasive Dentistry

Interdisciplinary Clinical and Scientific Approaches

Edited by
Aylin Baysan and Paul Anderson

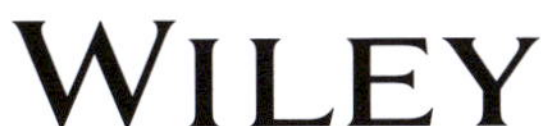

Registered Offices
John Wiley & Sons, Inc., 111 River Street, Hoboken, NJ 07030, USA
John Wiley & Sons Ltd, New Era House, 8 Oldlands Way, Bognor Regis, West Sussex, PO22 9NQ, UK

For details of our global editorial offices, customer services, and more information about Wiley products visit us at www.wiley.com.

The manufacturer's authorized representative according to the EU General Product Safety Regulation is Wiley-VCH GmbH, Boschstr. 12, 69469 Weinheim, Germany, e-mail: Product_Safety@wiley.com.

Wiley also publishes its books in a variety of electronic formats and by print-on-demand. Some content that appears in standard print versions of this book may not be available in other formats.

Library of Congress Cataloging-in-Publication Data Applied for

Paperback ISBN: 9781119215066
ePDF: 9781119215004
epub: 9781119215011

Cover Design: Wiley
Cover Image: © Ayiln Baysan and Paul Anderson

Set in 9.5/12.5pt STIXTwoText by Straive, Pondicherry, India

Printed in Singapore
M062874220725

Contents

1   Introduction to Minimally Invasive Dentistry: History of Minimally Invasive Dentistry and Key Concepts   *1*
Aylin Baysan and Kenneth Eaton

2   Where Are We with the Evidence for Minimally Invasive Dentistry?   *11*
Derek Richards and Valeria Marinho

List of Contributors

Bennett T. Amaechi
Department of Comprehensive Dentistry
University of Texas Health Science Center
at San Antonio, San Antonio
TX, USA

Paul Anderson
Institute of Dentistry
Queen Mary University of London
London, UK

Paul Ashley
Paediatric Dentistry, University College
London, London, UK

Aylin Baysan
School of Medicine and Dentistry
Hacettepe University
Ankara, Turkey

Lesley Ann Bergmeier
Institute of Dentistry
Queen Mary University of London
London, UK

Kenneth Eaton
Eastman Dental Institute
London, UK

Tarek El-Bialy
Katz Group Centre for Pharmacy and
Health Research University of Alberta
Edmonton, Alberta, Canada

John Featherstone
School of Dentistry, University of
California San Francisco
San Francisco, CA, USA

David Gillam
Institute of Dentistry, Queen Mary
University of London, London, UK

Sevil Gurgan
School of Medicine and Dentistry
Hacettepe University
Ankara, Turkey

Robert Hill
Institute of Dentistry
Queen Mary University of London
London, UK

Zeynep Bilge Kutuk
Hacettepe University
Ankara, Turkey

Valeria Marinho
Barts and the London, Queen Mary
University of London, London, UK

Nik Pandya
Queen Mary University of London
London, UK

Derek Richards
Dental Public Health
London, UK

Saroash Shahid
Institute of Dentistry
Queen Mary University of London
London, UK

Alastair J. Sloan
Cardiff University
Cardiff, UK

Wendy Turner
Queen Mary University of London
London, UK

Ferranti Wong
Queen Mary University of London
London, UK

Foreword

Having been a strong proponent of minimally invasive dentistry for many years, I am delighted to have been asked to prepare this Foreword. Also, being firmly of the view that all forms of interventive oral healthcare should be minimally invasive, underpinned by sound science and the best available evidence, and delivered as part of a holistic, patient-centred care, I am delighted to commend this book.

While it is recognized that 'more experimental research, and research of better methodological quality is needed' in the field of minimally invasive dentistry, this book makes a compelling case for the approaches advocated. With considerations ranging from saliva – 'a precious body fluid' – as a 'totally non-invasive mechanism for the protection and repair of the dental hard tissues', not to forget its importance in tooth surface loss and periodontal disease processes, to the impact of minimally invasive approaches on the socio-economic impact of oral and dental disease, this book sheds much-needed light on the enormous importance of minimally invasive dentistry, specifically in the future planning and provision of oral healthcare. In the meantime, this thought-provoking book should make readers consider their continuing use of unnecessarily interventive, traditional approaches in their clinical practice of dentistry. As such, this book will help drive the most welcome dynamic, paradigm shift in dentistry, whereby dentists are becoming as much oral physicians as dental surgeons, and dental teams no longer simply 'treat' but 'care' for their patients and, in the process, promote a better patient understanding of oral and dental diseases, personal engagement in achieving and maintaining oral health and more widespread appreciation of the importance of oral health to general health and well-being at all ages.

Reading the chapter on developments in dental biomaterials science, which facilitate the practice of minimally invasive dentistry, reinforces the view that many of the impressive materials available today are not being used to their best possible advantage – a problem caused by, amongst other things, teaching in dental schools lagging behind state-of-the-art practice, a reluctance by some oral healthcare professions to 'move with the times', and advances in dental biomaterials science being a less attractive topic for continuing professional development programmes than topics such as implant and aesthetic dentistry. Using the right materials, in the right place, at the right time can greatly enhance clinical outcomes.

The inclusion of chapters on Paediatric Dentistry and Orthodontics helps dispel regrettable misunderstandings that minimally invasive dentistry applies to adult dental care only.

Unnecessary, iatrogenic damage done to permanent teeth during childhood and adolescent years, apart from having possible adverse effects on young patients' attitudes to dental care, can lead to a lifetime of repair and replacement therapies, which drive the 'restorative downward spiral', resulting in the early loss of teeth, let alone a lifetime of spiralling costs of care – once a restorative patient, always a restorative patient. Minimally invasive dentistry should be firmly embedded in cradle-to-grave oral healthcare.

While one of the messages from this book is that the development of minimally invasive dentistry remains 'work in progress', colleagues are encouraged to keep on top of innovations as they occur, using this book as a 'stepping stone' in the journey to remain at the forefront of cutting-edge, minimally invasive dentistry. This book facilitates 'boldly going' where the practice of dentistry must be in years to come to best serve the interests of existing and future generations of patients.

Nairn Wilson DSc (*h.c.*), DDent (*h.c.*), PhD, MSc, BDS, FCGDent,
FDS, *RCS Edin, Eng (Hon) & RCPS Glasg (Hon)*,
FFD (*Hon*), FCDSHK (*Hon*), DRD, FHEA,
FICD, FACD, FADM, FPFA, FKC
Emeritus Professor of Dentistry, King's College London;
President Emeritus, College of General Dentistry

Preface

Minimally invasive dentistry (MID) has emerged as a cornerstone of innovative clinical practice, offering a tailored, patient-centered approach to oral health care. Grounded in the principles of early detection, prevention, tissue preservation and the use of advanced materials and technologies, MID represents a shift away from conventional, invasive methods towards more conservative, sustainable and biologically respectful strategies. As dental science continues to evolve, our methods are guided by research, clinical outcomes and ethical responsibility.

This book presents a comprehensive overview of minimally invasive dentistry strategies, with a focus on interdisciplinary sustainable clinical applications and scientifically supported guidance. The book is designed for clinicians, students and researchers who are seeking a deeper understanding of how to apply minimally invasive principles in real-world settings – across various dental specialties and in collaboration with broader healthcare disciplines.

Each chapter integrates current scientific literature with clinical decision-making, emphasising the importance of evidence-based practice in early detection, prevention, treatment planning and execution. Topics covered include caries risk assessment and management, preventive strategies, adhesive restorative techniques, bioactive materials and the role of emerging technologies. The book also explores how interdisciplinary collaboration whether with periodontists, endodontists, orthodontists, prosthodontists or medical professionals can enhance treatment outcomes and patient satisfaction. A central theme throughout this work is the importance of individualised care. Rather than relying on a one-size-fits-all model, minimally invasive dentistry encourages clinicians to make precise, patient-specific decisions that consider both biological and functional longevity. This approach is particularly relevant in the context of precision healthcare, where patients are increasingly informed and value treatments that are not only effective but also sustainable, conservative, functional and aesthetically rewarding. Furthermore, the integration of interdisciplinary approaches reflects the complexity of mouth care. Oral health is inseparably linked with systemic health, and comprehensive care often requires input from multiple fields. By fostering collaboration and promoting minimally invasive strategies, we can ensure sustainable outcomes for our patients.

In a nutshell, this book aspires to serve as both a reference and a source of inspiration for clinicians, researchers, students and policymakers who aim to combine scientific knowledge with clinical excellence. By embracing minimally invasive and interdisciplinary strategies, we can uphold the integrity of hard and soft dental tissues, improve patient experiences and contribute meaningfully to the advancement of twenty-first century precision dentistry.

About the Companion Website

This book is accompanied by a companion website:

www.wiley.com/go/baysan/minimally_invasive_dentistry 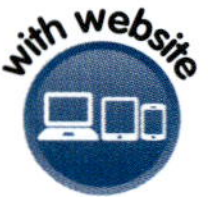

The website includes:

- Case Studies
- Multiple Choice Questions

1

Introduction to Minimally Invasive Dentistry: History of Minimally Invasive Dentistry and Key Concepts

Aylin Baysan and Kenneth Eaton

Key Topics

- Facts and figures: Demographics of dental disease
- Concept of Minimally Invasive Dentistry
- Principles of Minimally Invasive Dentistry with advantages and disadvantages
- History of Minimally Invasive Dentistry

Learning Objectives

- Be able to appreciate the facts and figures on demographics of dental disease
- Be able to appreciate the limited evidence on epidemiology of common dental diseases
- Be able to define the concept of Minimally Invasive Dentistry
- Be able to understand the principles with advantages and disadvantages
- Be able to understand the history of Minimally Invasive Dentistry and impact on clinical dentistry

Introduction

The World Health Organisation (WHO) Global Oral Health Status Report (2022) reported that oral diseases affect approximately 3.5 billion people worldwide. In this respect, it is estimated that 2 billion people present with dental caries in permanent teeth whilst 514 million children have carious lesions in primary teeth [1].

The Global Burden of Oral Conditions report revealed that untreated dental caries in permanent teeth was the most prevalent of all the 291 diseases and conditions investigated. With this respect, severe periodontitis was sixth most common and untreated dental caries in deciduous teeth was the tenth [2].

Minimally Invasive Dentistry: Interdisciplinary Clinical and Scientific Approaches, First Edition.
Edited by Aylin Baysan and Paul Anderson.
© 2026 John Wiley & Sons Ltd. Published 2026 by John Wiley & Sons Ltd.
Companion website: www.wiley.com/go/baysan/minimally_invasive_dentistry

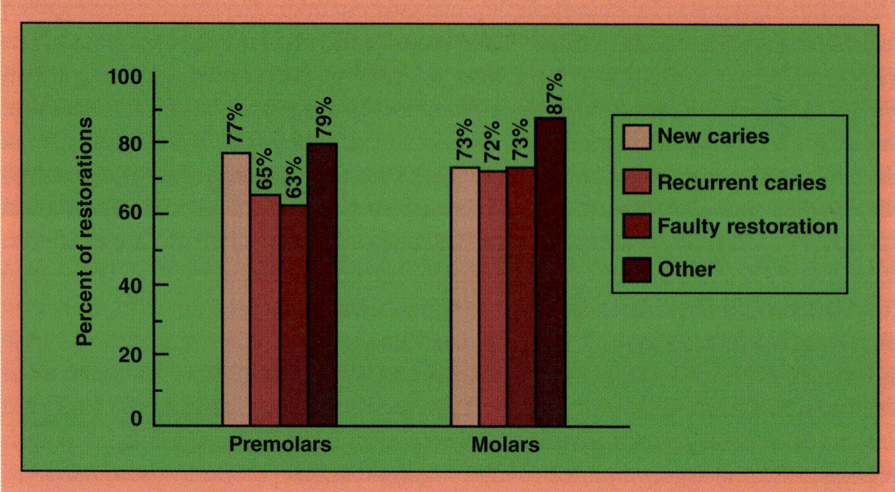

Figure 1.1 Percentage of restorations for which replacement with an increased number of surfaces according to tooth type and reason for replacement.

Following this evidence, the cost of the provision of oral care was reported to be £79 billion and that over two thirds of this cost related to the treatment of dental caries and its sequelae [3]. However, these costs could substantially be reduced if the population was educated in preventive practices and oral health care workers improved the early diagnosis of dental caries in their patients, such that enamel caries was treated with the application of fluoride and early dentinal caries with minimally invasive restorations. Elderton [4] reported a negative factor in replacing restorations which is the likelihood of increasing the size of potential new restorations. This author also emphasised the need for preventive advice and Minimally Invasive Dentistry (MID). Subsequently, Brantley et al. [5] illustrated the percentage of restorations and planned replacement with an increased number of surfaces (Figure 1.1). The reasons "new caries" and "other" (i.e., fracture, fracture risk, abutment, contact/contour problems led to the greatest proportion of increased surfaces for premolar teeth. The reason "other" was cited most frequently by dentists who recommended replacement of restorations in molar teeth with extensive restorations. However, "recurrent caries" and "faulty restoration" led to the increase in the number of surfaces for approximately one-half of premolar and molar restorations.

The Epidemiology of Dental Caries Worldwide

Dental caries is still a major oral health problem in most countries, affecting 60–90% of schoolchildren and the vast majority of adults. Despite recent improvements in oral health of sections of the population of developed countries, overall there appears to have been some deterioration, particularly amongst under-privileged groups in developed countries and in many developing countries [1]. It is also a most prevalent oral disease in several Asian and Latin-American countries, whilst interestingly dental caries is less common and less severe in most African countries. Frencken et al. [6], reported that untreated cavitated dentine carious lesions are the only single most common disease that affects humans worldwide.

There is evidence that the severity of cavitated dentine carious lesions amongst 5- and 12-year-old children declined over the last decades. However, the percentage of observed dental caries within these age groups is still high, with a low prevalence among 12-year-olds and among 35- to 44-year-olds in high-income countries [6].

However, the data on which the above trends have been reported must be treated with caution. International comparisons may be very unreliable due to a wide range of factors including, the threshold level for a diagnosis of caries, sampling techniques and the fact that some of the studies took place more than 15 years ago [3].

In the UK, since 1968 for adults and 1973 for children, national epidemiological surveys of oral health have taken place [7]. A remarkable improvement has been reported as far as the prevalence of dental caries in children and adults is concerned. In 1968, 37% of adults were edentulous and by 2009 this had fallen to 6% [8]. By 2013 the percentage of 12-year-old children with no obvious dental caries had risen to 66% (56% in 2003) [9]. However, within these overall improvements, there are still challenges for the management of dental caries.

More people over the age of 75 years are retaining teeth [7], which have often been restored with invasive procedures such as crowns, bridges, and dental implants. Unfortunately, due to the conditions such as rheumatoid arthritis, Alzheimer, and dementia, many are unable to maintain their oral health. In addition, reduced salivary flow affects the ability to buffer acids, produced by cariogenic bacteria, and secondary and/or root caries are more likely to ensue.

In spite of the overall reduction in the prevalence of dental caries in children, there has been a polarisation such that there has been no improvement, over the years, in dental caries in a minority of children, who invariably come from socio-economically deprived groups with the population [9]. Interestingly, extraction of teeth of those under 16 years of age, under general anaesthetic, was previously the most frequently performed hospital operation in the UK.

In order to promote the concepts of prevention for dental caries worldwide, the Alliance for a Cavity Free Future (ACFF) has been formed. The ACFF seeks to work with dental educators, clinicians, policymakers and patients to prevent dental caries and where/when these lesions occur, the ultimate aim is to diagnose and treat this disease, before there is dentinal involvement [10].

If dental caries is present, it is essential to assess its extent in a tooth. The simple diagnosis of caries present or absent is unable to help the practice of MID. A more detailed assessment with different grades is required. This concept has been incorporated in the International Caries Detection and Assessment System (ICDAS), which grades dental caries from 0 to 6 (Figure 1.2) [11]. Diagnosis of early dentinal caries (ICDAS Grade 3) can be an indication for the caries removal and the placement of a restoration following minimally invasive cavity preparation.

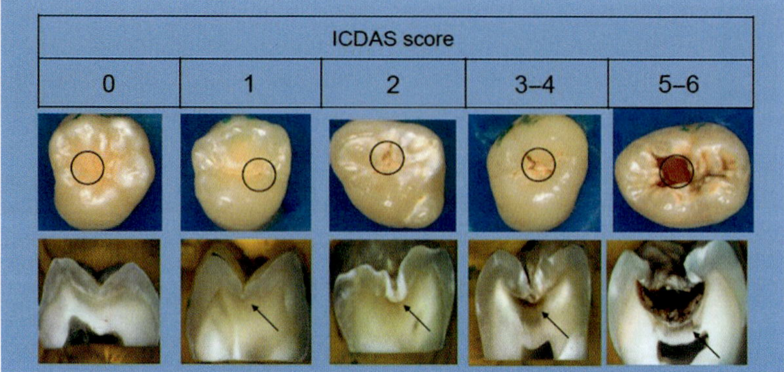

Figure 1.2 ICDAS clinical visual codes, based on evidence of the histological extent of carious lesions by staging the caries continuum. Source: Pitts and Ekstrand [11]/John Wiley & Sons, Inc.

The Epidemiology of Periodontitis Worldwide

As previously stated in 2010 the Global Burden of Disease study suggested that periodontitis was the sixth most prevalent disease on Earth. Periodontitis is a chronic, multifactorial inflammatory disease and is associated with diabetes, hypertension, and cardiovascular diseases. This disease is interestingly linked to behavioural and lifestyle factors (i.e., smoking habits, psychosocial stress, and nutrition) [12–14]. Frencken et al. [6] suggested that the prevalence and incidence of periodontitis are highly age dependent and that there is marked geographic variation. There are no meaningful gender differences and that the prevalence and incidence of periodontitis may have stagnated over the past 20 years (Figure 1.3).

In 2010, worldwide loss of productivity due to severe periodontitis was estimated to be US $54 billion *per* year. The global prevalence of periodontal disease is expected to increase in coming years due to growth in the aging population and increased retention of natural teeth due to a significant reduction in tooth loss in the older population.

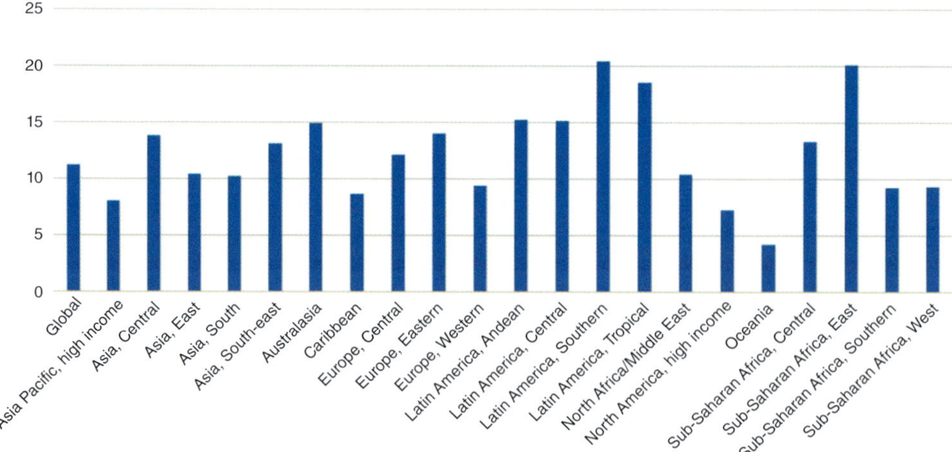

Figure 1.3 Prevalence of periodontitis globally. Source: Frencken et al. [6]/John Wiley & Sons.

However, even worse than epidemiological data for dental caries, national data for severity of periodontitis are unreliable as the thresholds for a case definition of periodontitis have varied widely from country to country [15] and also utilising the techniques for assessment [16].

Periodontal care is being provided in a variety of health systems around the world and given the global burden of disease, the active engagement of a motivated oral health professional team and patients play a key role for the management of this disease. However, as the complexity of treatment increases with disease progression, it is important to plan appropriate primary and secondary care in national health systems. Therefore, consensus on appropriate assessments and enhancement could be achieved and performed in every country for optimising the national oral healthcare strategies and services.

The Epidemiology of Tooth Wear

Tooth wear is an irreversible and cumulative condition. Tooth wear is predominantly related to multifactorial aetiology. Delayed or inadequate diagnosis with a lack of preventive intervention could lead to irreversible and advanced tissue loss. As a consequence, vitality of a tooth with function and aesthetics can be compromised. Despite the high prevalence observed in multiple countries, the information about incidence of tooth wear worldwide remains unclear.

There is some evidence with respect to tooth wear related to erosion worldwide. The global prevalence of dental erosion in children and adolescents aged between 8 and 19 years ranging from 7.2% [17] to 95.0% [18]. According to these authors, the variability in the obtained prevalence rates could be explained by using different indices to diagnose dental erosion, type of examined teeth, sample size, age, and geographic factors.

In this respect, Tooth Wear Index (TWI), which was adopted in most studies, could overestimate the prevalence, since it is not specific for detection of dental erosion [19]. In addition, geographic location seems to influence the prevalence rates observed in the literature, since cultural, ethnical, and dietary habits vary according to the regions [20].

There is a general trend to acknowledge that different aetiological factors to cause tooth wear cannot be determined and analysed separately. Therefore, considering the evaluation of exposed tooth tissue, the presence of enamel/dentine or only dentine exposed fails to explain the heterogeneity of the data presented in the literature.

The Epidemiology of Tooth Loss

The National Institutes of Health estimate that there are 158 million people without teeth worldwide and 120 million Americans are missing one or more teeth according to the Centers for Disease Control (CDC) NHANES data (Figure 1.4).

Data on tooth loss reflects not only dental disease worldwide, however this information will give an indication of patients' and dentists' attitudes, the dentist-patient relationship, the availability and accessibility of dental services, and the prevailing philosophies of dental care [21, 22].

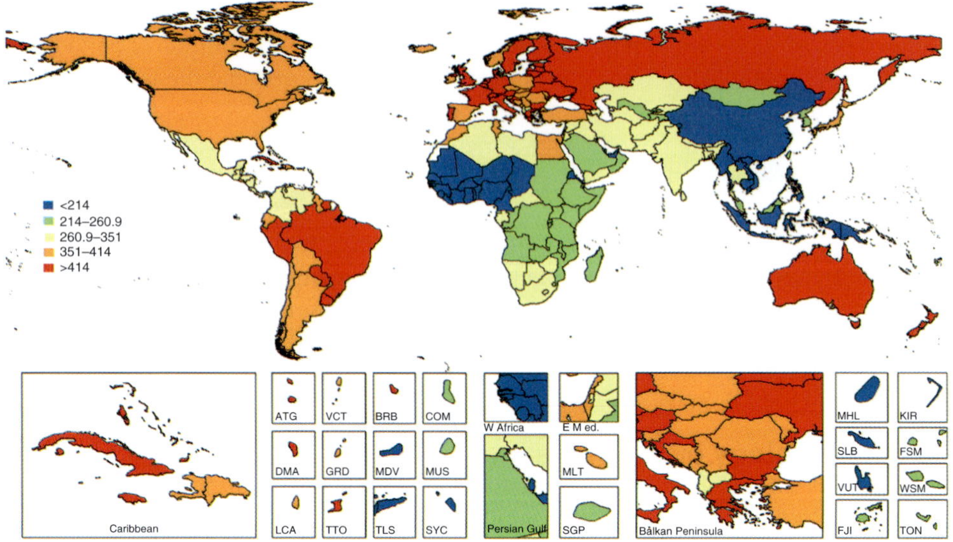

Figure 1.4 The worldwide distribution of severe tooth loss incidence *per* 100,000 persons [23].

The global age-standardised incidence rate of severe tooth loss in 2010 was 205 cases *per* 100,000 person-years (95% UI: 187, 226). There was a significant decrease of 45% from the 1990 incidence rate of 374 cases *per* 100,000 person-years (95% UI: 347, 406). Women generally showed higher age-standardised prevalence and incidence of severe tooth loss when compared to men. However, the gap between gender has reduced over time with only minor differences since 2010. In both genders, prevalence increased gradually with age, showing a steep increase around the seventh decade of life that was associated with a peak in incidence at 65 years old (Figure 1.5). These age patterns have not changed during the past two decades in spite of the gradual declines in prevalence and incidence within the same period.

Sound knowledge on current trends in tooth loss is vital for planning dental services and workforce as well as for updating the dental education worldwide. However, the epidemiology of tooth loss has not yet been fully analysed. In addition, Kudsi et al. [24] reported

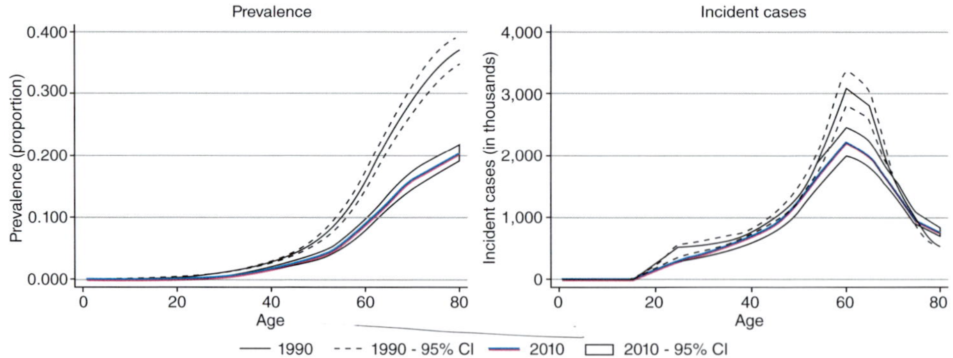

Figure 1.5 Prevalence (proportion) and number of incident cases of severe tooth loss in 1990 (light line) and 2010 (dark line) with 95% uncertainty intervals by age.

tooth loss and removable dentures could be associated with body image dissatisfaction and psychologic morbidity. Therefore, planning for patient-centred care is paramount prior to extracting any teeth and providing replacement options, especially removable dentures.

The Concept of Minimally Invasive Dentistry (MID)

The concept of MID supports a systematic understanding for the hard and soft tissues, including diagnosis, risk assessment, preventive treatment, and minimal tissue removal on dental treatment. The motivation for MID emerges from the fact that restorations are not for life. The main reasons for failure are secondary caries, tooth/restoration fracture, and decementation/debonding. To overcome these issues, there is an urgent need for establishing guidelines to maintain the oral health and retain the healthy natural hard and soft tissues as long as possible.

Therefore, the key concepts are:

- Correct early detection of disease
- Thorough risk assessment
- Patient education on awareness and knowledge of oral health
- Targeted preventive treatment to stop the disease
- Restoration of the lesion, if required, with as little removal of healthy tissue as possible
- The use of durable material if required
- The prevention of disease recurrence

Principles of Minimally Invasive Dentistry (MID) with Advantages and Disadvantages

To date, there is a lack of an evidence-based approach for MID. Therefore, there are advantages and disadvantages with this concept according to the literature to date (Table 1.1).

Table 1.1   The advantages and disadvantages of MI concept in clinical dentistry.

Advantages	Disadvantages
Patient's well-being	Lack of concrete evidence with multi-centred randomised clinical trials
Conservation of the hard and soft tissues	Limited indication in some cases
Cost effectiveness—long-term benefit	If not implied adequately, MID can be more damaging
Reduced need for the use of local anaesthetics	Remineralisation is only possible with non cavitated lesions
Hard and soft tissue engineering	Some minimal invasive methods have less survival rates
Routine reassessments and maintenance	Patient compliance orientated strategy

The History of Minimally Invasive Dentistry (MID)

MID has developed over the past 20 utilising the preventive measures to preserve natural tooth structures. The science for MID is advancing to enable individuals to retain more teeth for longer.

Interestingly, despite being blamed for the "extension for prevention" concept, Black published a series of papers and texts on dental materials and preparation and restoration techniques between 1869 and 1915 on minimal intervention strategies. Black was the first dentist to propose treating dental caries using minimal intervention based on the knowledge and materials available at that time.

The basic philosophy of MID recognises the fact that all restorations have a finite life and that large restorations (either composite or amalgam) have a shorter longevity than smaller ones. Black made a statement in 1891: "...And if the filling should serve for five, ten, or fifteen years, valuable teeth will have been saved to the patient that much longer by filling and afterward crowning, than by present crowning...." It was clear that Black encouraged the clinicians to choose the least invasive option since the more invasive option would usually be available for a later date.

MID became a popular approach following the enhancement of bonding principles within the hard tooth structure. In 1955, Buonocore described a technique for etching enamel surfaces to make them retentive for a restoration. In 1962, Bowen submitted a patent, entitled a "Dental filling material comprising vinyl silane treated fused silica and a binder consisting of BIS phenol and glycidyl acrylic," that enabled the restoration of a tooth with a tooth-coloured plastic better known today as Bis-GMA. These two developments led to the MID.

Subsequently, the MI philosophy was introduced by the application of silver fluoride diamine to dental caries in the early 1970s [25]. Newly developed, this cariostatic agent is the original preparation diammine silver fluoride ($Ag(NH3)2F$) (generally called: silver ammonia fluoride). For the purpose of caries prevention and the desensitisation of hypersensitive dentine, either fluoride or silver nitrate has been used.

Summary

A new paradigm using MI techniques for a more comprehensive and holistic approach to manage dental diseases can provide sustainable and focusing less on national/international resources by actively contributing to the improvement of patients' well-being and oral health for general health. In addition, MI strategies aim to reduce the replacement of dental restorations since every year, despite the effectiveness of preventive dentistry and dental health care, 75% of restorations fail and require replacement [26], which has an enormous socio-economic impact.

Overall, cumulative effects of dental diseases on oral health and also for general health strongly suggest prevention and patient-centred approaches using futuristic sustainable materials.

Further Reading

General

Adult Health Survey UK is an authoritative and free website based in the UK, written and reviewed by experts on dental public health, clinical academics, and other health professionals: https://digital.nhs.uk/data-and-information/publications/statistical/adult-dental-health-survey/adult-dental-health-survey-2009-first-release.

MI compendium (online resource).

WHO fact sheets (online resources).

References

1 World Health Organisation. https://www.who.int/news-room/fact-sheets/detail/oral-health.

2 Marcenes, W., Kassebaum, N.J., Bernabe, E., Flaxman, A., Naghavi, M., Lopez, A., and Murray, C.J. (2013). Global burden of oral conditions in 1990 – 2010: A systematic analysis. *J. Dent. Res.* 92: 592–597.

3 Patel, R. The state of oral health in Europe. Report Commissioned by the Platform for Better Oral Health in Europe 2012. https://www.oralhealthplatform.eu/ (accessed 20 September 2016).

4 Elderton, R.J. (1990). Clinical studies concerning re-restoration of teeth. *Adv. Dent. Res.* 4 (1): 4–9. doi: 10.1177/08959374900040010701.

5 Brantley, C.F., Bader, J.D., Shugars, D.A., and Nesbit, S.P. (1995). Does the cycle of rerestoration lead to larger restorations? *J. Am. Dent. Assoc.* 126 (10): 1407–1413. ISSN 0002-8177, doi: 10.14219/Jada.Archive.1995.0052. https://www.sciencedirect.com/science/article/pii/S0002817715612764.

6 Frencken, J.E., Sharma, P., Stenhouse, L., Green, D., Laverty, D., and Dietrich, T. (2017 March). Global epidemiology of dental caries and severe periodontitis – A comprehensive review. *J. Clin. Periodontol.* 44 (Suppl 18): S94–S105. doi: 10.1111/jcpe.12677.

7 Adult Oral Health Survey. https://dam.ukdataservice.ac.uk/media/428503/osullivanadhs.pdf.

8 White, D.A., Tsakos, G., Pitts, N., Fuller, E., Douglas, G.V.A., Murray, J.J., and Steele, J.G. (2013). Adult dental health survey 2009: Common oral health conditions and their impact on the population. *BDJ* 213: 573–574.

9 Health and Social Care Information Centre. Children's dental health survey: England, Wales and Northern Ireland 2013. www.hscic.gov.uk (accessed 20 September 2016).

10 Alliance for Caries Free Future. www.alliancefor.acariesfreefuture.org.

11 Pitts, N.B., and Ekstrand, K.R. (2013). International Caries Detection and Assessment System (ICDAS) and its International Caries Classification and Management System (ICCMS) – Methods for staging of the caries process and enabling dentists to manage caries. *Community Dent. Oral Epidemiol.* 41: e41–e52. © 2012 The Authors. Journal Compilation © 2012 Blackwell Munksgaard.

12 Sanz, M., Ceriello, A., Buysschaert, M., Chapple, I., Demmer, R.T., Graziani, F., Herrera, D., Jepsen, S., Lione, L., Madianos, P., Mathur, M., Montanya, E., Shapira, L., Tonetti, M.,

and Vegh, D. (2018). Scientific evidence on the links between periodontal diseases and diabetes: Consensus report and guidelines of the joint workshop on periodontal diseases and diabetes by the International Diabetes Federation and the European Federation of Periodontology. *J. Clin. Periodontol.* 45 (2): 138–149.

13 Sanz, M., Marco Del Castillo, A., Jepsen, S., Gonzalez-Juanatey, J.R., D'Aiuto, F., Bouchard, P., Chapple, I., Dietrich, T., Gotsman, I., Graziani, F., Herrera, D., Loos, B., Madianos, P., Michel, J.B., Perel, P., Pieske, B., Shapira, L., Shechter, M., Tonetti, M., and Wimmer, G. (2020). Periodontitis and cardiovascular diseases: Consensus report. *J. Clin. Periodontol.* 47 (3): 268–288.

14 Carra, M.C., Fessi, S., Detzen, L., Darnaud, C., Julia, C., Hercberg, S., Touvier, M., Andreeva, V.A., and Bouchard, P. (2021). Self-reported periodontal health and incident hypertension: Longitudinal evidence from the NutriNet-Santé e-cohort. *J. Hypertens.* 39 (12): 2422–2430.

15 Savage, A., Eaton, K.A., Moles, D.R., and Needleman, I. (2009). A systematic review of definitions of periodontitis and methods that have been used to identify this disease. *J. Clin. Periodontol.* 36: 455–467.

16 Leroy, R., Eaton, K.A., and Savage, A. (2010). Methodological issues in epidemiological studies of periodontitis - How can it be improved? *BMC Oral Health* 10: 1.

17 Vargas-Ferreira, F., Praetzel, J.R., and Ardenghi, T.M. (2011). Prevalence of tooth erosion and associated factors in 11–14-year-old Brazilian schoolchildren. *J. Public Health Dent.* 71: 6–12.

18 Al-Majed, I., Maguire, A., and Murray, J.J. (2002). Risk factors for dental erosion in 5–6 year old and 12–14 year old boys in Saudi Arabia. *Community Dent. Oral Epidemiol.* 30: 38–46.

19 van Rijkom, H.M., Truin, G.J., Frencken, J.E., Konig, K.G., vant Hof, M.A., Bronkhorst, E.M., and Roeters, F.J. (2002). Prevalence, distribution and background variables of smooth-bordered tooth wear in teenagers in the Hague, the Netherlands. *Caries Res.* 36: 147–154.

20 Kazoullis, S., Seow, W.K., Holcombe, T., Newman, B., and Ford, D. (2007). Common dental conditions associated with dental erosion in schoolchildren in Australia. *Pediatr. Dent.* 29: 33–39.

21 Baelum, V., van Palenstein Helderman, W., Hugoson, A., Yee, R., and Fejerskov, O. (2007). A global perspective on changes in the burden of caries and periodontitis: Implications for dentistry. *J. Oral Rehabil.* 34: 872–906.

22 Fejerskov, O., Escobar, G., Jossing, M., and Baelum, V. (2013). A functional natural dentition for all—and for life? The oral healthcare system needs revision. *J. Oral Rehabil.* 40: 707–722.

23 Kassebaum, N.J., Bernabé, E., Dahiya, M., Bhandari, B., Murray, C.J.L., and Marcenes, W. (2014 July). Global burden of severe tooth loss: A systematic review and meta-analysis. *J. Dent. Res.* 93 (7 Suppl): 20S–28S.

24 Kudsi, Z., Fenlon, M.R., and Baysan, A. (2022 September/October). Do tooth loss and dentures cause body image disturbance? *Int. J. Prosthodont.* 35 (5): 609–615. doi: 10.11607/ijp.7667. Epub 2022 May 25. PMID: 35649278.

25 Yamaga, R., Nishino, M., Yoshida, S., and Yokomizo, I. (1972 September). Diammine silver fluoride and its clinical application. *J. Osaka Univ. Dent. Sch.* 12: 1–20. PMID: 4514730.

26 Dental Practice-Based Research Network Collaborative Group. (2012). Repair or replacement of defective restorations by dentists. *J. Am. Dent. Assoc.* 143: 593–601.

2

Where Are We with the Evidence for Minimally Invasive Dentistry?

Derek Richards and Valeria Marinho

Key Topics

- Evidence-based approach in Minimally Invasive Dentistry (MID)
- Clinical experiences and evidence-based approach
- Searching the best evidence
- Cochrane reviews on MID approaches

Learning Objectives

- Understand the key elements of the evidence-based approach
- Describe the structure of a Population (or Problem) Intervention, Comparison and Outcome (PICO) question
- Identify a range of sources of primary and pre-appraised evidence
- Be aware of the findings of Cochrane reviews on MID resources

Introduction

There is a relatively recent history of use of MID through a variety of approaches across the prevention, diagnosis, control, and treatment of dental disease—in particular of minimally invasive strategies in caries management, already widely implemented in general dental practice.

The effects of MID approaches for caries and its consequences are assessed and summarised in Cochrane reviews compiling the evidence on this subject, which are forming the basis of the international evidence base for the appropriate use of MID approaches in caries prevention, detection, control, and repair.

The MID concept of care uses the least invasive interventions and minimal removal of tooth tissues to conserve teeth functional throughout life. MID care is relatively new and its

Minimally Invasive Dentistry: Interdisciplinary Clinical and Scientific Approaches, First Edition.
Edited by Aylin Baysan and Paul Anderson.
© 2026 John Wiley & Sons Ltd. Published 2026 by John Wiley & Sons Ltd.
Companion website: www.wiley.com/go/baysan/minimally_invasive_dentistry

field is wide, including the prevention, diagnosis, treatment, and control of dental disease (Fédération Dentaire Internationale (FDI) 2017).

Dental caries is the world's most prevalent chronic disease affecting around 60% to 90% of school-aged children and the vast majority of adults (Marcenes et al. 2013; Petersen and Lennon 2004). However, the changing epidemiology of dental caries and the current understanding of dental disease and its process, MID approaches are gaining popularity in modern dentistry throughout the world. Indeed, minimally invasive care in caries management in particular is being implemented in general practice (Holmgren et al. 2014) and its adoption explicitly recommended as a learning outcome for the dental team (GDC-UK 2015).

Cochrane reviews have become influential as a foundation for clinical practice and policy in dentistry by objectively appraising best available research evidence on a large number of dental procedures. The effects of various MID approaches mainly for caries prevention and management using the least invasive procedures and minimal removal of tooth tissues to conserve teeth functional have been assessed and summarised in Cochrane reviews, and this evidence is presented later.

With this respect, it should be noted that the evidence-based healthcare approach emerged during the 1990s with the first dental articles on the topic appearing toward the end of the decade (FDI 2017; Marcenes et al. 2013). However, the imperative to provide the best care and treatment for our patients is far older than this as demonstrated by the long history of the development of fair tests of treatment as illustrated on the James Lind Library website (www.jameslindlibrary.org).

Clinical Experiences and Patient Values

The evidence-based approach involves bringing together three key elements:

- the best available evidence,
- clinical experience, and
- the patient's values

in order to provide the most appropriate and effective care for the patient's clinical problem.

Evidence-Based Dentistry (EBD) was defined by the American Dental Association as

'an approach to oral healthcare that requires the judicious integration of systematic assessments of clinically relevant scientific evidence, relating to the patient's oral and medical condition and history, with the dentist's clinical expertise and the patient's treatment needs and preferences (American Dental Association 2018).'

Evidence

In considering what constitutes the best available evidence it is worth noting that the type of evidence required depends on the particular question that is being addressed. For example, when considering whether a particular treatment is beneficial or better than an alternative, good quality randomised controlled trials (RCTs) or systematic reviews of RCTs provide the best quality evidence. However, cross-sectional studies with consistently applied reference standards and blinding or systematic reviews of these studies are needed for diagnostic tests.

The 2011 Oxford Centre for Evidence Based Medicine's Levels of Evidence tables (www.cebm.net/category/ebm-resources/loe/) provides a useful summary of this approach and is helpful for busy clinicians. Although it is important to stress that the interpretation of the range of available evidence requires careful thought and good judgement.

Systematic reviews can be conducted to combine most types of study designs and generally provide better information than a single study and evidence from a number of high quality systematic reviews relevant to MID are summarised later.

Clinical Experience

As clinicians there are some procedure, we undertake every day while other we do infrequently. If we have chosen to specialise in one area of dentistry we can become very highly skilled in some clinical aspects while in others our expertise declines. Because of advances in materials and procedure, we often need to develop an understanding of new techniques and materials and there is often a learning curve. Consequently, when we are considering a new approach because of changing evidence we need to factor this into our decision-making.

Patients Values

The role of the patient is becoming increasingly important in health care decision-making and this was recognised in the early development of the evidence-based approach although it was submerged for a time by a greater focus on the evidence. Understanding the values that a patient places on their care forms and important part in clinical decision-making. For example, some patients will place greater value on appearance than functionally of their dentition while others take the opposite view. Understanding the patients' perspective is therefore an important element in making good evidence-based decisions.

The Evidence-based Approach

The evidence-based approach should be thought of as a structured approach to support the delivery of the best care for patients and consists of 5 stages:

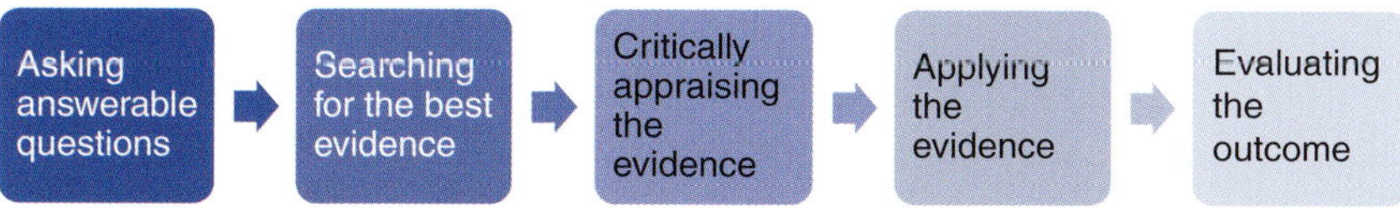

These five key elements were outlined in the 2005 Sicily statement on evidence-based practice, which was developed by an international working group representing both organisations and individual teachers and developers of evidence-based practice (Dawes et al. 2005) .

Asking Answerable Questions

Good clinical questions are generally built around the PICO format, articulated by Richardson in 1995 (Richardson et al. 1995). Table 2.1 demonstrates how this could be applied to produce a focused question.

The focused question could then be written as:

'In a patient with extensive caries in a permanent tooth would partial or stepwise caries removal compared with complete carious removal result in fewer pulpal exposures.'

For some questions, a time frame may be added for example as a variation on the above question creating a PICO question.

'In a patient with extensive caries in a permanent tooth would partial or stepwise caries removal compared with complete carious removal result maintain a viable pulp after 2 years'.

Searching for the Best Evidence

Ideally the clinician would search relevant databases in order to find the best evidence and appraise the evidence themselves. Some examples of biomedical databases are shown in Table 2.2, although this is just a small sample of the number that are available.

Searching for yourself is a good way to ensure that the evidence available is most appropriate for the patients' needs and matches your clinical skills. This is also important as new evidence is constantly being generated and published in the large number of dental and biomedical journals and other sources that are currently available. This constant stream of

Table 2.1 Developing a PICO question.

	Consider	Example
Population (or Problem)	How would you describe the patient or their problem?	Patient with extensive carious involvement of dentine in a permanent tooth
Intervention	What would be the main/most common (traditional) treatment approach?	Complete removal of caries
Comparison	What alternatives are available?	Partial or stepwise caries removal
Outcome	What are the important outcomes?	Preservation of pulp, lack of pain

Table 2.2 Examples of biomedical databases.

Name	Source URL
Cochrane Library	www.cochranelibrary.com
DIMDI– Medical Knowledge Online	https://www.bfarm.de/EN/Medical-devices/Portals/DMIDS/_node.html
EBSCO	www.ebscohost.com/aboutus
EMBASE	www.embase.com/
Clarivate Web of Science	https://clarivate.com/products/scientific-and-academic-research/research-discovery-and-workflow-solutions/webofscience-platform/
PubMed	https://pubmed.ncbi.nlm.nih.gov/
Scopus	https://www.elsevier.com/products/scopus

information is challenging for the practicing clinician to manage but fortunately a number of sources providing pre-appraised evidence and summaries of primary evidence are available which could be useful resources for practitioners.

Evidence-based Computerised Decision Support Systems

In some areas of health care evidence-based computerised decision support systems are available but these are in their relative infancy in dentistry. With the current pace of development of information technology, they are likely to have increasing impact in the future.

Evidence-based Guidelines

At present evidence-based guidelines provide some of the best summaries available and are available in some areas. Guidelines are available from a number of organisations, colleges, and specialist societies. Those produced by the American Dental Association, The National Institute for Health and Care Excellence (NICE), The Scottish Intercollegiate Guidelines Network (SIGN), and the Scottish Dental Clinical Effectiveness Programme (SDCEP) have some of the most robust evidence-based processes.

Systematic Reviews

After guidelines, systematic reviews provide the next most useful sources of evidence although in general they provide evidence on single specific interventions rather than wider topic areas that is often seen in guidelines. Clear guidelines on how to report systematic reviews are available from the PRISMA (Preferred Reporting Items for Systematic Reviews and Meta-Analyses) website (http://prisma-statement.org/) .

Systematic reviews produced that carefully follow the PRISMA approach are likely to provide better quality information while those produced by the Cochrane Collaboration follow strict evidence-based methodological approaches and of the highest standard. The Cochrane Oral Health Group has published a number of reviews relevant to MID, which are summarised later.

Individual Studies

If systematic reviews are not available, then high quality individual studies provide the next best source of information. When looking at individual studies guidance on the reporting of the broad range of study types is available from the The EQUATOR (Enhancing the QUAlity and Transparency Of health Research) Network (www.equator-network.org/). The EQUATOR Network is an international initiative that seeks to improve the reliability and value of published health research literature by promoting transparent and accurate reporting and wider use of robust reporting guidelines.

While all these resources are helpful in order to use them effectively an awareness of their structure and search systems is necessary.

As an alternative to a 'hopeful' search in a general database such a Medline (PubMed) or Google, a good strategy is to use the well-structured meta-search engine such as the TRIP database (www.tripdatabase.com/). This clinical search engine searches a broad range of databases and other sources and clearly identifies evidence by type, making it easy to identify the best available information on a given topic. The clear way in which any search findings are presented in the TRIP database facilitates the rapid identification of the level of evidence available for any given search topic.

Critical Appraisal

Having found relevant evidence it is important that it is assessed critically. This requires a systematic evaluation of the evidence source. Detailing how to critically appraise the range of study designs available is beyond the scope of this book. However, in essence critical appraisal needs to address a number of key features of each study.

1) Is the study addressing your clearly focused question?
2) Has the study used a valid methodology to answer the question?
3) What are the results and are they clinically important?
4) Are the results relevant to my patient or population?

These broad questions are relevant to all types of study designs but a number of organisations have developed critical appraisal worksheets to assist in the assessment of different types of study designs. The tools produced by the Critical Appraisal Skills Programme (CASP) are widely used in health care (https://casp-uk.net/) but a useful summary of most of the available tools can be found at the University of South Australia's Library (https://guides.library.unisa.edu.au/SystematicReviews/CriticalAppraisal).

Applying the Evidence

Once you have chosen to apply a particular evidence-based approach, it may seem to be a relatively straightforward step to use that approach. However, there are potential barriers that may or not be easily overcome (Antman et al. 1992). First you need to be able to undertake the procedure, which might require additional training. Then you need to act on your decision to undertake the procedure. Before you can do this the patient needs to consent, which is usually made easier by involving them actively in the decision-making. In some circumstances, the procedure might need patient compliance for the best possible outcome. Many of these barriers act during our normal interactions with patients and only become more obvious when adopting a new approach.

Evaluating the Outcome

The final stage of the evidence-based process is to evaluate how our conclusions and the treatment options developed for consideration of the evidence worked with our patients as opposed to those in the clinical studies. The can be done using standard clinical audit type approaches or peer review. This formal closing of the loop helps ensure that we are continuing to work toward achieving the best evidence-based clinical outcomes for our patients.

High Quality Evidence in Relation to MID

Twenty-five years ago, medical and dental health care practice largely rested on the opinion of experts whose recourse to research evidence was to support their pre-formed views. In many cases, through experience and perception and an appraisal of the literature, these opinions may well have been right. However, expert opinion has been shown to differ significantly from objective synthesis of the best research evidence compiled cumulatively in meta-analysis and in comprehensive systematic reviews (Glasziou and Haynes 2005; Evidence-Based Medicine Working Group 1992).

Much earlier than 25 years ago, Archie Cochrane (Cochrane 1972), in his book *Effectiveness and Efficiency*, explored for the first time the dangers of simply assuming, based on uncontrolled biased assessments, that contemporary medical practice was necessarily effective in combating illness. Cochrane made a strong case for the evaluation of new and existing interventions in RCTs, explaining how evidence from such trials could help in a more rational use of resources in the health services.

In 1993, in response to Cochrane's call for an organised summary of RCTs by healthcare specialty, the Cochrane Collaboration was established as an international non-profit organisation. It challenged those working in health care to put practice and policy on a footing of objectively synthesised research evidence in the form of Cochrane reviews (Chalmers 1993; Chalmers et al. 1992) (which, over the years, have been shown to be more rigorous than other systematic reviews) (Jadad et al. 1998; Glenny et al. 2003; Ijaz et al. 2010).

Cochrane reviews are different in many ways to either traditional reviews (broadly speaking, opinion pieces without a 'methods' section) or standard systematically conducted reviews (those with a workable 'methods' section published in article); all have been used as sources of evidence by dentists and policymakers, and often they concur.

For example, MID concept of care did not need a Cochrane review to know Atraumatic Restorative Treatment (ART) was a useful approach for the management of dental caries where access to resources are limited. However, it did need it to consistently answer the patient's direct question 'What are my chances of not getting pain or restoration failure with the use of ART in comparison with having conventional treatment applied to my teeth?' or the policymakers' 'How many people have to be given this particular treatment in order to avoid painful/costly outcomes?'

This section provides an overview of the evidence compiled in existing Cochrane reviews of minimal intervention options for managing dental caries and its consequences, which is forming the basis of the international evidence base for the use of MID approaches in dentistry. It describes key information highlighting the reviews' main questions, main findings, and conclusions for clinical practice (as well as methodological features and research implications). The aim is to facilitate the appropriate use of minimal intervention in practice, within various dental specialties, i.e., to be applicable to children, but also to adult patients.

The concept of MID dental caries management is to maintain as much healthy tooth structure as possible and help keep teeth functional for life. A recent FDI policy statement on Minimal Intervention Dentistry for managing dental caries describes the major MID components as: (i) early detection of carious lesions and assessment of caries risk and activity; (ii) remineralisation of demineralised enamel and dentine; (iii) optimal measurements to keep sound teeth sound; (iv) tailored dental recalls; (v) minimally invasive operative interventions to ensure tooth survival; and (vi) repairing rather than replacing defective restorations (FDI 2017). Available Cochrane reviews on minimal invasive procedures under any of these components are thus considered.

Cochrane Reviews on the Effects of Minimal Intervention Approaches in Caries Management

The Cochrane reviews on MID interventions for the management of dental caries in children and adults systematically compile the available evidence on the effects of various approaches of professionally applied interventions currently used in caries management (Dorri et al. 2015, 2017; Montedori et al. 2016; Innes et al. 2015; Ricketts et al. 2013). They are systematic reviews of RCTs mainly, produced under the auspices of the Cochrane Oral Health Group (COHG).

The recently published ART vs. Conventional treatment for caries management Cochrane review has 15 trials included, whereas 4 other MID caries management reviews—on laser for caries removal, micro-invasive treatment for caries, preformed crowns for carious primary teeth, and the 2013 review on operative caries management—have 9, 8, 5, and 8 RCTs included, respectively. Because the reviews are updated as new evidence emerges and in response to feedback, the Cochrane Library should be accessed for the most recent version of the complete reviews, which are published electronically in the Cochrane Database of Systematic Reviews (CDSR), in the Cochrane Library. It should also be accessed for protocols of relevant reviews in progress.

Five main questions have been addressed in these five reviews:

1) What is the effectiveness of a minimally invasive approach, namely ART compared with conventional treatment for managing dental caries in the primary and permanent teeth of children and adults? (Dorri et al. 2017)
2) What is the effectiveness of laser-based methods compared with conventional mechanical methods/drills for removing dental caries in the primary and permanent teeth of children and adults? (Montedori et al. 2016)
3) What is the effectiveness of micro-invasive treatments for managing proximal caries lesions in primary and permanent dentition in children and adults compared with other types of micro-invasive treatment, non-invasive measures (e.g., interdental cleaning using dental floss, application of fluoride varnish), invasive means (conventional restorations), placebo or no intervention? (Dorri et al. 2015)
4) What is the clinical effectiveness and safety of all types of preformed crowns for restoring primary teeth compared with conventional filling materials (such as amalgam, composite, glass ionomer cement, resin-modified glass ionomer, and compomers), other types of crowns or methods of crown placement, non-restorative caries treatment, or no treatment? (Innes et al. 2015)
5) What is the effectiveness of stepwise, partial or no dentinal caries removal compared to complete caries removal for the management of dentinal caries in both primary and permanent teeth in children and adults? (Ricketts et al. 2013)

All the reviews presented meta-analyses of the relevant experimental evidence with no language restrictions. The available five Cochrane reviews on MID interventions for the management of dental caries in children and adults objectively assessed and summarised about 45 trials, each review establishing important findings that primary studies were unable to show individually.

The Main Findings/Conclusions from Each Review Were

1) There is low-quality evidence to suggest that primary teeth treated with the **atraumatic restorative treatment (ART)** approach using high viscosity glass ionomer cement may be more likely than those receiving **conventional treatment** with the same material to result in restoration failure. In the treatment of primary teeth, ART may reduce pain experience compared with conventional treatment.

   The evidence available for evaluating the differences between ART and conventional treatments using other restorative materials or in permanent teeth is very low quality so we cannot draw any conclusions. None of the included studies reported on negative side effects or costs. Practitioners and patients should interpret these results with caution.

Although there is some evidence in favor of conventional treatment rather than ART in primary teeth, ART may still be considered as a treatment option where access to resources (e.g., dentists, rotary handpieces, and electricity) are limited (Dorri et al. 2017).

2) Despite the inclusion of a fair number of studies, only a few trials of low quality completely reported information on the primary outcome. There was not enough evidence to suggest that either **lasers or drills** were better at decay removal. Episodes of pain were significantly reduced in people treated with lasers. Some evidence in favor of laser therapy for need of anesthesia and patient discomfort was also found but, again, the body of evidence was of low quality. There was no difference in terms of side effects, such as inflammation or death of dental pulp, between the two interventions. The conclusion was that evidence was insufficient to support the use of laser as an alternative to conventional 'drilling and filling' for caries removal (Montedori et al. 2016).

3) Evidence of moderate quality suggests that **micro-invasive treatment of proximal caries lesions** arrests non-cavitated enamel and initial dentinal lesions (limited to outer third of dentine, based on radiograph) and is significantly more effective than **non-invasive professional treatment** (e.g., fluoride varnish, advice to floss) **or no treatment/placebo**. No studies compared micro-invasive with **invasive treatment**. For **comparisons of different types of micro-invasive treatments**, due to the small number of studies, it does remain unclear which micro-invasive technique offers the greatest benefit, or whether the effects of micro-invasive treatment confer greater or lesser benefit according to different clinical or patient characteristic. Overall however, clinicians could consider micro-invasive treatments a viable option for treating non-cavitated proximal lesions, taking into account clinical indication and the feasibility of different techniques (Dorri et al. 2015).

4) Based on moderate quality evidence, **crowns placed on primary molar** teeth with carious lesions, or following pulp treatment, are likely to reduce the risk of major failure/problems or pain in the long term compared with **fillings**; and **crowns fitted using the Hall Technique** (no injections or tooth trimming) may reduce discomfort at the time of treatment compared **with fillings**. Crowns may increase the risk of gingival bleeding but this result was unclear. The amount and quality of evidence for crowns compared with **non-restorative caries treatment**, and for **metal compared with aesthetic** crowns, is very low, and no reliable conclusions from these can be drawn. There are no RCTs comparing **crowns fitted conventionally** with using **the Hall Technique**. Some outcomes of interest were not measured in any of the studies: these included time to restoration failure or retreatment, patient satisfaction, and costs (Innes et al. 2015).

5) Based on moderate quality evidence for all comparisons, it was found that: when the **complete caries removal technique** was compared with **stepwise excavation**, the pulp or nerve of the tooth would have been exposed in 347 of every 1,000 teeth treated with complete caries removal, whereas when the stepwise excavation technique was used (Ricketts et al. 2013), this would have occurred in only 154 teeth per 1,000. When the **partial caries removal technique** was used, pulp or nerve would have been

exposed in 50 teeth out of 1,000 treated, whereas when the **complete caries removal** technique was used this figure would have been 219 teeth per 1,000 treated.

There was less nerve damage when part of the decay was left behind, compared with all the decay, for both primary and permanent teeth. There was no difference in the number of teeth with toothache with any of the techniques. One of the no dentinal caries removal techniques needed fewer replacement fillings, although there was no difference found when comparing any of the rest of the techniques to complete caries removal.

Cochrane Reviews on the Effects of Other MID Approaches (Consequences of Dental Caries)

There is another published Cochrane review addressing other MID interventions and comparisons—endodontic procedures for retreatment of periapical lesions (Del Fabbro et al. 2016).

This review includes 20 RCTs and assesses the effects of **surgical** compared with **non-surgical therapy for endodontic retreatment of teeth with apical periodontitis** (retreating patients for whom root canal therapy has failed) and also the effects of **surgical root-end resection** under various conditions (if using specific materials, devices and procedures might improve healing of the lesion or reduce patient discomfort after surgery).

It shows that there is lack of evidence that a surgical approach leads to better results compared with non-surgical retreatment at 1 year (or at 4 or 10 years) after intervention. However, participants treated surgically reported more pain and swelling during the first week after treatment. Healing at one-year follow-up seemed to be improved by the use of ultrasonic devices, instead of the traditional bur, for root-end preparation. There was some evidence of better healing at one-year follow-up when root-ends were filled with mineral trioxide aggregate compared with their being treated by smoothing of orthograde gutta percha root filling.

Use of a graft composed of a gel enriched with the patient's own platelets applied to the defect during the surgical procedure significantly reduced postoperative pain. Exposure to a low energy level laser did not apparently reduce pain at the surgical site.

A small gingival incision may preserve the gum between two adjacent teeth, improving the aesthetic appearance and causing less pain after surgery. There was no evidence that use of antibiotics reduces the occurrence of postoperative infection (although when the procedure is done well, infection is an extremely rare event). Different ways of enhancing the surgeon's view did not lead to different results at least one year after operation, and results of retreatment were independent of the radiographic technique used to make the diagnosis.

Overall, none of the review findings can be assumed to be conclusive, as the quality of the evidence was low to very low. Information is still insufficient to inform clinicians whether root canal retreatment or root-end resection should be used, and which procedures for root-end resection should be followed to achieve the best results for patients.

Summary

In this chapter, principles of evidence-based dentistry and MID approach using the evidence available in the literature were discussed. To date, there are some Cochrane reviews on MID approaches. Interestingly, Cochrane reviews on the effects of MID approaches for dental caries management provide some evidence on the relative effectiveness of a large number of treatment modalities. Overall estimates of effects are reported as the results of various trials addressing specific comparisons could be quantitatively combined in meta-analyses. However, owing to the relatively limited quantity of randomised evidence addressing the questions posed in six reviews, and also the limited quality of the evidence available, a common conclusion for further research from each is that more experimental research, and research of better methodological quality, is needed. In this regard, all Cochrane reviews include an 'authors' conclusions section, divided into 'implications for practice' and 'implications for research,' which are important sources of information for those making decisions and recommendations in these areas.

In addition, the general scarcity of information on various comparisons and outcomes considered relevant in each of these MID reviews for the management of dental caries suggests that further primary (RCT) research should include assessments and reporting of all potentially important benefits as well as harms and costs (Richards and Lawrence 1995).

It should also be stressed that findings from these Cochrane reviews are increasingly underpinning evidence-based recommendations/guidelines from professional bodies and health services in the United Kingdom and internationally. It is fair to suggest that such reliable summaries of the evidence available can and should be used widely, particularly by patients and dentists who have firsthand experience of the topics addressed in the reviews.

After all, Cochrane reviews are produced to improve decision making as well as the efficiency of use of resources in clinical dentistry and in health care (Richards and Lawrence 1995). Therefore when a research is designed to implement MID, study methodology need to be planned thoroughly and systematically to produce evidence and clinical experiences considering patients' values to provide good quality research.

Further Reading

In addition to the main sources of evidence noted above there are a number of publications that provide summaries or critical commentaries of the available literature, which can be useful for the busy clinician. Some of the known sources are:

The Dental Elf (www.nationalelfservice.net/dentistry/)
The Evidence-based Dentistry Journal
The Journal of Evidence-based Dental Practice
The Journal of the American Dental Association
University of Texas Health Science Center San Antonio School of Dentistry Oral Health
searchable Critically Appraised Topic library (https://cats.uthscsa.edu/).

References

American Dental Association. Policy statement on evidence-based dentistry. https://www.ada.org/en/about-the-ada/ada-positions-policies-andstatements/policy-on-evidence-baseddentistry (accessed 16 July 2018).

Antman, E.M., Lau, J., Kupelnick, B., Mosteller, F., and Chalmers, T.C. (1992). A comparison of results of meta-analyses of randomized control trials and recommendations of clinical experts: Treatments for myocardial infarction. *JAMA* 268: 240–248.

Chalmers, I. (1993). The cochrane collaboration: Preparing, maintaining and disseminating systematic reviews of the effects of health care. In: *Doing More Good than Harm: The Evaluation of Health Care Interventions* (ed. K.S. Warren and F. Mosteller), 156–163. New York: Annals of the New York Academy of Sciences.

Chalmers, I., Dickersin, K., and Chalmers, T.C. (1992). Getting to grips with archie cochrane's agenda. *BMJ* 305: 786–788.

Cochrane, A.L. (1972). *Effectiveness and Efficiency. Random Reflections on Health Services.* London: Nuffield Provincial Hospitals Trust.

Dawes, M., Summerskill, W., Glasziou, P., Cartabellotta, A., Martin, J., Hopayian, K., Porzsolt, F., Burls, A., Osborne, J., and Second International Conference of Evidence-Based Health Care Teachers and Developers (2005). Sicily statement on evidence-based practice. *BMC Med. Educ.* 5: 1. https://bmcmededuc.biomedcentral.com/articles/10.1186/1472-6920-5-1.

Del Fabbro, M., Corbella, S., Sequeira-Byron, P., Tsesis, I., Rosen, E., Lolato, A., and Taschieri, S. (2016). Endodontic procedures for retreatment of periapical lesions. *Cochrane Database Syst. Rev.* (10). Art. No.: CD005511. doi: 10.1002/14651858.CD005511.pub3.

Dorri, M., Dunne, S.M., Walsh, T., and Schwendicke, F. Micro-invasive interventions for managing proximal dental decay in primary and permanent teeth. Cochrane systematic review – intervention version published: 5 November 2015. https://www.cochranelibrary.com/cdsr/doi/10.1002/14651858.CD010431.pub2/full.

Dorri, M., Martinez-Zapata, M.J., Walsh, T., Marinho, V., Sheiham, A., and Zaror, C. (2017). Atraumatic restorative treatment versus conventional restorative treatment for managing dental caries. *Cochrane Database Syst. Rev.* 12: CD008072. doi: 10.1002/14651858.CD008072.pub2.

Evidence-Based Medicine Working Group. (1992). Evidence-based medicine. A new approach to teaching the practice of medicine. *JAMA* 268: 2420–2425.

Fédération Dentaire Internationale (FDI). (2017). FDI policy statement on minimal intervention dentistry (mid) for managing dental caries: Adopted by the general assembly: September 2016. *Poland. Int. Dent. J.* 67: 6–7.

GDC-UK. (2015). https://www.gdc-uk.org/docs/default-source/education-and-cpd/education-provider-guidance/standards-for-education-(revised-2015).pdf

Glasziou, P., and Haynes, B. (2005). The paths from research to improved health outcomes. *ACP J. Club* 142: A8–10.

Glenny, A.M., Esposito, M., Coulthard, P., and Worthington, H.V. (2003). The assessment of systematic reviews in dentistry. *Eur. J. Oral Sci.* 111: 85 92.

Holmgren, C., Gaucher, C., Decerle, N., and Doméjean, S. (2014). Minimal intervention dentistry II: Part 3. Management of non-cavitated (initial) occlusal caries lesions – noninvasive approaches through remineralisation and therapeutic sealants. *BDJ* 216: 237–243.

Ijaz, S., Croucher, R.E., and Marinho, V.C. (2010). Systematic reviews of topical fluorides for dental caries: A review of reporting practice. *Caries Res.* 44: 579–592.

Innes, N.P.T., Ricketts, D., Chong, L.Y., Keightley, A.J., Lamont, T., and Santamaria, R.M. Preformed crowns for decayed primary molar teeth. *Online Publication Date*: December 2015. https://doi.org/10.1002/14651858.CD003808.pub3.

Jadad, A.R., Cook, D.J., Jones, A., Klassen, T.P., Tugwell, P., Moher, M., and Moher, D. (1998). Methodology and reports of systematic reviews and meta-analyses: a comparison of Cochrane reviews with articles published in paperbased journals. *JAMA* 280: 278–280.

Marcenes, W., Kassebaum, N.J., Bernabe, E., Flaxman, A., Naghavi, M., Lopez, A., and Murray, C.J. (2013). Global burden of oral conditions in 1990–2010: A systematic analysis. *J. Dent. Res.* 92: 592–597.

Montedori, A., Abraha, I., Orso, M., D'Errico, P., Pagano, S., and Lombardo, G. Lasers for caries removal in deciduous and permanent teeth. *Online Publication Date*: September 2016. https://www.ncbi.nlm.nih.gov/pmc/articles/PMC6457657.

Petersen, P.E., and Lennon, M.A. (2004). Effective use of fluorides for the prevention of dentalcaries in the 21st century: The WHO approach. *Community Dent. Oral Epidemiol.* 32: 319–321.

Richards, D., and Lawrence, A. (1995). Evidence based dentistry. *Br. Dent. J.* 179: 270–273.

Richardson, W.S., Wilson, M.C., Nishikawa, J., and Hayward, R.S. (1995). The well-built clinical question: A key to evidence-based decisions [editorial]. *ACP J. Club* 123: A12–3.

Ricketts, D., Lamont, T., Innes, N.P.T., Kidd, E., and Clarkson, J.E. (2013). Operative caries management in adults and children. *Cochrane Database Syst. Rev.* (3). Art. No.: CD003808. https://www.cochranelibrary.com/cdsr/doi/10.1002/14651858.CD003808.pub3/pdf/full.

3

Molecular Dentistry: Role of Salivary Proteins in Dental Hard Tissue Protection

Paul Anderson

Key Topics

- Facts and figures: Overview of role of saliva
- Saliva and dental hard tissue mineral preservation
- The enamel-saliva continuum
- Molecular Dentistry and Minimally Invasive Dentistry (MID)

Learning Objectives

- Understand the importance and complexity of saliva in hard tissue mineral preservation
- Why saliva malfunction leads to complications in dental hard tissue mineral preservation
- The relationship between Molecular Dentistry and MID
- The requirements for MID artificial saliva

Introduction

In 2019, the Ig Nobel Prize was awarded to a paper that described the estimation of the daily volume of saliva production in 5 year olds (Watanabe et al. 1995). In 2018, Ig Nobel Prize for Chemistry was awarded for a paper describing the benefits of saliva for cleaning surfaces (Paula et al. 1990). This ability of saliva to clean surfaces was attributed to the fact that saliva contains amylase proteases, and illustrates just one of the many thousands of saliva's protein components, demonstrating that saliva is not only inorganic ions and water, but is a complex multifunctional biological system containing sophisticated biomolecules. An understanding of this many-function ability of saliva is required in order

Minimally Invasive Dentistry: Interdisciplinary Clinical and Scientific Approaches, First Edition.
Edited by Aylin Baysan and Paul Anderson.
© 2026 John Wiley & Sons Ltd. Published 2026 by John Wiley & Sons Ltd.
Companion website: www.wiley.com/go/baysan/minimally_invasive_dentistry

to develop novel biomimetic therapeutic strategies, particularly for the development of 'smart' artificial salivas. This is relevant for a 'molecular dentistry' based MID approach using molecular biomimicry, for the benefit of salivary-flow compromised patients.

Therefore, the first aim of this chapter is to describe the mineral protection role of those proteins amongst the many thousand salivary components that are mineral protecting proteins, and how consideration of their role is important for the development of novel saliva-based MID treatments, particularly, for salivary compromised patients. These proteins serve to directly protect the dental hard tissues from the hostile environment within the oral cavity. This natural function of saliva cannot be overstated, as it can be considered that saliva operates as the natural conservative dentist for both the protection and, for the repair, of the dental soft and hard tissues. In order to understand this role, and the potential for therapeutic benefit, it is necessary to discuss some underlying oral biological and chemical concepts in order to help in the understanding this role of saliva, highlighting the similarities of the molecular biology of saliva protein operation with the molecular biology of enamel formation itself.

Saliva has been described as a 'precious body fluid,' which, is at best, an understatement (DePaola 2008). Although 98% by volume water, saliva is immensely complex, and multifunctional. At the molecular level, saliva components include calcium ions, phosphate ions, and, more importantly, calcium-binding proteins. In essence these constituents are similar to the chemical components of enamel, but, at markedly different concentrations. Further, it must be noted that saliva has evolved *contemporaneously* with the dental hard tissues within the oral environment. It seems that all creatures that have true enamel (rather than fishes), also have saliva. So, it is likely, at the molecular level, the processes involved in enamel formation, and enamel preservation, are interlinked. The role of saliva in mineral preservation cannot be overemphasised. Therefore, as a clinical consequence, any form of saliva dysfunction, be it radiation induced, chemically or medically induced, dry mouth (xerostomia), or, diseased based, which negatively impacts salivary flow or quality, may lead to dental hard tissue mineral destruction. So, a further aim of this chapter is to highlight the direct impact of lack of saliva on dental hard tissue mineral destruction (Robinson et al. 1995).

Protein Control of Enamel Formation

During amelogenesis, enamel mineral is formed in the extra-cellular matrix adjacent to the Tome's process of the ameloblast cells. Ameloblast cells export calcium and phosphate ions from within the cell into the extra-cellular matrix (ECM). The pH of the ECM is basic, and therefore, calcium hydroxyapatite crystal nuclei form. However, ameloblasts also secrete a range of proteins, including the protein amelogenin which is a calcium hydroxyapatite-binding protein involved in enamel mineral formation. The biomineralisation role of amelogenin in enamel formation was first described by Fincham, who suggested that this protein binds to the two crystallographic side faces of precursor hydroxyapatite crystals, but not the end face (Fincham and Belcourt 1985). By binding to these chemically similar side-face, but not to the end face of the crystal (001), *only* long-axis (c-axis) growth of the crystal is allowed, ensuring that the forming crystallites grow by extending length, but not widthways. The enamel crystallites therefore are formed as very long elongated crystals extending from the enamel-dentine junction (EDJ) to the enamel surface. Only at the later stages of amelogenesis, once the full-length enamel crystal is formed, the amelogenin proteins are destroyed by MMP20 proteases, and amelogenin then loses its face-specific hydroxyapatite binding functionality, allowing the growing enamel crystallites to grow widthways, into each other until full mineralisation is achieved. It was reported (Kawasaki and Weiss 2006) that amelogenin is a member of a family of calcium binding proteins, which all have evolutionary links to a common calcium-binding precursor protein, that has subsequently evolved into a series of related calcium binding proteins, including the salivary protein statherin, and the milk protein casein.

The Inorganic Chemistry of Dental Hard Tissue Mineral Loss

The mineral structures of dental hard tissues are composed of a form of a calcium-deficient hydroxyapatite, which is a highly insoluble calcium orthophosphate (Elliott 1994). The solubility behaviour of calcium orthophosphates is complex, and depends not only on the local concentrations of hydrogen ions (i.e., the pH), but also the concentration of calcium ions (Anderson et al. 2001). Although phosphate ions are also involved, and need to be present in excess, that a solution is undersaturated or supersaturated with respect to calcium hydroxyapatite can be calculated from the solution's pH and calcium concentration alone using the calcium hydroxyapatite solubility product, and the necessary ion-pair formation constants (Leung and Darvell 1991). Figure 3.1 shows the solubility isotherm of

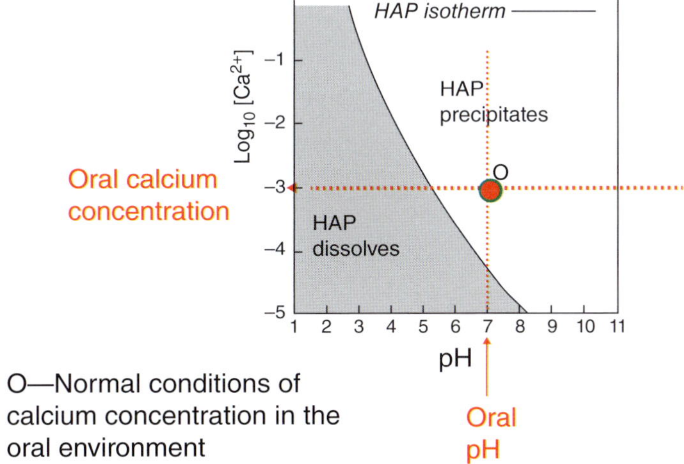

Figure 3.1 Plot of the solubility isotherm of calcium hydroxyapatite. Area in grey represents pH and calcium ion concentration conditions under which calcium hydroxyapatite will 'demineralise'. Area in white represents the combination of pH and calcium ion concentration conditions under which calcium hydroxyapatite will 'remineralise'.

calcium hydroxyapatite which can be calculated using speciation calculation software (Chemist (MicroMath, Missouri, USA)) (Hassanali et al. 2017).

The solution conditions (i.e., calcium concentration and proton concentration represented as pH) are shown on the plot as the axes. Conditions above the solid line (the solubility isotherm) represent thermodynamic conditions when precipitation (i.e. 'remineralisation') should take place. Whereas, conditions below the line represent thermodynamic conditions when dissolution (i.e. 'demineralisation') should occur. Point O represents normal oral pH and calcium concentration conditions. It is generally considered that the concentrations of calcium, phosphate, and hydrogen ions in saliva at normal resting conditions are about 1.7 mmol L^{-1}, 10.0 mmol L^{-1}, and 1.0×10^{-7} mol L^{-1} (pH 7), respectively. Under these conditions, chemical speciation calculations suggest there should be precipitation of hydroxyapatite mineral, as normal resting adult saliva is massively supersaturated with respect to calcium hydroxyapatite. However, in the oral cavity, this inorganic chemistry predicted precipitation of mineral does not happen. This is because these salivary proteins 'manage' the balance between the free and the bound calcium ions in saliva, ensuring that sufficient calcium ions are bound to proteins, and therefore are excluded from the speciation calculations, as the actual effective calcium ion concentration is much much lower. So, precipitation of calcium hydroxyapatite does not occur, and therefore the oral cavity is not coated with calcium hydroxyaptite. On the other hand, if the oral pH decreases, then demineralisation should occur. However, the mineral manageing salivary proteins are stimulated to release calcium ions by a complex pH switching mechanisms as the proteins change conformation, thereby reducing the thermodynamic driving force for demineralisation. The principal protein involved in this calcium ion management function is the salivary protein statherin.

The inorganic chemistry of calcium hydroxyapatite means that the dental hard tissue mineral react with free protons (from acids), be this via metabolic by-products of oral bacterial as in caries, or, acids from other sources, as in erosion (e.g., drinks, foodstuffs, gastric juices). At the molecular level, as far as the enamel mineral in the form of calcium hydroxyapatite is concerned, the source of protons (acid) is unimportant. But, should the oral pH drop markedly, say during a cariogenic or erosive challenge, the chemical conditions are no longer supersaturated with respect to enamel mineral, and enamel surfaces become undersaturated (assuming that the calcium concentrations do not change). Chemical speciation calculations which are used to calculate inorganic chemical thermodynamics, show that as the pH decreases, the pH value at which the chemical conditions changes from supersaturation to undersaturation is about 5.5, termed the 'critical pH' (Dawes 2004). The actual calculated value of critical pH for any individual will depend on a variety of chemical thermodynamic values used in the calculation , including the solubility product of calcium hydroxyapatite, and of course the actual values of a particular individual's calcium ion concentration. Salivary calcium concentration values differ significantly between individuals, which will mean a different values for critical pH for different individuals (Anderson et al. 2001). Of course, pH is a logarithmic scale, so a decrease in pH from 7.0 to 5.5 represents an (approximately) 31 times increase in proton concentration. A drop from to pH 7 to 4, as during a carious challenge, means a 1,000 times increase in proton concentration, and therefore more undersaturation. The greater the degree of undersaturation, the greater the driving force for the dissolution reaction.

All chemical reactions in solutions are reversible. So, during a carious challenge for example, as the local pH rises again above 5.5, the chemical conditions reverse, and the chemical environment adjacent to the enamel surface will become supersaturated with respect to hydroxyapatite once again, and precipitation condition resume. Thus, this continuous de-and remineralisation cycling of oral pH means that there is constant alternation of mineral precipitation and mineral loss at the enamel surface. At the molecular level, as the oral pH changes from above to below the critical pH at an enamel surface, and back, there is constant a reversal between undersaturation and supersaturation. However, this is only as long as there are sufficient calcium ions (and phosphateions) present. These ions are also provided by saliva. This results in a constant reversal of conditions between mineral loss, and mineral gain, represented in many textbooks diagram as a dynamic balance (Figure 3.2a, b, and c). This ion concentration driven dynamic balance is considered to maintain the chemical balance and therefore maintenance of the mineral. However, this reversibility is chemical only, and does not mean that the physical structure of enamel in terms of the original enamel crystal shapes will also be maintained.

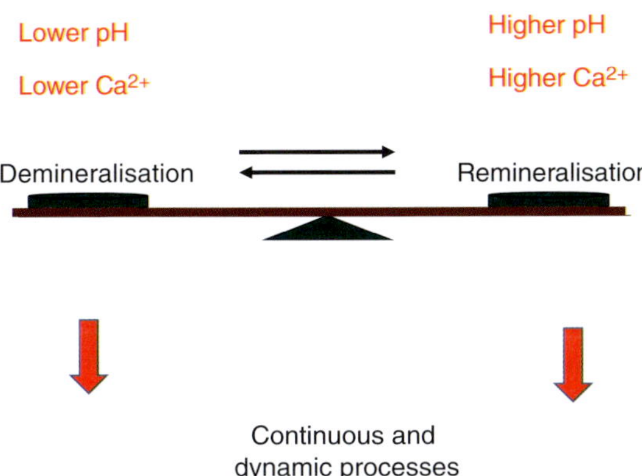

Figure 3.2a The Dynamic Balance: Equilibrium no caries.

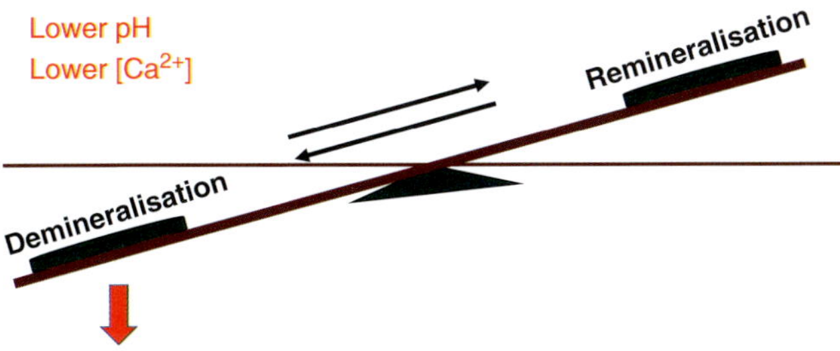

Figure 3.2b The Dynamic Balance: Low pH Low calcium concentration: Demineralisation.

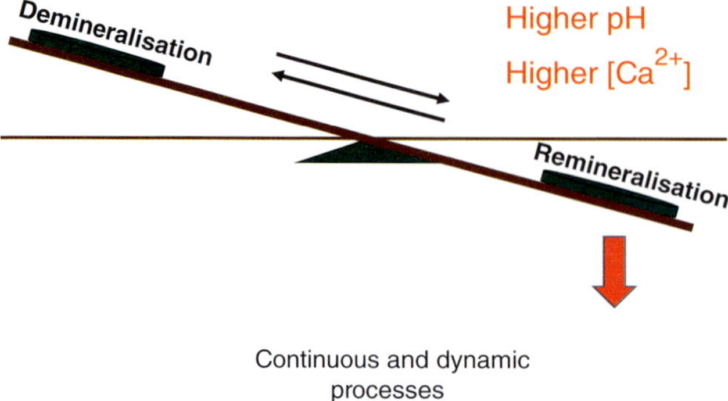

Figure 3.2c The Dynamic Balance: High pH High calcium concentration: Remineralisation.

The Role of the Organic Proteins of Saliva in Enamel Mineral Preservation

However, although the inorganic chemistry can be given as a simple explanation, oral biological processes cannot be described simply in terms of inorganic chemistry alone; biological macromolecules including salivary proteins are fundamentally involved. This includes the role of salivary proteins in the dental hard tissue protection process. Saliva contains many thousands of organic components (Castagnola et al. 2017), some of which are proteins directly involved in the mineral preservation process. Four salivary proteins have been identified in the mineral preservation process, although it is likely that more will be identified in future. These proteins are associated with enamel pellicle formation, which is the thin organic 'skin' of proteins that bind directly to the enamel surfaces (Hannig 2011). These proteins not only prevent spontaneous precipitation of hydroxyapatite mineral within the oral environment, but, also directly aid in mineral preservation. The enamel pellicle proteins bind to an enamel surface in a particular order (Hannig 2011). The first protein in the enamel pellicle (or that closest to the enamel surface) is statherin, which has been shown to bind directly to the 001 face of hydroxyapatite crystals (Masica and Gray 2009), and is the most rapidly and strongest binding protein to the enamel surface. As described earlier, statherin is a member of a group of calcium binding proteins that have been shown to have evolved from a single ancient enamel matrix protein. Although the exact mechanism by which this demineralisation inhibition function is achieved is not known, it is the statherin protein binding to the particular crystal faces of enamel crystallites which are exposed at the enamel surface (the 001) that is crucially involved in preventing dissolution pits co-alescing, thereby inhibiting progression of dissolution, and therefore reducing the rate of enamel demineralisation (Tang et al. 2004).

Thus, statherin (and therefore the enamel pellicle) can be described as a 'smart system', i.e., it responds appropriately to the external environment. It has two separate molecular-level functions. Free unbound to a surface in saliva, statherin binds free calcium ions preventing precipitation at normal oral pH levels. However, when the oral pH becomes acidic, statherin provides additional free calcium ions. Secondly, when bound to hydroxyapatite surfaces, statherin inhibits the reaction mechanism between protons and hydroxyapatite mineral, protecting the enamel surface.

Therefore, dental hard tissue mineral loss cannot simply be described in terms of inorganic chemistry alone. Demineralisation and remineralisation are 'managed' in the oral cavity by the function of salivary proteins which form the enamel pellicle, which demonstrates the dual role benefit for the protection of the these tissues. Therefore, the demineralisation and remineralisation in enamel are better described as bio-demineralisation and bio-remineralisation, respectively (Anderson and Al-Jawad 2015).

Biomineralisation and Bio-demineralisation/remineralisation

Biomineralisation is the control of inorganic crystal growth by proteins. Biomineralisation is responsible (for example), for the formation of complex and exquisite shapes of calcium carbonate based structures such as sea shells, as well as many complex inorganic structures in biology ranging from diatoms to magnetic-field detecting guidance systems in birds (Lowenstam and Weiner 1989). Enamel formation is also a biomineralisation process. The fundamental tenant of biomineralisation is that proteins control inorganic crystal growth by inhibiting growth of specific crystallographic faces of crystals, in this case hydroxyapatite crystals, at controlled times throughout the amelogenesis process. By this highly precise positional and temporal molecular control mechanism, ultra-engineered highly specific shapes of inorganic crystals can be grown to form very exquisite and complex structures as required for biological systems. For example, single enamel crystallites are highly elongated, extending the entire length from the enamel-dentine junction to the enamel surface. This complex molecular-level architecture gives bulk enamel its unique mechanical properties, requiring precision crystallite orientation control.

Both proteins statherin and amelogenin, bind quite precisely to the calcium hydroxyapatite crystal in a 'lock and key' manner, but, to different crystallographic faces. These binding sites are molecular charge and *stearic* specific interactions, where the molecular orientation of the specific amino acid residues in each protein is critical. It is also likely that protein conformation in each case is determined by the inorganic structure of the hydoxyapatite face. However, for both processes, by binding to a particular face of hydroxyapatite, the growth of enamel crystals can be inhibited. In amelogenesis, the amelogenin protein binds to the side (the a and b) faces of the hydroxyapatite crystal (Figure 3.3), only allowing growth of the crystal along the c axis. Whereas, for the salivary pellicle proteins, including statherin, the binding is to the end face (001) of the crystal, reducing the rate of demineralisation on the (001) face (that face that is exposed to the oral environment), but allowing precipitation to the side faces of the hydroxyapatite crystal. So, both amelogenesis, and bio-demineralisation and remineralisation events are protein-controlled biomineralisation processes, but occurring at different hydroxyapatite crystal surfaces.

Molecular level protein controlled amelogenesis (amelogenin), and protein controlled de-remineralisation (statherin) demonstrate how biomineralisation phenomena influences what happens at the whole tooth level.

Overall, the destruction of enamel mineral during caries and erosion involves biomolecules, as well as acids, and inorganic mineral ions in the oral environment, which is awash with saliva. Although caries and erosion are often described as occurring as a result of an ion inbalance during low and high pH episodes, both these processes also involve salivary components, including the proteins which manage the local calcium concentration, and, inhibit the interaction of acids with hydroxyapatite surfaces.

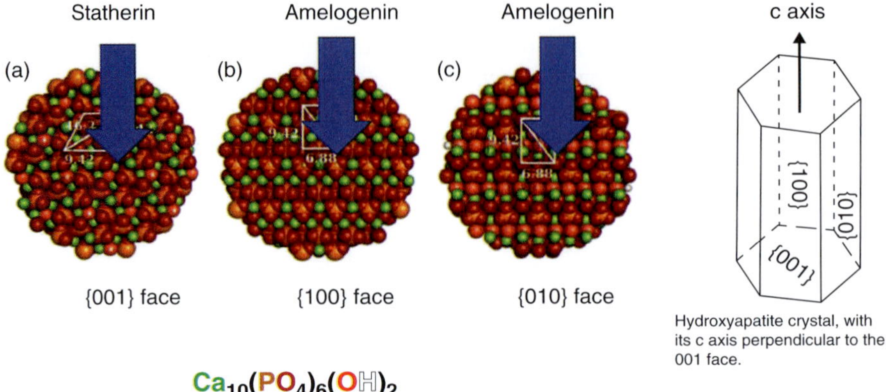

Figure 3.3 Statherin and Amelogenin binding at different crystallographic faces of hydroxyapatite. Statherin binds to the top {001} face, which is the long c-axis of the crystal that extends from the EDJ to the surface. Whereas, amelogenin binds to the side {100} and {010} faces of the hydroxyapatite crystal.

The Potential Roles of Protein Engineered Salivas in Minimally Invasive Dentistry

Saliva provides a totally non-invasive mechanism for the direct protection and the repair of the dental hard tissues, via biomineralisation process which at the molecular level, are similar to the processes of enamel formation. Therefore, a successful MID salivary-based repair mechanisms should aim to replicate this role of saliva. For erupted enamel, the ameloblasts have long gone, so a therapeutic repair mechanism which is identical to enamel formation is not possible, unlike most cellular repair processes of other hard and soft tissues in human and other biological systems. However, the salivary glands cells secrete proteins which effect a similar but not identical molecular protection mechanism to amelogensis but which operates directly on already formed enamel. This process is similar to enamel formation, in that it is a biomineralisation role, but one which the salivary gland secretions exert control of dental hard tissue protection, maintenance, and repair. However, if salivary glands become damaged or destroyed through disease, or other events, this will negatively impact on this dental hard tissue maintenance function of saliva. For patients with a complete absence of saliva, rampant caries occurs quite quickly because the extensive tissue protection function of the 'precious body fluid' are lost. Chemically, this is not only the loss of supply of the enamel mineral constituent calcium and phosphate ions, but also the loss of supply of the salivary pellicle proteins involved in the calcium ion management and the demineralisation inhibition processes of saliva. Further, reductions in saliva volume, and in composition will also contribute to increased susceptibilities to caries diseases and erosion.

Artificial salivas are an important therapeutic intervention for patients with either little or no salivary flow, or, poor quality saliva. Dry mouth is a condition that has severe impact on the quality of life of patients (Sreebny and Vissink 2010). However, many commercial artificial salivas do not contain the complex mineral protection proteins that are part of the organic components of natural saliva. Many are little more than aqueous substitutes, and many others have been developed to aid swallowing and therefore include rheological polymers. These coat the oral soft tissues, but offer no biomineralisation controlled protection for the dental hard tissues. More sophisticated formulations also include calcium and phosphate ions. However, they do not contain the biomolecules that are needed to control the growth of hydroxyapatite in the enamel crystallites. Consequently, calcium phosphate precipitation may occur, but this will be uncontrolled and haphazard mineral precipitation. The architecture of hydroxyapatite-like crystallites within natural enamel is complex. Therefore biomineralisation is needed to control the 'regrowth' of damaged enamel crystallites in an orientated fashion. Saliva contains molecules which control the crystal growth of hydroxyapatite. This is a similar process to the role of amelogenin proteins within amelogenesis, i.e., *inhibit* the growth of particular hydroxyapatite crystallite faces. Under cariogenic or erosive demineralisation conditions, salivary proteins inhibit the demineralisation of the oral cavity facing surfaces of the enamel crystallites, those surfaces that are subject to acids. Under remineralisation conditions in the oral cavity, these same proteins prevent growth of the outward facing face, and promote the growth of the two faces side faces of existing enamel crystallites. Therefore, an MID salivary-based biomimetic treatment needs to include the two contradictory roles of salivary proteins. Although salivary proteins mimic the biomineralisation role of amelogenesis protcins, i.e., inhibiting the growth of particular faces, the crystallographic faces concerned in each case are different. Therefore, the proteins that are incorporated into functionality salivas must be salivary protein emulating (statherin in particualr), rather than amelogenin emulating proteins.

New therapeutic systems are required, based on the salivary protein mimicking functionality, which control orientated enamel crystallite formation. Elsharkawy et al. (2018) have recently described an elastin-like polymer that contains statherin-like amino acid residues, which can stimulate the formation of oriented crystal growth of calcium hydroxyapatite, suitable for the replacement of diseased enamel with orientated hydroxyapatite crystals. It may be that protein-engineered statherin-like proteins with highly specific binding properties can be developed that will be an even better impact at protecting demineralising hydroxyapatite surfaces.

Overall Conclusion

In conclusion, the natural MID functions and roles of saliva have been reported, in terms of both its inorganic, and organic components. The future direction for artificial salivas for enamel regeneration by biomimickery of the original enamel formation process have been suggested.

References

Anderson, P., and Al-Jawad, J. (2015). Biomineralization and biodemineralization of enamel. In: *Handbook of Oral Biomaterials* (ed. J. Matinlinna), 33487–2742. Boca Raton, FL: CRC Press. ISBN 978981446312.

Anderson, P., Hector, M.P., and Rampersad, M.A. (2001). Critical pH in resting and stimulated whole saliva in groups of children and adults. *Int. J. Paediatr. Dent.* 11: 266–273. doi: 10.1046/j.1365-263X.2001.00293.x.

Castagnola, M., Scarano, E., Passali, G.C., Messana, I.,, Cabras, T., Iavarone, F., Di Cintio, G., Fiorita, A., De Corso, E., and Paludetti, G. (2017). Salivary biomarkers and proteomics: Future diagnostic and clinical utilities. *Acta Otorhinolaryngol. Ital.* 37 (2): 94–101. doi: 10.14639/0392-100X-1598.

Dawes, C. (2004). What is the critical Ph and Why does a tooth dissolve in acid? *J. Can. Dent. Assoc.* 69: 722–724.

DePaola, D.P. (2008). Saliva The precious body fluid. *J. Am. Dent. Assoc.* 139: 5S–6S.

Elliott, J.C. (1994). *Structure and Chemistry of the Apatites and Other Calcium Orthophosphates Elliott J.C.* Elsevier Science. ISBN 10 0444815821 Studies in Inorganic Chemistry (Book 18).

Elsharkawy, S., Al-Jawad, M., Mehta, K., Tejeda-Montes, E., Agarwal, S., Shuturminska, K., Rice, A., Tarakina, N., Wilson, R.M., Bushby, A.J., Rodriguez-Cabello, J.C., Hernandez, A.D.R., Stevens, M.M., Anderson, P., and Mata, A. (2018). Nucleation and crystal growth of stiff hierarchically-ordered apatite crystals. *Nat. Commun.* 9: 2145. doi: 10.1038/s41467-018-04319-0.

Fincham, A.G., and Belcourt, A.B. (1985). Amelogenin biochemistry: Currentconcepts. In: *The Chemistry and Biology of Mineralized Tissues* (ed. W.T. Butler), 240–247. Birmingham: Ebsco Media.

Hannig, M. (2011) Protective nature of the salivary pellicle. *Int. Dent. J.*52: 417–423. doi: 10.1111/j.1875-595X.2002.tb00731.x.

Hassanali, L., Wong, F.S., Lynch, R.J.M., and Anderson, P. (2017). A novel kinetic method to measure apparent solubility product of Bulk Human Enamel. *Front. Physiol.* 8: 714. doi: 10.3389/fphys.2017.00714. https://lscpagepro.mydigitalpublication.com/publication/?i=627902&article_id=3507824&view=articleBrowser.

Kawasaki, K., and Weiss, K.M. (2006). Evolutionary genetics of vertebrate tissue mineralization: The origin and evolution of the secretory calcium-binding phosphoprotein family. *J. Exp. Zool.* 306B: 295–316. doi: 10.1002/jez.b.21088.

Leung, V.W.-H., and Darvell, B.W. (1991). Calcium phosphate system in saliva-like media. *J. Chem. Soc., Faraday Trans.* 87: 1759.

Lowenstam, H.A., and Weiner, S. (1989). *On Biomineralization.* New York: Oxford University Press.

Masica, D.L., and Gray, J.J. (2009). Solution- and adsorbed-state structural ensembles predicted for the statherin-hydroxyapatite system. *Biophys. J.* 96 (8): 3082–3091. doi: 10.1016/j.bpj.2009.01.033.

Paula, M.S., Romao, A.M.A., and Cesar, A.N.V. (1990). Human saliva as a cleaning agent for dirty surfaces. *Stud. Conserv.* 35 (3): 153–155. doi: 10.1179/sic.1990.35.3.153.

Robinson, C., Kirkham, J., and Shore, R.J. (1995). *Dental Enamel Formation to Destruction.* Boca Raton, Fla, USA: CRC Press.

Sreebny, L.M., and Vissink, A. (2010). *Dry Mouth: The Malevolent Symptom: A Clinical Guide.* Ames, Iowa: Wiley-Blackwell.

Tang, R., Wang, L., Orme, C.A., Bonstein, T., Bush, P.J., and Nancollas, G.H. (2004). Dissolution at the nanoscale: Self-Preservation of biominerals. *Angew. Chem. Int. Ed.* 43: 2697–2701. doi: 10.1002/anie.200353652.

Watanabe, S., Ohnishi, M., Imai, K., Kawano, E., and Igarashi, S. (1995). Estimation of the total saliva volume produced per day in five-year-old children. *Archs. Oral Biol.* 8: 781–782. doi: 10.1016/0003-9969(95)00026-L.

4

Dental Caries Risk Assessment and Early Caries Detection

Bennett T. Amaechi

Key Topics

- What is caries risk assessment?
- What are the purposes of risk assessment?
- How do you determine the caries risk status of a patient?
- What are the required conditions for detecting early caries lesion?
- What are the criteria for detecting early caries lesions and assessing their activity status?
- What are the different staging of caries process as it relates caries diagnosis and risk assessment?

Learning Objectives

- Understand and appreciate the importance of caries risk assessment as part of caries management strategy
- Be able to analyze and appraise the risk indicators of dental caries
- Be able to assess patient's caries risk status based on risk indicators
- Have understanding of the different criteria for detection of early caries in various surfaces of a tooth
- Gain the full knowledge of the application caries risk assessment in clinical practice

Introduction

Dental caries, as a very complex disease that affects most individuals during their lifetime, continues to be a global unmet oral health problem that negatively impacts quality of life and overall health of individuals, with 60–90% of school children and nearly 100% adults being affected worldwide (Dye et al. 2007, 2010; WHO). Dental caries is a multifactorial

Minimally Invasive Dentistry: Interdisciplinary Clinical and Scientific Approaches, First Edition.
Edited by Aylin Baysan and Paul Anderson.
© 2026 John Wiley & Sons Ltd. Published 2026 by John Wiley & Sons Ltd.
Companion website: www.wiley.com/go/baysan/minimally_invasive_dentistry

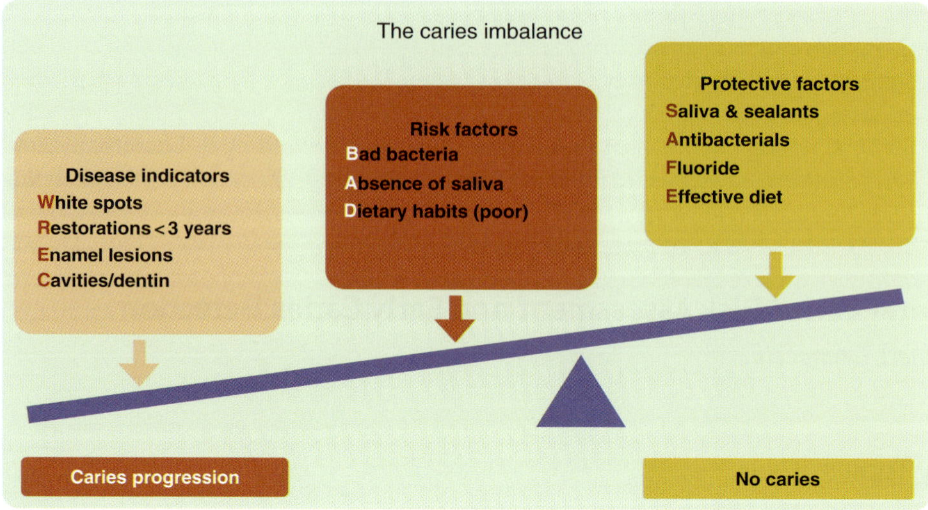

Figure 4.1 The Caries Imbalance. Source: Featherstone (2003) and American Dental Association (2016).

disease, the development and progression of which involves an interaction between the pathological (risk) factors and the preventive (protective) factors. Caries lesion develops when the pathological factors that increase caries risk outweigh the protective factors that decrease caries risk, tilting the caries balance toward caries development (Figure 4.1) (Featherstone 2003). Thus, dental caries is a preventable disease, and can be prevented in an individual by strategies that permits the protective factors to replace or overcome the risk factors. However, the caries risk factors varies among individuals, so caries prevention can only be achieved in an individual if the risk factors associated with that individual are identified early and risk appropriate management is implemented. Besides, patients are taking control of their health and treatment; identifying the risk factors associated with an individual patient would enable the person to establish and maintain own lifelong oral health and well-being by controlling his/her risk factors. Therefore risk assessment is a key and essential component of Minimal Intervention (MI) dentistry that stresses a preventive philosophy, with individualised caries risk assessment; accurate and early detection of caries lesions and assessing their activity status; and efforts to arrest or remineralise non-cavitated lesions and treat cavitated lesions by tooth-preserving operative care (Tyas et al. 2000; Fontana and Gonzalez-Cabezas 2012). A MI approach to caries management is the corner-stone of the modern comprehensive personalised caries care plan (Figure 4.2), described as the **ICCMS™ 4D approach caries management** (Determine patient's caries risk, Detect and assess caries lesions, Decide on a personalised treatment plan, and Do caries management), which aims to personalise caries management with the goal of maintaining health by preserving tooth structure and restoring only when indicated, and in which every component of the management plan is risk-based and as such it is referred to as risk management (Pitts et al. 2013, 2018; Ismail et al. 2015).

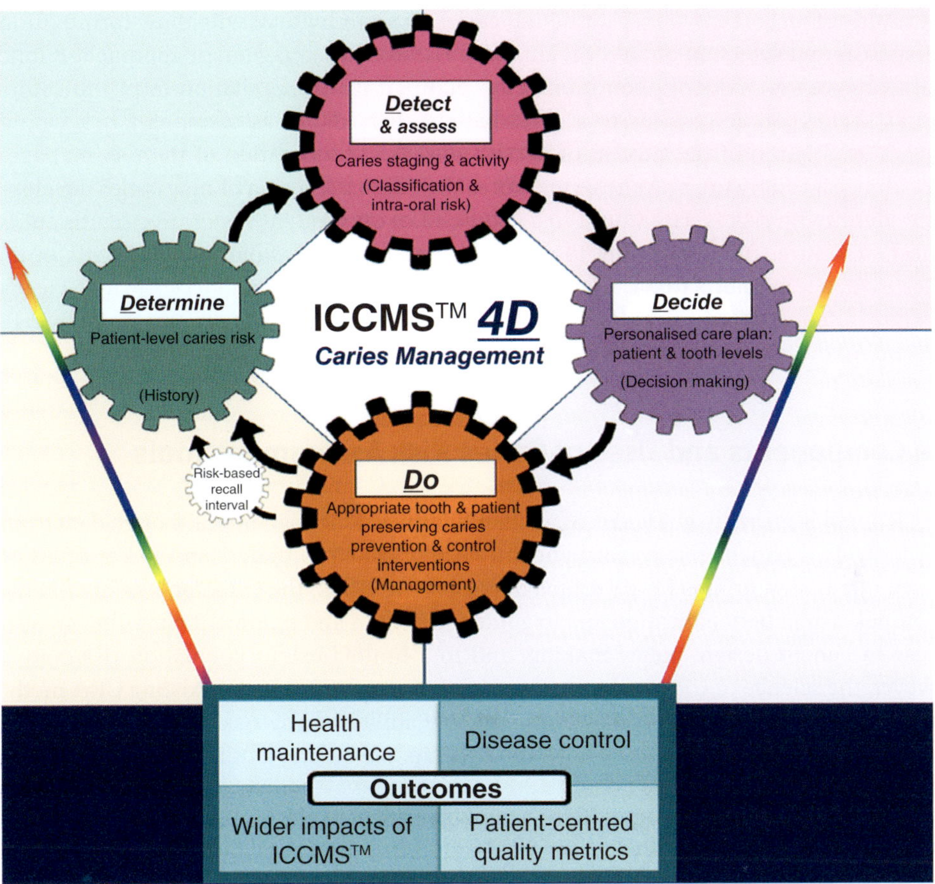

Figure 4.2 The International Caries Classification and Management System (ICCMS™) 4D approach of caries management (Determine patient's caries risk, Detect and assess caries lesions, Decide on a personalised treatment plan, and Do caries management). Source: Pitts et al. (2013, 2018) and Ismail et al. (2015).

What Is Caries Risk Assessment and Its Benefits?

Let's start by defining caries risk first. Caries risk may be defined as the probability of an individual developing a certain number of caries lesions reaching a given stage of disease progression during a specified period (Reich et al. 1999). Therefore Caries Risk Assessment (CRA) is a logical systematic approach of assessing the risk/susceptibility of the individual patient for future development of dental caries by identifying the individual etiologic factors contributing to the existing caries lesions and exacerbating risk. It provides a basis to explain to the patient how to prevent the disease and to communicate and facilitate needed change in behaviour to prevent future disease. It assists the oral health-care practitioner/team to determine the appropriate interventions (non-invasive as well as operative) and recall consultation strategies suitable for an individual patient.

Indications of an increased risk for dental caries in an individual will allow formulation of diagnosis and selection of an individualised risk-based management approach. Public health interventions should continue to be planned using population-level indicators such as socio-economic status in a child patient. Periodic re-assessmentof risk would allow an evaluation of the success of, or the need for, modification of the risk management plan, especially the preventive measures. Besides prevention of new caries development, identifying risk is paramount to a successful treatment, as restorative treatment is subject to failure, frequently due to caries lesions around restorations (Ricketts et al. 2013). Evidence supports that Caries Management by Risk Assessment (CAMBRA) leads to better outcomes (Domejean et al. 2015; Chaffee and Featherstone 2015). With risk assessment, the overall prognosis can be determined.

The Components and Uses of Caries Risk Assessment Tools

The CRA tool is meant to guide risk assessment for individual patients, although data from such individual patient risk assessment can be aggregated to understand risk profiles of defined population groups for programs development. Thus, the CRA tool is not only for the purposes of patient education and to guide prevention and treatment planning but also for use in benefit design, policy making, and to a limited extent population risk status. However, the science of CRA to date is mostly subjective, and so is the existing CRA methods. It is pertinent to mention that the predictive ability of any risk factor and thus the validity of any CRA tool will vary with the baseline prevalence of disease in the defined population in which it is being used.

Considering that caries is a multifactorial disease, the format and components of existing CRA tools varies among developers and depends on the information the tool is tailored to collect. In general, CRA tools uses three important groups of predictive factors; caries risk factors, caries risk indicators, and caries protective factors, to assess caries risk in children and/or adults. Several CRA tools and guidelines are available and have been evaluated on children and adults (Domejean et al. 2011; Hansel Petersson et al. 2016; Petersson and Twetman 2015; Gao et al. 2013; Petersson et al. 2010; Mejare et al. 2014; Chaffee et al. 2017). Recognising that the relative importance of the risk and protective factors varied by age, some of the CRA systems have different tools for children 0–5 years old (Table 4.1) (Kleemola-Kujala and Räsänen 1982; American Academy of Pediatric Dentistry 2014) and other individuals 6 years and above (Table 4.2) (Leroy et al. 2012; American Dental Association 2016). However, the same factors are broadly applicable across all children, so recently one tool was developed for all children below 18 years of age (Table 4.3). A standard CRA tool should consist of three major sections (Kleemola-Kujala and Räsänen 1982; American Academy of Pediatric Dentistry 2014; Leroy et al. 2012; American Dental Association 2016).

The first part is the '*subjective or patient-level*' risk assessment section (Table 4.4), which is a brief questionnaire that collects the information given by the patient on his/her:

- medical health, including use of medications affecting caries risk, head and neck radiation, etc.;

- dietary habits;
- oral hygiene behaviour (dental plaque control);
- use of fluoride and other anticaries agents;
- mother's or caregiver's caries experience (for children); and
- socioeconomic status, including access to dental care.

Contrary to some recommendations that patients can fill this questionnaire in the waiting room, it is highly advised that this questionnaire must be administered by a dental personnel, such as a dental assistant or hygienist, since the patient's response to some questions may necessitate follow-up questions on factors that might exacerbate risk.

Table 4.1 Assessment tool for risk of new caries lesion for children 0–5 years old.

Factors	High Risk	Moderate Risk	Low Risk
Biological			
Mother/primary caregiver has active caries	Yes		
Parent/caregiver has low socioeconomic status	Yes		
Child has >3 between meal sugar-containing snacks or beverages per day	Yes		
Child is put to bed with a bottle containing natural or added sugar	Yes		
Child has special health care needs		Yes	
Child is a recent immigrant		Yes	
Protective			
Child receives optimally-fluoridated drinking water or fluoride supplements			Yes
Child has teeth brushed daily with fluoridated toothpaste			Yes
Child receives topical fluoride from health professional			Yes
Child has dental home/regular dental care			Yes
Clinical Findings			
Child has > I decayed/missing/filled surfaces	Yes		
Child has active white spot lesions or enamel defects	Yes		
Child has elevated mutans streptococci levels	Yes		
Child has plaque on teeth		Yes	

Circling those conditions that apply to a specific patient helps the practitioner and parent understand the factors that contribute to or protect from caries. Risk assessment categorization of low, moderate, or high is based on preponderance of factors for the individual. However, clinical judgement may justify the use of one factor (e.g., frequent exposure to sugar-containing snacks or beverages, more than one dmfs) in determining overall risk.

Overall assessment of the child's dental caries risk: High ☐ Moderate ☐ Low ☐

Source: American Academy of Pediatric Dentistry (2014).

Table 4.2 Assessment tool for risk of new caries lesion for individuals 6 years and above (Leroy et al. 2012; American Dental Association 2016).

Caries Risk Assessment Form (Age > 6)

Patient Name:

Birth Date: Date:

Age: Initials:

		Low Risk	Moderate Risk	High Risk
Contributing Conditions		**Check or Circle the conditions that apply**		
I.	**Fluoride Exposure** (through drinking water, supplements, professional applications, toothpaste)	☐ Yes	☐ No	
II.	**Sugary Foods or Drinks** (including juice, carbonated or non-carbonated soft drinks, energy drinks, medicinal syrups)	Primarily at mealtimes ☐		Frequent or prolonged between meal exposures/day ☐
III.	**Caries Experience of Mother, Caregiver and/or other Siblings** (for patients age 6-14)	No carious lesions in last 24 months ☐	Carious lesions in last 7-23 months ☐	Carious lesions in last 6 months ☐
IV.	**Dental Home**: established patient of record, receiving regular dental care in a dental office	☐ Yes	☐ No	
General Health Conditions		**Check or circle the conditions that apply**		
I.	**Special Health Care Needs** (developmental, physical, medical or mental disabilities that prevent or limit performance of adequate oral health care by themselves or caregives)	☐ No	☐ Yes (over age 14)	☐ Yes (ages 6-14)
II.	**Chemo/Radiation Therapy**	☐ No		☐ Yes
III.	**Eating Disorders**	☐ No	☐ Yes	
IV.	**Medications that Reduce Salivary Flow**	☐ No	☐ Yes	
V.	**Drug/Alcohol Abuse**	☐ No	☐ Yes	
Clinical Conditions		**Check or circle the conditions that apply**		
I.	**Cavitated or Non-Cavitated** (incipient) **Carious Lesions or Restorations** (visually or radiographically evident)	No new carious lesions or restorations in last 36 months ☐	1 or 2 new carious lesions or restorations in last 36 months ☐	3 or more carious lesions or restorations in last 36 months ☐
II	**Teeth Missing Due to Caries in past 36 months**	☐ No		☐ Yes

III	**Visible Plaque**	☐ No	☐ Yes		
IV	**Unusual Tooth Morphology** that compromises oral hygiene	☐ No	☐ Yes		
V	**Interproximal Restorations - 1 or more**	☐ No	☐ Yes		
VI	**Exposed Root Surfaces** Present	☐ No	☐ Yes		
VII	**Restorations with Overhangs** and/or **Open Margins; Open Contacts** with Food impaction	☐ No	☐ Yes		
VIII	**Dental/Orthodontic Appliances** (fixed or removable)	☐ No	☐ Yes		
XI	**Severe Dry Mouth (Xerostomia)**	☐ No			☐ Yes
	Overall assesment of dental caries risk:	☐ Low		☐ Moderate	☐ High

Patient Instructions:

Source: American Dental Association (2016).

Table 4.3 Assessment toll for risk of new caries lesion in children below 18 years.

Pt. Name:		Assessment Date:	
Age*:			
Protective Factors			
Brushes twice a day with toothpaste containing fluoride		Yes	No
Predominantly drinks fluoridated water/beverages made form fluoridated water		Yes	No
Receives professionally applied fluoride		Yes	No**
Uses over the counter fluoride mouth rinse (over age 6 years)		Yes	No**
Uses at-home prescription fluoride products (over age 6 years)		Yes	No**

** Additional fluoride exposure may not be needed for all children but can lower risk for children deemed to be at risk for Caries

Risk Factors			
Consumes more than 3 sugary beverages or snacks between meals each day (or infants put to bed with a bottle containing beverage with sugar)		No	Yes
Physical or behavioural health issues that impede home care		No	Yes
Clinically little saliva or dry mouth due to medical condition or medication		No	Yes
Recent caries experience (Moderate or advanced lesion(s) since last assessment (or in the last 3 years)		No	Yes
Parents or siblings have cavitated lesion(s) in the last year (consider for children under age 14 years)		No	Yes
Visible plaque		No	Yes
Un-coalesced, and unsealed pits & fissures		No	Yes
Orthodontic or prosthodontics appliances that impede oral hygiene		No	Yes
Disease Indicators			
Active initial lesion(s) (i.e., enamel lesions, white spots)		No	Yes
Active moderate or advanced lesion(s)		No	Yes

Table 4.4 ICCMS[TM] Patient Level (Subjective) Risk Assessment Model.

Patient Level	**Medical health**

Medical health

Current use of medications, recreational drugs, or systemic conditions that may cause hyposalivation. 85% of the medications patients are taking causes hyposalivation, especially in adult patients, and as such significantly increases caries risk (Tenovuo 1997). These subjects lack the protective qualities of saliva, of which the flow rate and buffering capacity may be the most important. Buffering capacity has also been shown to positively correlate to caries risk (Dyasanoor and Saddu 2014; Voelker et al. 2013). An unstimulated saliva flow assessment provides the most accurate clinical assessment of saliva volume, so measuring salivary flow, particularly unstimulated, is useful because a low flow rate may help to explain multiple lesions.

Head and neck radiation

Patients undergoing radiotherapy for head and neck cancer are categorised as high risk for developing caries because of the side effects or sequelae of the treatment regimens (Glenny et al. 2010; Alaki et al. 2013). The symptoms include (but are not limited to) xerostomia or hyposalivation, mucositis (affecting eating and oral hygiene practices) and altered taste sensation (which may result in patients utilising inappropriate or cariogenic means of addressing the issue).

Dietary habits

The role of diet in dental caries is irrefutable. Based on the evidence from systematic reviews and several well-conducted cohort studies (Kramer et al. 2007; Leong et al. 2013; Lim et al. 2008), it can be concluded that there is a significant association between higher risk of dental caries and high exposure to sugared beverages and snacks. Therefore, consumption of sugared beverages and snacks needs to be included as a part of a patient's caries risk assessment. A brief assessment of the diet with the goal of identifying frequency and type of fermentable carbohydrates exposure is usually enough to determine the main dietary culprits. Focus should be on patterns of in between meals consumption of fermentable carbohydrates and sipping of any beverage with sugar.

Oral hygiene behaviors

Poor oral hygiene status as evidenced by accumulated plaque on the dentition can be predictive of caries development and, hence, is a useful risk indicator. In study, plaque visible on the labial surface of anterior teeth without additional aids or disclosing solution in young children demonstrated a sensitivity of 83% and specificity of 92% as a good predictor of caries development, with 91% of children correctly classify with regard to future caries risk using the plaque accumulation alone (Alaluusua Malmivirta 1994). Similarly in adults, visible heavy plaque increased risk for future caries development (Domejean et al. 2011). Multiple other studies demonstrated oral hygiene, in particular toothbrushing, to be an important risk indicator in children (Tagliaferro et al. 2008; Mascarenhas 1998; Mathiesen et al. 1996). In assessing oral hygiene practices, ICCMS[TM] recommends evaluating the frequency and time spent during tooth brushing and flossing, and timing (after meals, before bedtime) (Pitts et al. 2013, 2018; Ismail et al. 2015).

Fluoride exposure

Patients under certain conditions can be considered to have inadequate fluoride exposure if they have the following profiles (Marinho et al. 2003, 2004; Walsh et al. 2010; Twetman 2009; Griffin et al. 2007) No daily use of fluoridated toothpaste (less than 2x daily)

- For children: tooth brushing with non-fluoridated toothpaste
- Concentration of fluoridated toothpaste less than 1000 ppm of fluoride.

Table 4.4 (Continued)

Mothers or caregivers' caries experience (for children)

It is well accepted that development of early childhood caries is influenced by environmental factors beyond individual-level factors, including a mother or caregiver's dental health. Several mother-child dyad studies reported that there is a significant correlation between mothers and children's caries status (Smith et al. 2002; Reisine et al. 2008; Ismail et al. 2009; Weintraub et al. 2010; Dye et al. 2011), thus suggesting a mother's (or caregiver's) caries status can be a predictor for child's caries development.

Socioeconomic status (SES)

SES is an indicator for various exposures and behaviors that impact caries risk. Significant evidence exists to support a strong correlation between SES and caries experience (Costa et al. 2012; Schwendicke et al. 2015; Kallestal and Wall 2002; Al Agili and Griffin 2015; Chaffee et al. 2016; Polk et al. 2010). Hence, SES is often used as a risk indicator to target public health interventions (e.g., school-based sealant programs). Many studies have shown that social deprivation can predispose to caries (Beal 1996; Hunt 1990). The dentist may notice high caries rates in siblings, and the patient or parent may possess little knowledge of dental disease. Concern about dental health may be low and dental visits irregular. Data from the Global Oral Health Data Bank, maintained by the World Health Organization (WIIO), suggested that developing countries, where caries prevalence was low initially, experience a high level of caries prevalence as they are industrialised and exposed to refined 'cariogenic' foods (Petersen et al. 2005).

Source: Pitts et al. (2013, 2018) and Ismail et al. (2015) with permission of ICCMS™.

The second part is the '*objective or intraoral*' risk assessment (Table 4.5), which contains information gathered about the patient by the dental practitioner through clinical examination and biological testing (if applicable), and is composed of:

- existing active caries
- previous caries experience (restorations)
- oral hygiene conditions (thick, undisturbed, and sticky biofilm)
- saliva properties and conditions (dry mouth)
- exposed root surfaces
- appliances that may increase development of the biofilm
- PUFA (*Exposed Pulp, Ulceration associated with retained root fragments or sharp edges caused by carious destruction, Fistula, and Abscess*)
- other oral conditions that might predispose the patient to caries risk.

The risk predicting factors assessed in these first two sections of the CRA tool are depicted in Figure 4.3, and their implications in caries risk status of a patient are described in Tables 4.4 and 4.5. This list of predictive factors may be adjusted based on the age the patients.

The third part of the CRA tool is the '*Decision-making: weighting of factors and risk status classification*' section. In this section the information gathered in the first two sections are synthesised to identify the overall risk level (low, moderate, high) of the patient. Most CRA tools and caries management systems, such as the International Caries Classification and

Table 4.5 ICCMS™ Intraoral Level (Objective) Risk Assessment Model.

Intraoral Level	**Active caries lesions**

Intraoral Level

Active caries lesions

The presence of active caries lesions is an indication that the patient is actively developing new caries, which may progress from initial caries to visible cavitation. This immediately places the patient at a high caries risk status.

Caries experience

This includes any restorations, extractions or teeth missing due to caries. Increased caries risk is associated with the presence of restorations (or extractions) (Kidd and O'Hara 1990; Boyd and Richardson 1985; Goldberg et al. 1981; Hamilton et al. 1983). There is evidence that the presence of marginal ditching places teeth at increased caries risk (Hamilton et al. 1983; Ando et al. 2005). The extent of marginal deficiencies will range from those barely perceptible on visual examination alone to those that will readily admit a ball-ended probe. Since an increased width of the marginal deficiency may be a risk factor for the likelihood of developing caries it may be important to have a threshold at which the deficiency is recorded as present or absent. The ICCMS™ recommends that if a ball-ended probe is part of the examination kit, two categories of ditching could be recorded according to whether or not the probe can full enter into the gap between tooth and restoration.

Thick, sticky, and undisturbed biofilm

Dental plaque is the risk factor for dental caries (Fejerskov and Manji 1990). There is plethora of evidence supporting the causal relationship between accumulation of a thick layer of biofilm or in stagnation areas and increased caries risk (Ekstrand et al. 1998, 2008; Ferreira et al. 2005; Skrīvele et al. 2013; Quaglio et al. 2006). Biofilm is a mass of bacteria enmeshed in exopolysaccharides, and dental caries is now considered an endogenous infection caused by a change in the oral microbial ecology (microbiome) resulting in the selection of bacterial species that have the potential to ferment sugars and starch, with consequent release of organic acid that causes tooth demineralisation (Li et al. 2007; Teanpaisan et al. 2012).

Dry mouth

There is an increased caries risk associated with xerostomia/hyposalivation. The level of evidence supporting the causal relationship between xerostomia/hyposalivation and increased caries risk is based a small number of case-control or cohort studies (Saini et al. 2005; Murray 2014).

Exposed root surfaces

Increased risk of root caries is associated with the number of exposed root surfaces. The level of evidence supporting the causal relationship between root caries and exposed root surfaces is supported by one systematic review, and a small number of case-control or cohort studies (Chi et al. 2013; Ritter et al. 2012).

Appliances that may increase development of the biofilm

Increased caries risk is associated with the use of an oral appliance including partial dentures. The level of evidence supporting the causal relationship between use of the oral appliances and increased caries risk is based on a small number of case-control or cohort studies, as well as expert opinions (Hadler-Olsen et al. 2012; Lorov et al. 2007; Martignon et al. 2010; Ogaard 1989; Richter et al. 2011; van der Veen et al. 2010; Zimmer and Rottwinkel 2004).

Table 4.5 (Continued)

PUFA

(Exposed Pulp, Ulceration associated with retained root fragments or sharp edges caused by carious destruction, Fistula, and Abscess) Increased caries risk is associated with a higher PUFA score. The level of evidence supporting the causal relationship between an increasing PUFA score and increased caries risk is based on only one study (Bagińska et al. 2013).

Source: Pitts et al. (2013, 2018) and Ismail et al. (2015) with permission of ICCMS™.

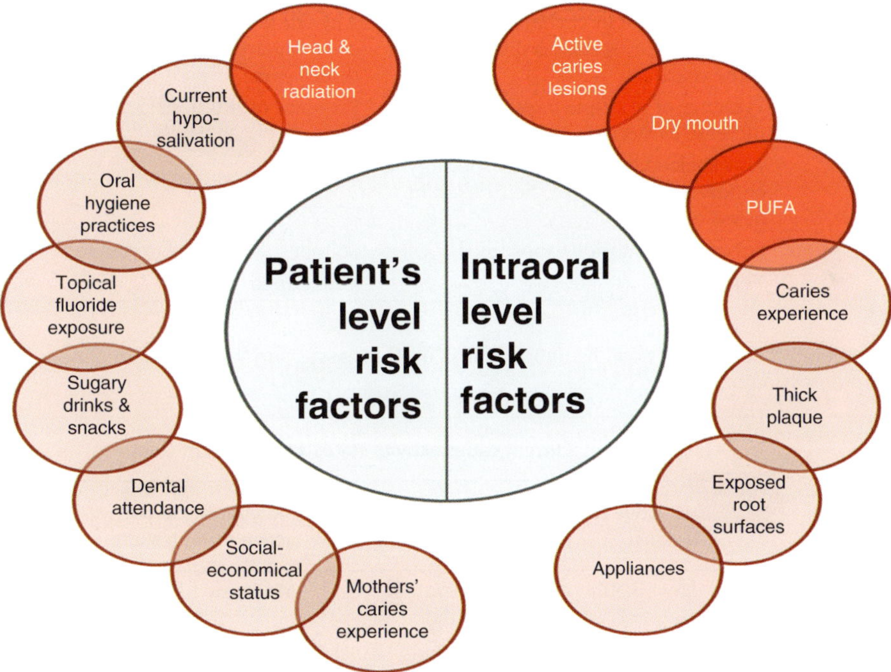

Figure 4.3 The patient-level and intraoral level caries risk predictors. Those in red would automatically put the patient at high caries risk. Source: Ismail et al. (2015).

Management System (ICCMS™) (Pitts et al. 2013, 2018; Ismail et al. 2015), classify caries risk status into 3 categories: low, moderate, and high risk. A suggested guide for assigning a risk status to a patient is shown in Table 4.6.

The Caries Risk Likelihood Matrix

The decision of the risk or susceptibility of an individual to develop new caries lesions or the progression of existing lesions is not limited to establishment of the caries risk status of the person. A final step in risk assessment, recommended by the ICCMS™, is the use of a second assessment tool, *'Likelihood matrix'* shown in Table 4.7. In this step, the established caries risk status of the patient is used in combination with the presence/absence of active

Table 4.6 Guide for deciding the Caries Risk Status of an individual patient.

Caries risk categories	Age group	
	Younger than 6 years	**6 years or older**
Low	No white spot or cavitated primary or secondary caries lesions during the last three years, and no factors that may increase caries risk	
Moderate	No white spot or cavitated primary or secondary caries lesions during the last three years, but presence of at least one factor that may increase caries risk	
High	Any white spot or cavitated primary or secondary caries lesions during the last three years	Any white spots or cavitated primary or secondary caries lesions in the last three years.
	Presence of multiple factors that may increase caries risk	Presence of multiple factors that may increase caries risk.
	Low socioeconomic status, especially in children too young for their risk to be based on caries history.	
	Suboptimal fluoride exposure	Suboptimal fluoride exposure.
	Xerostomia	Xerostomia.

Table 4.7 ICCMS™ Caries Risk and Likelihood Matrix used for assessing the likelihood of new lesions or progression of existing caries.

		Current caries activity status at the patient level		
		No active caries lesions*	Initial stage active caries lesions	Moderate-or extensive-stage active caries lesions
Risk status	Low risk	Low likelihood	Moderate likelihood	Moderate likelihood*
	Moderate risk	Low likelihood	Moderate likelihood	High likelihood
	High risk	Moderate likelihood	High likelihood	High likelihood

Source: Pitts et al. (2018).

caries lesions to determine the 'likelihood' of the individual developing new caries lesions and/or the progression of existing caries lesion. This helps the practitioner/dental team to correctly identify those patients with a risk of increased progression of the severity of the existing caries lesions (Pitts et al. 2018).

Identification of Factors Predictive of Risk

The probability of an individual developing new dental caries in future or progression of existing lesions (caries risk status) is collectively predicted by the factors involved in the etiology of the caries disease process being experienced by the individual (risk factors), his/her exposure to biologic or therapeutic factors or measures that can collectively offset the challenge presented by risk factors (protective factors), and the clinical observations that tell about his/her past caries history and activity, which are indicators or clinical signs that there is disease present or that there has been recent disease (disease indicators). These three groups of factors shown in Figure 4.1 are the predictive factors of the caries risk status of an individual patient (Featherstone 2003; American Dental Association 2016). The influence of individual factors within these groups on the caries risk status of a patient are described in Tables 4.4 and 4.5 to guide the dental team for assessing the risk predictors. It is recommended that the risk predictors should be assessed using both interview data and clinical observations (Pitts et al. 2013, 2018; Ismail et al. 2015).

Caries Detection, Activity Assessment, Staging, and Diagnosis in Caries Risk Assessment

The best predictor of future caries in permanent teeth in adults, as established in a systematic review, is the past caries experience of the individual (Zero et al. 2001). This has been found to be the only consistently reliable caries indicator (Beck et al. 1992; Disney et al. 1990). Thus, the detection of caries lesions, the classification of the severity of the lesion, and determination of the activity status of the lesion, through clinical examination, are part of caries risk assessment process (Pitts et al. 2013, 2018; Ismail et al. 2015). The most important and complicated being the detection of early caries, which would facilitate minimal intervention in management of individual lesions, considering the well-established fact that when caries is detected at an early stage, the dentist can employ an effective prophylactic intervention that could reverse or arrest the lesion before the need for operative intervention (MI philosophy). The age long conventional caries detection methods are visual and radiographic examinations, and are discussed below.

Visual Caries Detection

The first clinical sign of caries (early caries) is a chalky and matte (rough) whitish surface, hence white spot lesion (Figure 4.4), which microscopically is a porous surface that can easily be stained into brown or black discoloration by chromogens from foods, and as such a caries lesion can be seen either as a white or brown/black spot lesion. Considering that visual examination has been found to be of low sensitivity and specificity with regards to early caries detection, the following conditions are necessary to optimise visual detection to improve its accuracy.

Clean tooth surface is necessary to reveal those early stage caries lesions that might be covered by bacterial plaque. This can be achieved by removing any film of bacterial plaque with the explorer or best detection should be carried out immediately following professional cleaning.

Dry tooth surface achieved by thoroughly drying with air water syringe for at least 5 seconds to facilitate detection of very early stage lesions is required. Saliva on tooth surface masks the very early stage caries lesion, due to the optical phenomenon resulting from

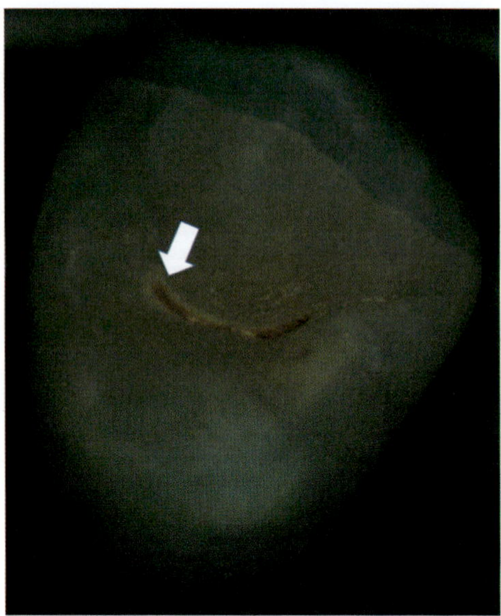

Figure 4.4 The first clinical sign of caries (early caries) is a chalky and matte (rough) whitish surface, and as such is referred to as white spot lesion (arrowed).

differences in refractive indices of water (1.33), enamel (1.62), and air (1.0). A white spot lesion is a porous surface, and the pores are filled with water in the presence of saliva. Due to the closeness of the refractive indices of water and enamel, an early white spot lesion cannot be distinguished from a sound enamel surface in the presence of saliva. However, when a white spot lesion is thoroughly dried, air replaces the saliva in the pores, making the lesion frostier and clearly seen. Besides, drying the tooth surface aids the decision on treatment and prognosis. An early lesion visible on a wet tooth surface indicates that demineralisation is over halfway through the enamel, possibly extending into dentin, while a lesion that becomes visible only after thorough air-drying is less than halfway through enamel (van Amerongen et al. 1992; Ekstrand et al. 1997, 1998). The later condition has a better prognosis of possible complete reversal on application of a therapeutic agent, while the former condition may only be arrested (Ekstrand et al. 1998).

Sharp probe or explorers are no longer accepted for detecting early lesions on any surface, including pit and fissures. The explorer can damage a white spot lesion by breaking through the relatively intact surface zone, cavitating an intact lesion that would otherwise be remineralised. Besides, vigorous use of a sharp explorer can cause a cavity that will subsequently trap dental plaque and encourage lesion progression. Explorers can also give false positive impression of the presence of demineralisation when it sticks (catch) in the pit or fissure. Detection of early caries lesions should rely on sharp eyes and a Community Periodontal Index of Treatment Need (CPITN) probe (ball-ended) or the blunt end of the explorer. In general, the use explorer is limited to cleaning plaque and debris from tooth surface, feeling the texture (roughness) of white spot lesions, feeling margins and defects to confirm and assess cavitations, and feeling the hardness of root surfaces to detect and assess root caries.

Table 4.8 Caries Diagnosis with staging and activity status per lesion.

ICCMS ™ combined categories	Activity status	
	Active lesions	**Inactive lesions**
ICCMS^{TM} Sound	**No lesion**	**No lesion**
ICCMS^{TM} Initial	**Initial active**	**Initial inactive**
ICCMS^{TM} Moderate	**Moderate active**	**Moderate inactive**
ICCMS^{TM} Extensive	**Extensive active**	**Extensive inactive**

Source: Courtesy: ICCMS™ Pitts et al. (2013, 2018) and Ismail et al. (2015).

Magnification using magnifying devices such as a head-worn prism loupe or a surgical microscope improves the accuracy of visual caries detection by 50% (Forgie et al. 2002), and good *Lighting* aids vision. Caries detection should be a stepwise process to permit the detection and assessment of the stage and activity status of the detected lesion before the final diagnosis, which must specify the severity stage and activity status of the lesion as shown in Table 4.8. Such descriptive diagnosis would aid the selection of the most appropriate intervention for each lesion after caries risk assessment. When looking at a tooth surface for detecting possible caries, questions of these nature should run through the examiners mind.

- Is there a change from normal appearance of enamel or root surface (presence of a lesion)? Figure 4.5 will help the examiner detect and classify a root caries.
- Is the change consistent with the appearance of carious white (or brown/black) spot lesion or developmental hypomineralisation? Table 4.9 will help the examiner distinguish white spot due to caries from developmental hypomineralisation.
- If caries, is it cavitated (loss of surface integrity) or non-cavitated?
- If non-cavitated, is it active or inactive (arrested?). Table 4.10 will help the examiner distinguish between active and inactive early caries.
- If non-cavitated and associated with pit or fissure, is there a shadowing underneath the surrounding enamel.

Detecting Early Lesions on Buccal, Lingual and Root Surfaces

Gingival margins are the typical locations of active early caries lesions on smooth, free surfaces of enamel. These active initial enamel lesions, which are commonly located in plaque stagnation areas, present chalky white and dull (matte) surfaces when air-dried, feels rough when the blunt tip of the probe is moved gently across the surface, and are usually covered by visible plaque (Figure 4.4) (Nyvad and Fejerskov 1997; Nyvad et al. 1999, 2003). An inactive or arrested enamel lesion may be white or brown with a plaque-free shiny surface that is mainly smooth but sometimes rough (Nyvad and Fejerskov 1997; Nyvad et al. 1999, 2003). They should be distinguished from developmental hypomineralisation as shown in Table 4.9.

A caries lesion on a root surface is seen as a clearly demarcated, light brown, dark brown, or black discoloured area on the root surface or at the cemento-enamel junction (Banting 2001).While an active root caries may feel soft or leathery with a rough and matte surface

Root Caries Staging and Activity Classification

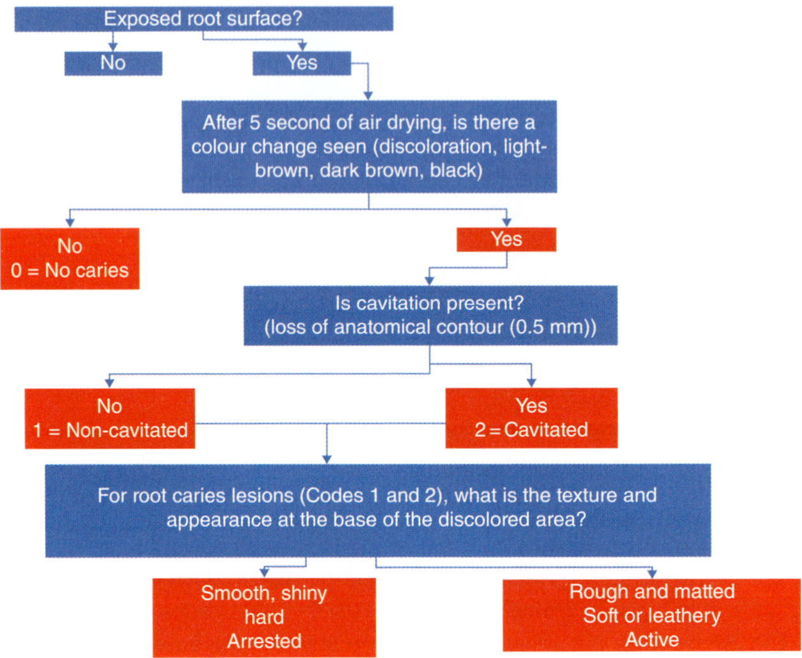

Figure 4.5   Root caries staging and activity status (with permission from ICCMS™). Source: Ismail et al. (2015).

Table 4.9   Differences between white spots due to caries and developmental hypomineralisation.

Characteristics	Caries	Developmental hypomineralisation
Appearance/Lustre	Opaque, chalky and matte surface when air-dried	Glossy (shiny) and less opaque surface when air-dried
Texture	Feels rough when the tip of a WHO probe (ball-ended) or blunt explorer is moved gently across the surface	Feels smooth when the tip of a WHO probe or blunt explorer is moved gently across the surface
Colour	White or may be discolored by extrinsic stain	No extrinsic discoloration
Location	Located in plaque stagnation areas	Located mainly in self-cleansing areas
Distribution	Not applicable	Bilateral or multiple corresponding teeth

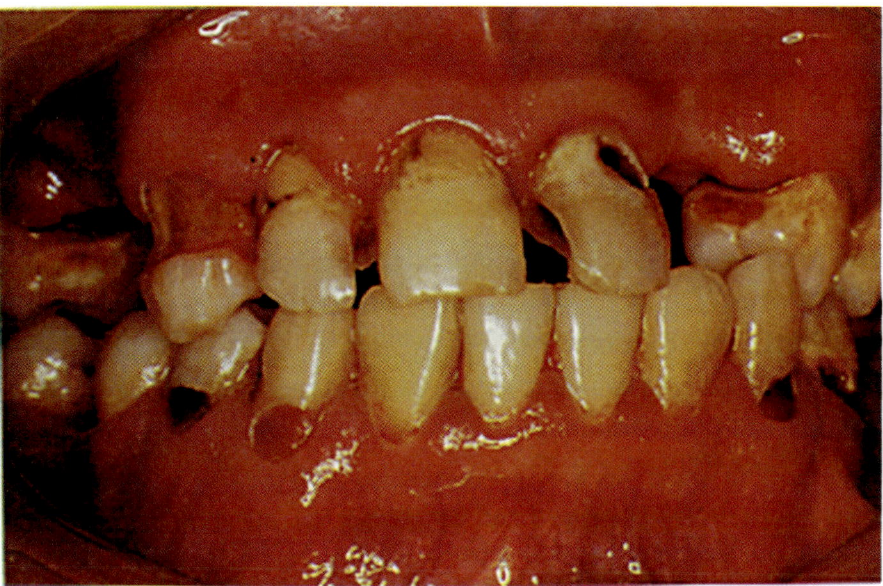

Figure 4.6 Root caries.

when felt with the WHO probe, an arrested/inactive root lesion feels hard in texture with smooth and shiny surface (Banting 2001). An early root surface lesion is considered cavitated if there is loss of anatomical contour or if the depth of the cavity is equal or greater than 0.5 mm when measured with the ball of the WHO probe (Figure 4.6). The diameter of the ball is 0.5 mm, so if the cavity accommodates the ball, then the depth is ≥ 0.5 mm. If there is no loss of surface integrity or if the depth of the cavity is less than 0.5 mm (not accommodating the ball), the lesion is non-cavitated (Banting 2001). Figure 4.5 can be used as guide for decision-making on root caries.

Detecting Early Caries in Pits and Fissures on Tooth Surface

The main requirement for detecting the presence of a non-cavitated caries in pits and fissures is sharp eyes, good lighting, dry clean teeth, and preferably a magnification device such as a prism loupe. Opaque (chalky) matte texture of enamel adjacent to a stained pit or fissure may indicate the presence of active caries underneath the pit or fissure. Shadowing or greyish discolouration underneath the adjacent translucent enamel along the pits or fissures may indicate possible undermining of enamel by caries (hidden caries) (Figure 4.7). Lesions underneath (along the walls) the stained pits or fissures would be discoloured by stain that diffused into the lesion through the porous lesion surface, so that an examiner looking perpendicular through the translucent adjacent healthy enamel along the pit and/or fissure would observe these stained 'wall' lesions as discoloration extending (underneath the translucent enamel) beyond the confines of the pit and/or fissure in the form of 'bottle-brush appearance' (Figure 4.7). When there is no caries underneath a stained pit

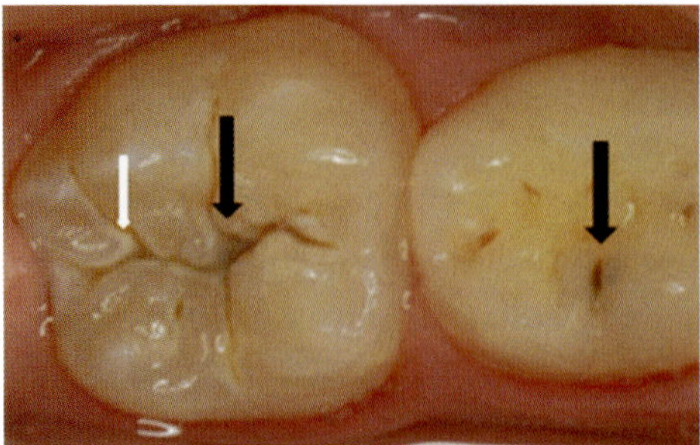

Figure 4.7 Shadowing or greyish discolouration (black arrows) underneath the adjacent translucent enamel along the pits or fissures may indicate possible undermining of enamel by caries (hidden caries). Note the white spot lesion (white arrow).

and/or fissure, the discoloration will remain within the confines of the pit and/or fissure. It has been reported that any sign of visible cavitation in the occlusal surface corresponds to progression of the lesion into the dentin (van Amerongen et al. 1992; Ekstrand et al. 1995, 1997).

Detecting Lesions on Tooth Proximal Surfaces

Detection of early proximal lesions in anterior teeth can easily be accomplished by fibre-optic transillumination technique using a stand-alone transilluminator, otherwise the fibre-optic light source at the handpiece coupler of the dental operatory is particularly appropriate and convenient (Mitropoulos 1985). Also available for this purpose are multiple commercial Near-infrared (NIR) light transillumination camera systems such as CariVu (Dexis, Hatfield, PA) which uses NIR occlusal transillumination with 780-nm light (Kuhnisch et al. 2015; Söchtig et al. 2014) and the Vistacam IX (PROXI) from Durr Dental (Bietigheim-Bissingen, Germany) which uses NIR reflectance at 850 nm. These clinical imaging systems are based on the principle that light intensity can be reduced by absorption (e.g., photons are lost to the hard tissue or the caries lesion) or scattering, in which the direction of the photons is changed without loss of energy. With NIR light transillumination, each tooth tissue (enamel or dentin) will be uniformly illuminated, with enamel appearing to be transparent while dentin scatters light more strongly, thus the two tissues can be distinguished (Staninec et al. 2010; Wu and Fried 2009). When tooth tissue is demineralised at the earliest stage of caries, this results in a higher scattering coefficient (Darling et al. 2006), thus reducing light intensity, and as such the presence of caries shows as a dark area at the marginal ridge for proximal caries or at occlusal surface for occlusal caries (Figure 4.8) (Söchtig et al. 2014).

In the posterior teeth, extensive active proximal lesions can be revealed by shadowing or greyish discoloration of the undermined occlusal enamel ridge; otherwise, when there is contact between proximal surfaces, the bite-wing radiograph is the most accurate method for detecting demineralisation. The radiograph should be examined carefully to determine whether caries lesions are present in the outer enamel, at the dentin-enamel junction, in the outer half of dentin, or in the inner half of dentin to facilitate appropriate treatment

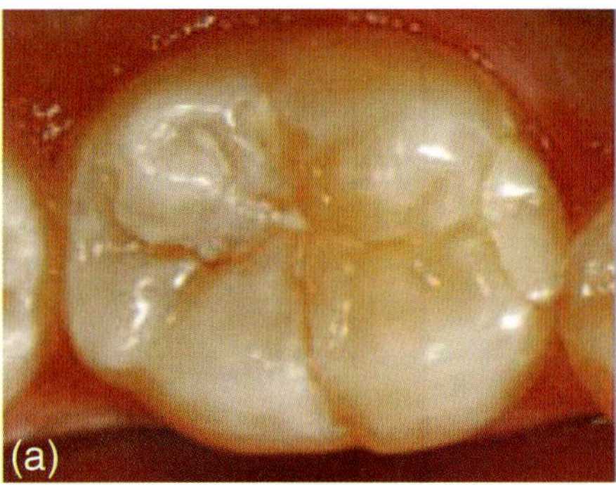 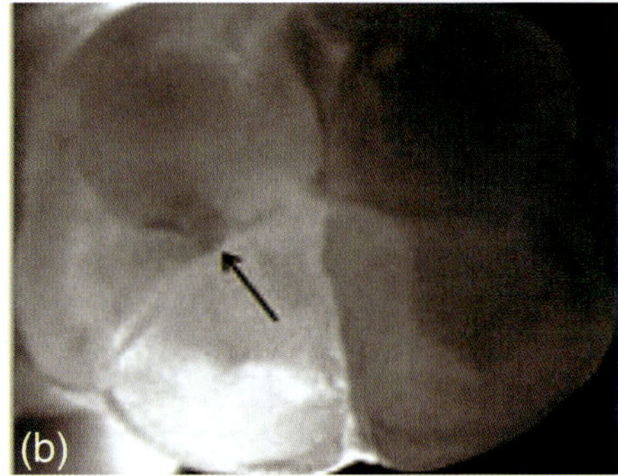

Figure 4.8 (a) A clinically sound occlusal tooth surface with hidden occlusal caries lesion revealed by a near-infrared (NIR) light transillumination device as a (b) circumscribed area of significant changed occlusal translucence (arrowed). Source: Bennett T. Amaechi/Elsevier B.V.

decision with minimal intervention. The use of an orthodontic separator has been advocated in some cases to allow the dentist to see more clearly and to gently feel for a break in the enamel surface (Rimmer and Pitts 1990).

Detecting Early Caries around Restorations

Detection criteria for primary caries developing around the margins of a restoration, commonly referred to as secondary or recurrent caries, are identical to those for primary caries at other tooth surfaces. An opaque chalky (frosty) and matte lesion around a restoration can be confirmed to be active lesion and may signal lesion extension beneath the restoration. There is evidence that the presence of marginal ditching around restorations places teeth at increased caries risk (Hamilton et al. 1983; Ando et al. 2005), and as such is an indication of caries beneath the restoration. However, since the extent of marginal deficiencies will range from those barely perceptible on visual examination alone to those that will readily admit a ball-ended probe, it may be important to have a threshold at which the deficiency is recorded as present or absence of secondary caries. Thus, the dentist can check that the restoration is secure in the cavity by pushing it with an explorer; a loose restoration ensures plaque stagnation and active caries is likely to be present.

Assessing Caries Lesion Activity

Caries development and progression is a dynamic process with alternating periods of activity and inactivity, and it has been demonstrated that caries lesions can be arrested at any stage of lesion development provided that clinically plaque-free conditions are maintained. Thus, a caries lesion detected in a clinical examination has the probability of being active (progressing) or arrested (inactive). Hence, it becomes necessary to determine the activity status of any lesion detected in clinical examination, considering reports has shown that a

Table 4.10 Important predictors for assessing caries activities.

Indicators	Activity	Inactivity
Location	Plaque stagnation area	Non-PSA
Plaque coverage	Sticky/visible plaque	No plaque
Gingival status	Inflammation	Healthy
Colour	White	Brown
Tactile: Enamel	Rough	Smooth
Tactile: Dentine	Soft	Hard
Lustre	Matt	Shiny

greater percentage of lesions that were considered active at baseline progressed to cavitation (Ferreira Zandona et al. 2012). It has been demonstrated that the clinical characteristics of a lesion can provide some indication of the probability of a lesion progressing toward cavitation (Ferreira Zandona et al. 2012; Varma et al. 2008; Ekstrand et al. 2007) thus the predictors shown in Table 4.10 can aid a clinical examiner to distinguish between an active and an inactive early caries lesion, although it is still subjective. In general, an active caries lesion appears chalky (frosty) and dull when air-dried, and feels rough when the tip of the explorer (probe) is moved gently across the surface, while an inactive lesion appears shiny when air-dried and feels rough or smooth depending on how long it has lasted (Ferreira Zandona et al. 2012; Varma et al. 2008; Ekstrand et al. 2007).

Staging of the Caries Process

The most established and recognised effort to classify the stages in the continuum of caries development and progression was the development of the International Caries Detection and Assessment System II (ICDAS II) to facilitate caries epidemiology, research, and appropriate clinical management (Pitts et al. 2013).The ICDAS scoring criteria (Table 4.11), which allow a 7-point staging of caries process, create the opportunity for inclusion of non-cavitated (early) caries lesions during initial and subsequent caries examination, thus enabling monitoring of lesion progression and comparison over time. ICDAS is a two stages, two-digit coding system comprising of a digit for the restoration or sealant status of the tooth surface, followed by a digit for the caries severity (Table 4.11).

However, the seven-point staging system was later consolidated into a globally accepted ICCMS™ four colour-coded stages of caries process (sound surface, initial, moderate, and advanced caries) for clinical practice and IT-based level systems as well as the appropriate management of individual caries lesions (Figure 4.9) (Pitts et al. 2013, 2018; Ismail et al. 2015; Young et al. 2015). In this system, lesions classified as the ICDAS II codes 1 and 2 becomes initial caries, 3 and 4 becomes moderate caries, while 5 and 6 becomes advanced (severe) caries. The addition of colour coding is envisaged to facilitate communications between the patients and the dental team. However, it is pertinent to mention that the separation of non-cavitated caries (white- or brown-spot lesion) into ICDAS II codes 1 and 2 is

Table 4.11 ICDAS criteria for visual examination of caries lesions, including two-digit coding for restoration and caries severity.

First digit = Restoration and sealant codes	Second digit = Caries severity codes
0 = Not sealed or restored	0 = Sound tooth surface
1 = Partial sealant	1 = First visual change (opacity or discoloration) in enamel hardly visible on the wet surface but distinctly visible after air drying.
2 = Full sealant	
3 = Tooth colored restoration	2 = Distinct visual change (opacity or discoloration) in enamel, visible without air drying
4 = Amalgam restoration	
5 = Stainless steel crown	3 = Enamel breakdown, no dentin visible
6 = Porcelain, gold, PFM crown or veneer	4 = Dentin shadow (not cavitated into dentin)
7 = Lost or broken restoration	5 = Distinct cavity with visible dentin
8 = Temporary restoration	6 = Extensive distinct cavity with visible dentin

PFM, Porcelain fused to metal.
Source: Pitts et al. (2013, 2018) and Ismail et al. (2015).

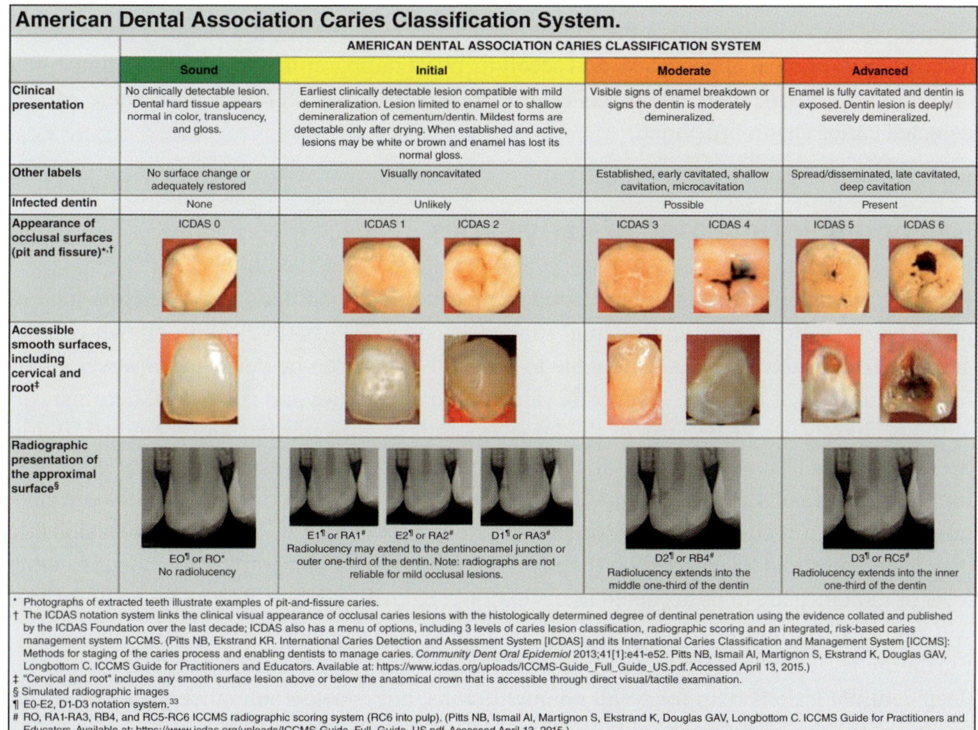

American Dental Association Caries Classification System.

	AMERICAN DENTAL ASSOCIATION CARIES CLASSIFICATION SYSTEM			
	Sound	**Initial**	**Moderate**	**Advanced**
Clinical presentation	No clinically detectable lesion. Dental hard tissue appears normal in color, translucency, and gloss.	Earliest clinically detectable lesion compatible with mild demineralization. Lesion limited to enamel or to shallow demineralization of cementum/dentin. Mildest forms are detectable only after drying. When established and active, lesions may be white or brown and enamel has lost its normal gloss.	Visible signs of enamel breakdown or signs the dentin is moderately demineralized.	Enamel is fully cavitated and dentin is exposed. Dentin lesion is deeply/severely demineralized.
Other labels	No surface change or adequately restored	Visually noncavitated	Established, early cavitated, shallow cavitation, microcavitation	Spread/disseminated, late cavitated, deep cavitation
Infected dentin	None	Unlikely	Possible	Present
Appearance of occlusal surfaces (pit and fissure)[*],[†]	ICDAS 0	ICDAS 1 ICDAS 2	ICDAS 3 ICDAS 4	ICDAS 5 ICDAS 6
Accessible smooth surfaces, including cervical and root[‡]				
Radiographic presentation of the approximal surface[§]	EO[¶] or RO[*] No radiolucency	E1[¶] or RA1[#] E2[¶] or RA2[#] D1[¶] or RA3[#] Radiolucency may extend to the dentinoenamel junction or outer one-third of the dentin. Note: radiographs are not reliable for mild occlusal lesions.	D2[¶] or RB4[#] Radiolucency extends into the middle one-third of the dentin	D3[¶] or RC5[#] Radiolucency extends into the inner one-third of the dentin

[*] Photographs of extracted teeth illustrate examples of pit-and-fissure caries.
[†] The ICDAS notation system links the clinical visual appearance of occlusal caries lesions with the histologically determined degree of dentinal penetration using the evidence collated and published by the ICDAS Foundation over the last decade; ICDAS also has a menu of options, including 3 levels of caries lesion classification, radiographic scoring and an integrated, risk-based caries management system ICCMS. (Pitts NB, Ekstrand KR. International Caries Detection and Assessment System [ICDAS] and its International Caries Classification and Management System [ICCMS]: Methods for staging of the caries process and enabling dentists to manage caries. *Community Dent Oral Epidemiol* 2013;41[1]:e41-e52. Pitts NB, Ismail AI, Martignon S, Ekstrand K, Douglas GAV, Longbottom C. ICCMS Guide for Practitioners and Educators. Available at: https://www.icdas.org/uploads/ICCMS-Guide_Full_Guide_US.pdf. Accessed April 13, 2015.)
[‡] "Cervical and root" includes any smooth surface lesion above or below the anatomical crown that is accessible through direct visual/tactile examination.
[§] Simulated radiographic images
[¶] E0-E2, D1-D3 notation system.[33]
[#] RO, RA1-RA3, RB4, and RC5-RC6 ICCMS radiographic scoring system (RC6 into pulp). (Pitts NB, Ismail AI, Martignon S, Ekstrand K, Douglas GAV, Longbottom C. ICCMS Guide for Practitioners and Educators. Available at: https://www.icdas.org/uploads/ICCMS-Guide_Full_Guide_US.pdf. Accessed April 13, 2015.)

Figure 4.9 ADA Caries Classification System 2015. Source: Young et al. (2015)/with permission from Elsevier.

Table 4.12 Diagnostic Stages of Caries based upon Clinical and Radiographic Status.

Clinical Caries Classification (C) for a tooth surface	Radiographic Caries Classification (R) for a tooth surface			
	R_{sound}	$R_{initial}$	$R_{moderate}$	$R_{Advanced}$
C_{Sound}	Sound	Initial	Moderate	Advanced
$C_{Initial}$	Initial	Initial	Moderate	Advanced
$C_{Moderate}$	Moderate	Moderate	Moderate	Advanced
$C_{Advanced}$	Advanced	Advanced	Advanced	Advanced

Source: Pitts et al. (2013, 2018) and Ismail et al. (2015).

not only based on clinical appearance of the lesion in relation to moisture on the surface, it has diagnostic, treatment, and prognostic values. Histologically, enamel demineralisation in ICDAS code 1 lesions is limited to the outer half of the enamel layer, and these lesions have higher chances of complete reversal with remineralisation therapy, while the demineralisation in code 2 lesion has involved the entire enamel layer and outer third of the dentin layer, with higher chances of being arrested rather than reversal (van Amerongen et al. 1992; Ekstrand et al. 1997, 1998).

The ICCMS™ further developed the four-stage system, making the stage of each lesion to be based on both the clinical appearance of the lesion and the radiographic depth toward the pulp of the radiolucency in the tooth tissue as follows. Firstly, the stage of the lesion is decided by its clinical appearance, and secondly by its radiographic appearance (Figure 4.9) (Young et al. 2015), then using the matrix shown in Table 4.12, the final stage of any detected caries lesion is decided.

Radiographic Detection of Early Caries

Bitewing radiography has long been used to detect clinically hidden caries lesions such as initial (early) caries lesions in proximal surfaces (Kidd and Pitts 1990). With bitewing radiographs early proximal lesions amenable to preventive care can be detected; however, it has been found to be of minimal diagnostic value for enamel caries and superficial dentinal caries on occlusal surfaces because of the large amounts of surrounding sound enamel. But in deeper occlusal lesions reaching the dentin, radiographs show a high specificity. Although useful for proximal surfaces, the ability of bitewing radiograph to distinguish between cavitated and non-cavitated enamel lesions is limited, thus it may be necessary to establish a diagnostic threshold level based on the depth of radiolucency in a pulpal direction (i.e., what level of radiolucency to be accepted as cavitation) (Bakhshandeh et al. 2011). This threshold will aid in determining the appropriate treatment to be applied for a particular lesion. Furthermore, it is pertinent to mention that the probability of having a cavity is greater for deep dentinal lesions than for small enamel lesions, but considerable uncertainty exists for lesions at the dentin-enamel junction (Figure 4.10) (Lunder 1996; Pitts and Rimmer 1992). Following detection of a caries lesion using a bitewing radiography, the practitioner would go further to stage the detected lesion using the ICCMS™ four-stage system described above and shown in Figure 4.9 (Pitts et al. 2013, 2018; Ismail et al. 2015; Young et al. 2015).

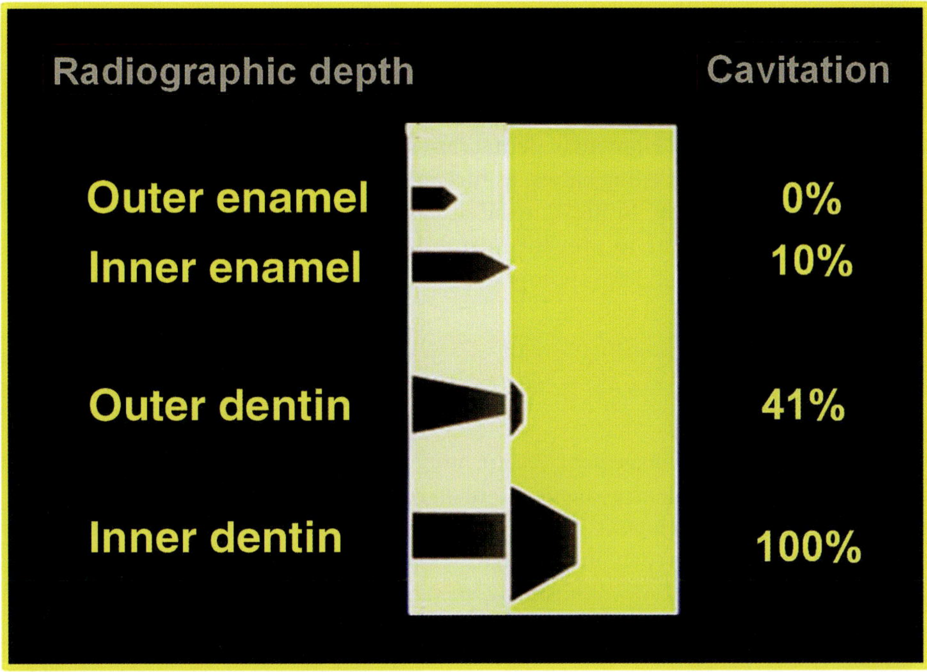

Figure 4.10 Prediction of proximal caries lesion cavitation based on the depth of radiolucency in bitewing radiograph. Source: Based on Pitts and Rimmer (1992).

Diagnosis of Dental Caries

Following the staging of the detected early caries, the dental practitioner can come to a final caries diagnosis with staging and activity status of each lesion as shown in Table 4.8 (Pitts et al. 2013, 2018; Ismail et al. 2015). Such descriptive diagnosis would aid in designating the caries risk status of the patient and the selection of the most appropriate intervention for each lesion after caries risk assessment.

Clinical Application of Caries Risk Assessment

To discuss how to apply these concepts in clinical practice, the use of case scenarios can help to demonstrate the importance of risk assessment in the management of caries disease in an individual, and also the need of assessing caries for the individual and not just assessing caries for the tooth. The following two patients/cases demonstrate the application of the caries management thought process at a patients' level and at a tooth level.

Summary

This chapter describes the intimate connection between early caries detection and CRA, and their role in minimal intervention dentistry. Although the detection and diagnosis of initial lesions remains a challenge for practitioners, it is an essential step in assessing the caries risk status of an individual patient, considering that the prediction of future caries risk is still based largely on a patient's past caries experience. CRA is the corner stone of minimal intervention dentistry, which is a major component of comprehensive personalised caries care plan. CRA is a logical systematic approach of assessing the risk of the individual patient for future development of dental caries by identifying the individual etiologic factors contributing to the existing caries lesions and exacerbating risk. It provides a basis for patient education on how to prevent the disease and to communicate and facilitate needed change in behaviour to prevent future disease. It assists the oral healthcare practitioner/team to determine the appropriate interventions and recall consultation strategies suitable for an individual patient.

Further Reading

Caries risk assessment and management. (2016). http://www.ada.org/en/member-center/oralhealth-topics/caires-risk-assessment-and-management. (accessed 13 June 2017).

Hayes, M., Da Mata, C., McKenna, G., Burke, F.M., and Allen, P.F. (2017). Evaluation of the Cariogram for root caries prediction. *J. Dent.* 62: 25–30.

Pitts, N.B., Ekstrand, K.R., ICDAS Foundation. (2013). System (ICCMS) – methods for staging of the caries process and enabling dentists to manage caries. *Community Dent. Oral Epidemiol.* 41: e41–52.

Pitts, N.B., Ismail, A.I., Martignon, S., Ekstrand, K., Douglas, G.V., and Longbottom, C. ICCMS Guide for Practitioners and Educators. Available at https://www.icdas.org/uploads/ICCMS-Guide_Full_Guide_UK.pdf (accessed January 2018).

Tellez, M., Gomez, J., Pretty, I., Ellwood, R., and Ismail, A.I. (2013). Evidence on existing caries risk assessment systems: Are they predictive of future caries? *Community Dent. Oral Epidemiol.* 41: 67–78.

Yip, K. (2012). Smales R.Oral diagnosis and treatment planning: part 2. Dental caries and assessment of risk. *Br. Dent. J.* 213 (2): 59–66. https://www.nature.com/articles/sj.bdj.2012.615.

References

Al Agili, D.E., and Griffin, S.O. (2015). Effect of family income on the relationship between parental education and sealant prevalence, national health and nutrition examination survey, 2005-2010. *Prev. Chronic Dis.* 12: E138.

Alaki, S.M., Ashiry, E.A., Bakry, N.S., Baghlaf, K.K., and Bagher, S.M. (2013). The effects of asthma and asthma medication on dental caries and salivary characteristics in children. *Oral Health Prev. Dent.* 11: 113–120.

Alaluusua, S., and Malmivirta, R. (1994). Early plaque accumulation–a sign for caries risk in young children. *Community Dent. Oral Epidemiol.* 22: 273–276.

American Academy of Pediatric Dentistry. Guideline on caries-risk assessment and management for infants, children, and adolescents. 2014; http://www.aapd.org/policies. (accessed 13 March 2018).

American Dental Association. (2016). *Center for Scientific Information*, ADA science institute.

Ando, M., Gonzalez-Cabezas, C., Isaacs, R.L., Eckert, G.J., and Stookey, G.K. (2005). Evaluation of several techniques for the detection of secondary caries adjacent to amalgam restorations. *Caries Res.* 38: 350–356.

Bagińska, J., Rodakowska, E., Wilczyńska-Borawska, M., and Jamiołkowski, J. (2013). Index of clinical consequences of untreated dental caries (PUFA) in primary dentition of children from north-east Poland. *Adv. Med. Sci.* 21: 1–6.

Bakhshandeh, A., Ekstrand, K.R., and Qvist, V. (2011). Measurement of histological and radiographic depth and width of occlusal caries lesions: A methodological study. *Caries Res.* 45: 547–555.

Banting, D.W. (2001). The diagnosis of root caries. *J. Dent. Educ.* 65: 991–996.

Beal, J.F. (1996). Social factors and preventive dentistry. In: *Prevention of Oral Disease* (ed. J.J. Murray), 216–233. Oxford: Oxford University Press.

Beck, J.D., Weintraub, J.A., Disney, J.A., Graves, R.C., Stamm, J.W., Kaste, L.M., and Bohannan, H.M. (1992). University of North Carolina caries risk assessment study: Comparisons of high risk prediction, any risk prediction, and any risk etiologic models. *Community Dent. Oral Epidemiol.* 20: 313–321.

Boyd, M.A., and Richardson, A.S. (1985). Frequency of amalgam replacement in general dental practice. *J. Can. Dent. Assoc.* 10: 763–766.

Chaffee, B.W., and Featherstone, J.D. (2015). Long-term adoption of caries management by risk assessment among dental students in a university clinic. *J. Dent. Educ.* 79 (5): 539–547.

Chaffcc, B.W., Featherstone, J.D., Gansky, S.A., Cheng, J., and Zhan, L. (2016). Caries risk assessment item importance: Risk designation and caries status in children under age 6. *JDR Clin. Trans. Res.* 1: 131–142.

Chaffee, B.W., Featherstone, J.D.B., and Zhan, L. (2017). Pediatric caries risk assessment as a predictor of caries outcomes. *Pediatr. Dent.* 39: 219–232.

Chi, D.L., Berg, J.H., Kim, A.S., and Scott, J. (2013). Correlates of root caries experience in middle-aged and older adults in the northwest practice-based research collaborative in evidence-based dentistry research network. *J. Am. Dent. Assoc.* 144: 507–516.

Costa, S.M., Martins, C.C., Bonfim, M.L.C., Zina, L.G., Paiva, S.M., Pordeus, I.A., and Abreu, M.H.N.G. (2012). A systematic review of socioeconomic indicators and dental caries in adults. *Int. J. Environ. Res. Public Health* 9: 3540–3574.

Darling, C.L., Huynh, G.D., and Fried, D. (2006). Light scattering properties of natural and artificially demineralized dental enamel at 1310 nm. *J. Biomed. Opt.* 11: 34023.

Disney, J.A., Graves, R.C., Stamm, J.W., Bohannan, H.M., and Abernathy, J.R. (1990). The university of North Carolina caries risk assessment study. II. Baseline caries prevalence. *J. Public Health Dent.* 50: 178–185.

Domejean, S., Leger, S., Rechmann, P., White, J.M., and Featherstone, J.D. (2015). How do dental students determine patients' caries risk level using the Caries Management By Risk Assessment (CAMBRA) system? *J. Dent. Educ.* 79: 278–285.

Domejean, S., White, J.M., and Featherstone, J.D.B. (2011). Validation of the CDA CAMBRA caries risk assessment – A six year retrospective study. *J. Calif. Dent. Assoc.* 39: 709–715.

Dyasanoor, S., and Saddu, S.C. (2014). Association of xerostomia and assessment of salivary flow using modified schirmer test among smokers and healthy individuals: A preliminutesary study. *J. Clin. Diagn. Res.* 8: 211–213.

Dye, B.A., Arevalo, O., and Vargas, C.M. (2010). Trends in paediatric dental caries by poverty status in the United States, 1988-1994 and 1999-2004. *Int. J. Paediatr. Dent.* 20: 132–143.

Dye, B.A., Tan, S., Smith, V., Lewis, B.G., Barker, L.K., Thornton-Evans, G., Eke, P.I., Beltran-Aguilar, E.D., Horowitz, A.M., and Li, C.-H. (2007). Trends in oral health status: United States, 1988–1994 and 1999–2004. *Natl. Health Stat.: Vital Health Stat.* 11: 1–92.

Dye, B.A., Vargas, C.M., Lee, J.J., Magder, L., and Tinanoff, N. (2011). Assessing the relationship between children's oral health status and that of their mothers. *J. Am. Dent. Assoc.* 142: 173–183.

Ekstrand, K.R., Bruun, G., and Bruun, M. (1998). Plaque and gingival status as indicators for caries progression on approximal surfaces. *Caries Res.* 32: 41–45.

Ekstrand, K.R., Kuzmina, I., Bjorndal, L., and Thylstrup, A. (1995). Relationship between external and histologic features of progressive stages of caries in the occlusal fossa. *Caries Res.* 29: 243–250.

Ekstrand, K.R., Martignon, S., Ricketts, D.J., and Qvist, V. (2008). Detection and activity assessment of primary coronal caries lesions: A methodologic study. *Oper. Dent.* 32: 225–235.

Ekstrand, K.R., Martignon, S., Ricketts, D.J., and Qvist, V. (2007). Detection and activity assessment of primary coronal caries lesions: A methodologic study. *Oper. Dent* . 32: 225–235.

Ekstrand, K.R., Ricketts, D.N.J., and Kidd, E.A.M. (1997). Reproducibility and accuracy of three methods for assessment of demineralization depth on the occlusal surface: An *in vitro* examination. *Caries Res.* 31: 224–231.

Ekstrand, K.R., Ricketts, D.N.J., Kidd, E.A.M., Qvist, V., and Schou, S. (1998). Detection, diagnosing, monitoring and logical treatment of occlusal caries in relation to lesion activity and severity: An *in vivo* examination with histological validation. *Caries Res.* 32: 247–254.

Featherstone, J.D. (2003). The caries balance: Contributing factors and early detection. *J. Cal. Dent. Assoc.* 31: 129–133.

Fejerskov, O., and Manji, F. (1990). Reactor paper: Risk assessment in dental caries. In: *Risk Assessment in Dentistry* (ed. J.D. Bader), 215–217. Chapel Hill: University of North Carolina Dental Ecology.

Ferreira Zandona, A., Santiago, E., Eckert, G.J., Katz, B.P., Pereira de Oliveira, S., Capin, O.R., Mau, M., and Zero, D.T. (2012). The natural history of dental caries lesions: A 4-year observational study. *J. Dent. Res.* 91: 841–846.

Ferreira, M.A., Mendes, N.S., Ferreira, M.A., and Mendes, N.S. (2005). Factors associated with active white enamel lesions. *Int. J. Paediatr. Dent.* 15: 327–334.

Fontana, M., and Gonzalez-Cabezas, C. (2012). Minimal intervention dentistry: Part 2. Caries risk assessment in adults. *Br. Dent. J.* 213: 447–451.

Forgie, A.H., Pine, C.M., and Pitts, N.B. (2002). The use of magnification in a preventive approach to caries detection. *Quintessence Int.* 33: 13–16.

Gao, X., Di, W.I., Lo, E.C., Chu, C.H., Hsu, C.Y., and Wong, M.C. (2013). Validity of caries risk assessment programmes in preschool children. *J. Dent.* 41: 787–795.

Glenny, A.M., Gibson, F., Auld, E., Coulson, S., Clarkson, J.E., Craig, J.V., et al. (2010). The development of evidence-based guidelines on mouth care for children, teenagers and young adults treated for cancer. *Eur. J. Cancer* 46: 1399–1412.

Goldberg, J., Tanzer, J., Munster, E., Amara, J., Thal, F., and Birkhed, D. (1981). Cross-sectional clinical evaluation of recurrent enamel caries, restoration of marginal integrity, and oral hygiene status. *J. Am. Dent. Assoc.* 102: 635–641.

Griffin, S.O., Regnier, E., Griffin, P.M., and Huntley, V. (2007). Effectiveness of fluoride in preventing caries in adults. *J. Dent. Res.* 86: 410–415.

Hadler-Olsen, S., Sandvik, K., El-Agroudi, M.A., and Ogaard, B. (2012). The incidence of caries and white spot lesions in orthodontically treated adolescents with a comprehensive caries prophylactic regimen–A prospective study. *Eur. J. Orthod.* 34: 633–639.

Hamilton, J.C., Moffa, J.P., Ellison, J.A., and Jenkins, W.A. (1983). Marginal fracture not a predictor of longevity for two dental amalgam alloys: A ten year study. *J. Prost. Dent.* 50: 200–222.

Hansel Petersson, G., Akerman, S., Isberg, P.E., and Ericson, D. (2016). Comparison of risk assessment based on clinical judgement and Cariogram in addition to patient perceived treatment need. *BMC Oral Health* 17: 13.

Hunt, R.J. (1990). Behavioural and sociodemographic risk factors for caries. In: *Risk Assessment in Dentistry* (ed. J.D. Bader), 29–34. Chapel Hill: University of North Carolina Dental Ecology.

Ismail, A.I., Pitts, N.B., Tellez, M., Authors of International Caries Classification and Management System (ICCMS), Banerjee, A., Deery, C., Douglas, G., Eggertsson, H., Ekstrand, K., Ellwood, R., Gomez, J., Jablonski-Momeni, A., Kolker, J., Longbottom, C., Manton, D., Martignon, S., McGrady, M., Rechmann, P., Ricketts, D., Sohn, W., Thompson, V., Twetman, S., Weyant, R., Wolff, M., and Zandona, A. (2015). The International Caries Classification and Management System (ICCMS) An example of a caries management pathway. *BMC Oral Health* 15 (Suppl 1): S9.

Ismail, A.I., Sohn, W., Lim, S., and Willem, J.M. (2009). Prediction of dental caries progression in primary teeth. *J. Dent. Res.* 88: 270–275.

Kallestal, C., and Wall, S. (2002). Socio-economic effect on caries. Incidence data among Swedish 12–14-year-olds. *Community Dent. Oral Epidemiol.* 30: 108–114.

Kidd, E.A., and Pitts, N.B. (1990). A reappraisal of the value of the bitewing radiograph in the diagnosis of posterior approximal caries. *Br. Dent. J.* 169: 195–200.

Kidd, E.A.M., and O'Hara, J.W. (1990). The caries status of occlusal amalgam restorations with marginal defects. *J. Dent. Res.* 69: 1275–1277.

Kleemola-Kujala, E., and Räsänen, L. (1982). Relationship of oral hygiene and sugar consumption to risk of caries in children. *Community Dent. Oral Epidemiol.* 10: 224–233.

Kramer, M.S., Vanilovich, I., Matush, L., Bogdanovich, N., Zhang, X., Shishko, G., Muller-Bolla, M., and Platt, R.W. (2007). The effect of prolonged and exclusive breast-feeding on dental caries in early school-age children. *Caries Res.* 41: 484–488.

Kuhnisch, J., Sochtig, F., Pitchika, V., Laubender, R., Neuhaus, K.W., Lussi, A., and Hickel, R. (2015). In vivo validation of nearinfrared light transillumination for interproximal dentin caries detection. *Clin. Oral Investig.* 20: 821–829.

Leong, P.M., Gussy, M.G., Barrow, S.L., De Silva-Sanigorski, A., and Waters, E. (2013). A systematic review of risk factors during first year of life for early childhood caries. *Int. J. Paediatr. Dent.* 23: 235–250.

Leroy, R., Bogaerts, K., Martens, L., and Declerck, D. (2012). Risk factors for caries incidence in a cohort of Flemish preschool children. *Clin. Oral Investig.* 16: 805–812.

Li, Y., Ge, Y., Saxena, D., and Caufield, P.W. (2007). Genetic profiling of the oral microbiota associated with severe early childhood caries. *J. Clin. Microbiol.* 45: 81–87.

Lim, S., Sohn, W., Burt, B.A., Sandretto, A.M., Kolker, J.L., Marshall, T.A., and Ismail, A.I. (2008). Cariogenicity of soft drinks, milk and fruit juice in low-income African-American children: A longitudinal study. *J. Am. Dent. Assoc.* 139: 959–967.

Lovrov, S., Hertrich, K., and Hirschfelder, U. (2007). Enamel demineralization during fixed orthodontic treatment–incidence and correlation to various oral hygiene parameters. *J. Orofac. Orthop.* 68: 353–363.

Lunder, N. (1996). Von der Fehrb F R. Approximal cavitation related to bite-wing image and caries activity in adolescents. *Caries Res.* 30: 143–147.

Marinho, V.C., Higgins, J.P., Sheiham, A., and Logan, S. (2004). Combinations of topical fluoride (toothpastes, mouthrinses, gels, varnishes) versus single topical fluoride for preventing dental caries in children and adolescents. *Cochrane Database Syst. Rev. CD002781.*

Marinho, V.C.C., Higgins, J.P.T., Logan, S., and Sheiham, A. (2003). Fluoride toothpastes for preventing dental caries in children and adolescents. *Cochrane Database Syst. Rev.* 1: CD002278.

Martignon, S., Ekstrand, K.R., Lemos, M.I., Lozano, M.P., and Higuera, C. (2010). Plaque, caries level and oral hygiene habits in young patients receiving orthodontic treatment. *Community Dent. Health* 27: 133–138.

Mascarenhas, A.K. (1998). Oral hygiene as a risk indicator of enamel and dentin caries. *Community Dent. Oral Epidemiol.* 26: 331–339.

Mathiesen, A.T., Ogaard, B., and Rolla, G. (1996). Oral hygiene as a variable in dental caries experience in 14-year-olds exposed to fluoride. *Caries Res.* 30: 29–33.

Mejare, I., Axelsson, S., Dahlen, G., Espelid, I., Norlund, A., Tranæus, S., and Twetman, S. (2014). Caries risk assessment. A systematic review. *Acta Odontol. Scand.* 72: 81–91.

Mitropoulos, C.M. (1985). The use of fibre-optic transillumination in the diagnosis of posterior-proximal caries in clinical trials. *Caries Res.* 19: 379–384.

Murray, T.W. (2014). Epidemiology of oral health conditions in older people. *Gerodontology* (Suppl. 1): 9–16.

Nyvad, B. and Fejerskov, O. (1997). Assessing the stage of caries lesion activity on the basis of clinical and microbiological examination. *Community Dent. Oral Epidemiol.* 25: 69–75.

Nyvad, B., Machiulskiene, V., and Baelum, V. (1999). Reliability of a new caries diagnostic system differentiating between active and inactive caries lesions. *Caries Res.* 33: 252–260.

Nyvad, B., Machiulskiene, V., and Baelum, V. (2003). Construct and predictive validity of clinical caries diagnostic criteria assessing lesion activity. *J. Dent. Res.* 82: 117–122.

Ogaard, B. (1989). Prevalence of white spot lesions in 19-year-olds: A study on untreated and orthodontically treated persons 5 years after treatment. *Am. J. Orthod. Dentofacial Orthop.* 96: 423–427.

Petersen, P.E., Bourgeois, D., Ogawa, H., Estupinan-Day, S., and Ndiaye, C. (2005). The global burden of oral diseases and risks to oral health. *Bull. World Health Organ.* 83: 661–666.

Petersson, G.H., and Twetman, S. (2015). Caries risk assessment in young adults: A 3 year validation of the Cariogram model. *BMC Oral Health* 15: 17.

Petersson, G.H., Isberg, P.E., and Twetman, S. (2010). Caries risk assessment in school children using a reduced Cariogram model without saliva tests. *BMC Oral Health* 10: 5.

Pitts, N.B., and Rimmer, P.A. (1992). An in vivo comparison of radiographic and directly assessed clinical caries status of posterior approximal surfaces in primary and permanent teeth. *Caries Res.* 26: 146–152.

Pitts, N.B., Ekstrand, K.R., and Foundation, I. (2013). International Caries Detection and Assessment System (ICDAS) and its International Caries Classification and Management.

Pitts, N.B., Ismail, A.I., Martignon, S., Ekstrand, K., Douglas, G.A.V., and Longbottom, C. ICCMS guide for practitioners and educators. Available at https://www.icdas.org/uploads/ICCMS-Guide_Full_Guide_UK.pdf (accessed January 2018).

Polk, D.E., Weyant, R.J., and Manz, M.C. (2010). Socioeconomic factors in adolescents' oral health: Are they mediated by oral hygiene behaviors or preventive interventions? *Community Dent. Oral Epidemiol.* 38: 1–9.

Quaglio, J.M., Sousa, M.B., Ardenghi, T.M., Mendes, F.M., Imparato, J.C., and Pinheiro, S.L. (2006). Association between clinical parameters and the presence of active caries lesions in first permanent molars. *Braz. Oral Res.* 4: 358–363.

Reich, E., Lussi, A., and Newbrun, E. (1999). Caries-risk assessment. *Int. Dent. J.* 49: 15–26.

Reisine, S., Tellez, M., Willem, J., Sohn, W., and Ismail, A. (2008). Relationship between caregiver's and child's caries prevalence among disadvantaged African Americans. *Community Dent. Oral Epidemiol.* 36: 191–200.

Richter, A.E., Arruda, A.O., Peters, M.C., and Sohn, W. (2011). Incidence of caries lesions among patients treated with comprehensive orthodontics. *Am. J. Orthod. Dentofacial Orthop.* 139: 657–664.

Ricketts, D., Lamont, T., Innes, N.P., Kidd, E., and Clarkson, J.E. (2013). Operative caries management in adults and children. *Cochrane Database Syst. Rev.* 3: CD003808.

Rimmer, P.A., and Pitts, N.B. (1990). Temporary elective tooth separation as a diagnostic aid in general practice. *Br. Dent. J.* 169: 87–92.

Ritter, A.V., Preisser, J.S., and Chung, Y. (2012). X-ACT collaborative research group. Risk indicators for the presence and extent of root caries among caries active adults enrolled in the Xylitol for Adult Caries Trial (X-ACT). *Clin. Oral Investig.* 16: 1647–1657.

Saini, T., Edwards, P.C., Kimmes, N.S., Carroll, L.R., Shaner, J.W., and Dowd, F.J. (2005). Etiology of xerostomia and dental caries among methamphetamine abusers. *Oral Health Prev. Dent.* 3: 189–195.

Schwendicke, F., Dorfer, C.E., Schlattmann, P., Foster Page, L., Thomson, W.M., and Paris, S. (2015). Socioeconomic inequality and caries: A systematic review and meta-analysis. *J. Dent. Res.* 94: 10–18.

Skrīvele, S., Care, R., and Bērziņa, S. (2013). Caries and its risk factor s in young children in five different countries. *Stomatologija* 15: 39–46.

Smith, R.E., Badner, V.M., Morse, D.E., and Freeman, K. (2002). Maternal risk indicators for childhood caries in an inner city population. *Community Dent. Oral Epidemiol.* 30: 176–181.

Söchtig, F., Hickel, R., and Kühnisch, J. (2014). Caries detection and diagnostics with nearinfrared light transillumination: Clinical experiences. *Quintessence Int.* 45: 531–538.

Staninec, M., Lee, C., Darling, C.L., and Fried, D. (2010). In vivo near-IR imaging of approximal dental decay at 1310 nm. *Lasers Surg. Med.* 42: 292–298.

Tagliaferro, E.P., Ambrosano, G.M., Meneghim Mde, C., and Pereira, A.C. (2008). Risk indicators and risk predictors of dental caries in schoolchildren. *J. Appl. Oral Sci.* 16: 408–413.

Teanpaisan, R., Chaethong, W., Piwat, S., and Thitasomakul, S. (2012). Vertical transmission of mutans streptococci and lactobacillus in Thai families. *Pediatr. Dent.* 34: e24–9.

Tenovuo, J. (1997). Salivary parameters of relevance for assessing caries activity in individuals or populations. *Community Dent. Oral Epidemiol.* 25: 82–86.

Twetman, S. (2009). Caries prevention with fluoride toothpaste in children: An update. *Eur. Arch. Paediatr. Dent.* 10: 162–167.

Tyas, M.J., Anusavice, K.J., Frencken, J.E., and Mount, G.J. (2000). Minimal intervention dentistry: A review. FDI commission project 1–97. *Int. Dent. J.* 50: 1–12.

van Amerongen, J.P., Penning, C., Eam, K., and Ten Cate, J.M. (1992). An in vitro assessment of the extent of caries under small occlusal cavities. *Caries Res.* 26: 89–93.

van der Veen, M.H., Attin, R., Schwestka-Polly, R., and Wiechmann, D. (2010). Caries outcomes after orthodontic treatment with fixed appliances: Do lingual brackets make a difference? *Eur. J. Oral Sci.* 118: 298–303.

Varma, S., Banerjee, A., and Bartlett, D. (2008). An in vivo investigation of associations between saliva properties, caries prevalence and potential lesion activity in an adult UK population. *J. Dent.* 36: 294–299.

Voelker, M.A., Simmer-Beck, M., Cole, M., Keeven, E., and Tira, D. (2013). Preliminary findings on the correlation of saliva pH, buffering capacity, flow, consistency and streptococcus mutans in relation to cigarette smoking. *J. Dent. Hyg.* 87: 30–37.

Walsh, T., Worthington, H.V., Glenny, A.-M., Appelbe, P., Marinho, V.C.C., and Shi, X. (2010). Fluoride toothpastes of different concentrations for preventing dental caries in children and adolescents. *Cochrane Database Syst. Rev. CD007868.*

Weintraub, J.A., Prakash, P., Shain, S.G., Laccabue, M., and Gansky, S.A. (2010). Mothers' caries increases odds of chilren's caries. *J. Dent. Res.* 89: 954–958.

World_health_organization oral health, fact sheet no. 318. Available at: http://www.who.int/mediacentre/factsheets/fs318/en.

Wu, J., and Fried, D. (2009). High contrast near-infrared polarized reflectance images of demineralization on tooth buccal and occlusal surfaces at lambda = 1310 nm. *Lasers Surg. Med.* 41: 208–213.

Young, D.A., Nový, B.B., Zeller, G.G., Hale, R., Hart, T.C., and Truelove, E.L. (2015). The American dental association caries classification system for clinical practice: A report of the American dental association council on scientific affairs. *J. Am. Dent. Assoc.* 146: 79–86.

Zero, D., Fontana, M., and Lennon, A.M. (2001). Clinical applications and outcomes of using indicators of risk in caries management. *J. Dent. Educ.* 65: 1126–1132.

Zimmer, B.W., and Rottwinkel, Y. (2004). Assessing patient-specific decalcification risk in fixed orthodontic treatment and its impact on prophylactic procedures. *Am. J. Orthod. Dentofacial Orthop.* 126: 318–324.

5

Management of Dental Caries: Minimally Invasive Dentistry vs. Conventional Strategies

John Featherstone

Key Topics

- Clinical challenges to manage dental caries
- Caries risk assessment and the process
- Levels of therapy needed according to the caries risk assessment
- Case studies illustrating caries risk levels
- Anticaries agents and their advantages with limitations
- Bioactive materials and Minimally Invasive Dentistry (MID)
- High risk patients and conventional treatment

Learning Objectives

- Be able to understand the process of caries risk assessment
- Be able to define the different categories of caries risk
- Be able to assess the levels of therapy needed according to the outcome of the caries risk assessment
- Be able to appreciate the importance of early caries detection in relation to retention of teeth for a long time
- Be able to understand the restorative cycle of conventional treatment with high caries risk individuals

Introduction

In the 21st century, dental caries, as a disease, is not eradicated, but rather only controlled to a certain extend (Petersen 2003). Dental caries is still one of the most common and costly chronic diseases affecting the general population, both children and adults. Minimal intervention strategies to manage dental caries can have an enormous socio-economic impact.

Minimally Invasive Dentistry: Interdisciplinary Clinical and Scientific Approaches, First Edition.
Edited by Aylin Baysan and Paul Anderson.
© 2026 John Wiley & Sons Ltd. Published 2026 by John Wiley & Sons Ltd.
Companion website: www.wiley.com/go/baysan/minimally_invasive_dentistry

Despite our knowledge of the basic concepts of dental caries, progress still needs to be made in the management of the disease. It has long been known that not all lesions progress to cavitation (Backer Dirks 1966). The challenge has been to determine which white-spot lesions will progress to cavitation within enamel whilst in dentine, and how much dentine lesions could be left in deep carious lesions. As described in detail below, recent approaches have concentrated on managing the disease to prevent further progress, and to halt or reverse the non-cavitated lesions.

Mount and Hume (Baysan and Lynch 2001) suggested that minimal restorative work can successfully be done based upon the principle of removing only carious tissue that is necessary to gain access to the carious lesions and remove areas that are infected and broken down to the point where remineralisation is no longer possible. In addition to this, the decision to repair rather than replace a restoration always must be based on the patient's risk of developing caries, the professional's judgment of benefits vs. risks and conservative principles of cavity preparation. For high and extreme caries risk individuals (see below), the risk level must be lowered at the same time that the restorative work is being done or restorations may be only a temporary fix.

It is now recognised that the most desirable treatment for dental caries is remineralisation (Featherstone 2004) since the ultimate aim is to preserve the tooth structure in an appropriate approach. Remineralisation is the natural repair process of non-cavitated lesions that can be arrested, or even reversed. However, if the bacterial challenge is high the amount of acid produced, when fermentable carbohydrates are ingested, can overcome the effects of remineralisation and lesions can progress to cavitation.

Clinical Challenges to Manage Dental Caries

Dental caries is a difficult disease to treat since it is caused by multiple species of bacteria, so it can not be considered as a simple bacterial infection. It is best considered as a balance between pathological factors and protective factors (Featherstone 2000, 2004). Management of dental caries can be enhanced by either reducing the pathological factors or enhancing the protective factors, or a combination of both (Featherstone 2000).

The three major pathological factors are: 1) cariogenic bacteria, 2) frequent ingestion of fermentable carbohydrate, and 3) severely impaired salivary function (hyposalivation). The three major protective factors are: 1) normal salivary function; 2) fluoride, calcium, and phosphate for remineralisation; and 3) antibacterial therapy to reduce the bacterial cariogenic challenge. The caries balance can be visualised as in Figure 5.1.

Placing restorations can restore the function of the tooth, but it does not affect the levels of cariogenic bacteria in the rest of the mouth (Feathestone et al. 2012). Therefore, successful management of dental caries requires management of the disease with chemical therapy, coupled with minimal intervention restorative work. Assessment of the level of risk for future occurrence of dental caries lesions is therefore very important as the first step in managing dental caries. The level of chemical therapy is determined by the risk level for each individual patient. The procedure for determining caries risk status is described in practical terms in the following section below.

In reality, once a tooth is in the vicious circle of the 'restorative cycle', it is a process in which small and innocent restorations lead to larger restorations involving more dentine,

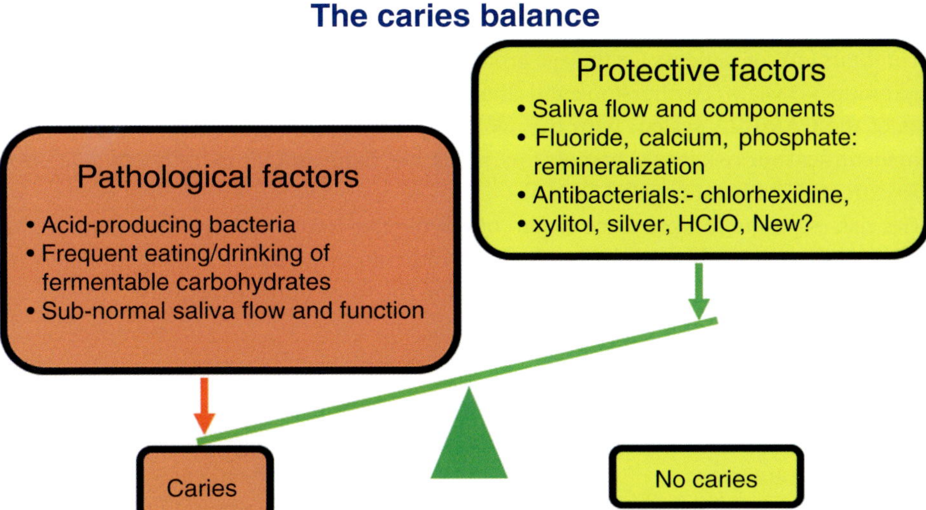

Figure 5.1 The caries balance showing the balance between pathological factors and protective factors. The balance can either be toward progression or reversal of the disease. Updated from Featherstone (2000).

which in turn are replaced repeatedly, until the dental pulp becomes involved. This requires endodontic treatment or extractions, then fixed/removable prosthesis or dental implants. The expectation of the survival/success of restorations depend on multiple factors such as patient related, general and local factors. In this equilibrium, the quality of life for patients is compromised. Therefore, early intervention based upon the caries risk status can break this cycle and preserve the teeth far into the future. Early detection of dental caries and assessment of risk can be used to successfully provide preventive and interventive therapy. Thus, minimally invasive or noninvasive strategies can manage dental caries and ultimately provide effective retention of teeth (Featherstone and Doméjean 2012).

Fluoride is the most widely accepted and effective prevention agent, at the levels of both populations and individuals. However, fluoride therapy alone is insufficient to deal with the bacterial challenge in high and extreme caries risk individuals, as described below. Not every single patient requires the same management strategy. A tailored approach to manage dental caries is one of the main cornerstones to MID.

Caries Risk Assessment and the Process

The assessment of caries risk for each individual patient is essential as the basis for the management of the disease we call dental caries. Caries risk is the likelihood of the patient having new caries lesions (white spots, cavities, etc.) in the near future. There are many caries risk assessment forms and procedures in the recent literature, and some are commercially available. However, there are only two systems that have been validated by long-term patient outcomes research (Featherstone et al. 2021a). One is the Cariogram system from Sweden and the other is the CAMBRA® (Caries Management by Risk Assessment) system that was developed at the University of California, San Francisco, in conjunction with several other universities and the California Dental Association (Featherstone et al. 2007; Ramos-Gomez et al. 2007; Featherstone and Chaffee 2018). The CAMBRA system has been validated three times in thousands of patients for the age group 6 years through adult and most recently for the age group 0–5 years (Featherstone and Chaffee 2018). The following step-by-step guide is for use of the CAMBRA system with the age group 6 years through adult. The CAMBRA system identifies four risk levels, namely low, moderate, high, and Please ad a new reference here as extreme (Featherstone et al. 2021b).

Caries risk assessment takes place as part of the regular comprehensive oral exam in the following sequence, leading to formulating an individualised caries management treatment plan that includes chemical therapy. Here are the steps in the process:

1) Take dental and medical history.
2) Conduct a clinical examination.
3) Detect caries lesions early enough to reverse or prevent progression.
4) Assess the caries risk as low, high, moderate, or extreme utilizing data from 1, 2, 3, and a short questionnaire.
5) Produce a treatment plan that includes chemical therapy appropriate to the caries risk level.
6) Use chemical therapy that includes fluoride and/or antibacterial agents based upon risk level.
7) Use minimally invasive restorative procedures to conserve tooth structure and function.
8) Recall and review at intervals appropriate to the caries risk status.
9) Reassess caries risk level at recall and modify the treatment plan as necessary.

Steps 1, 2, and 3 are done in conventional dentistry and form the basis of the caries risk assessment. Steps 2 and 3 provide a list of what are called 'disease indicators', which are simply clinical signs of the presence of caries, most likely ongoing over time.

The next step is the questionnaire that has a few simple questions to attempt to determine the cause of the ongoing disease, or to determine whether it is under control, or that the person is at low risk. The first part of the questionnaire is a list of 'biological and environmental risk factors'. These include the pathological factors described above. The second part of the questionnaire is a list of 'protective factors'. Only those factors that have been shown to be statistically significantly related to ongoing caries risk or reversal are included here (Featherstone and Chaffee 2018). See Table 5.1 for a visual summary of all three categories as a Caries Risk Assessment (CRA) form.

Disease Indicators

Disease indicators are the clinically observed results of previous and/or ongoing dental caries destruction of the tooth mineral.

a) Observed cavitation or radiographic evidence of progression into the dentin
b) White spot lesions on smooth surfaces
c) Radiographic evidence of non-cavitated demineralisation into the enamel
d) Existing restorations placed due to caries in the last 3 years for a new patient, or in the last year for a patient of record.

Table 5.1 Caries risk assessment components to be used as a caries risk assessment form. Refer to the text for details and instructions for use.

Caries risk component			
Disease indicators	**Check if yes**		
1. New cavities or lesion into dentin (radiographically)			
2. New white spot lesions on smooth surfaces			
3. New non-cavitated lesions in enamel (radiographically)			
4. Existing restorations in last 3 years (new patient) or the last year (patient of record)			
Biological or environmental risk factors	**Check if yes**		
1. Heavy plaque on the teeth			
2. Frequent snacking (>3 times daily)			
3. Hyposalivatory medications			
4. Reduced salivary function (low flow rate)			
5. Deep pits and fissures			
6. Recreational drug use			
7. Exposed tooth roots			
8. Orthodontic appliances			
Protective factors	**Check if yes**		
1. Fluoridated water			
2. Fluoridated toothpaste once a day			
3. Fluoridated toothpaste 2X daily or more			
4. 5000 ppm fluoridated toothpaste			
5. Fluoridated varnish last 6 months			
6. 0.05% sodium fluoride mouthrinse daily			
7. 0.12% or 0.2% chlorhexidine gluconate mouthrinse daily 7 days monthly			
8. Normal salivary function			
	Column 1	**Column 2**	**Column 3**
Final score: **Yes in column 1 indicates high or extreme risk** **Yes in columns 2 and 3: consider the balance**			

For a new patient visit, one or more of these disease indicators signals at least 'high caries risk'. For a patient of record at a follow-up visit any new appearance of a–d above signals at least 'high caries risk'. If hyposalivation is present, in addition (see below), this signals 'extreme risk'.

Biological and Environmental Risk Factors

The following are biological and environmental risk factors that have been shown to be statistically related to caries risk:

a) Heavy plaque on the teeth. This simple measure has been shown over and over to be a strong indicator of cariogenic bacterial activity, and strongly related to ongoing caries. At the time of writing there is no validated chairside test commercially available for measuring cariogenic bacterial levels. When this becomes available it would be added to this list

b) Frequent snacking on fermentable carbohydrates, at least 3 times daily outside of meal times

c) Use of medications that induce hypopsalivation

d) Reduced salivary function (low flow rate) by observation (dry mouth appearance and symptoms) or by measurement (stimulated flow rate less than 0.5 mL/minute)—**hyposalivation**

e) Deep pits and fissures

f) Daily or regular use of recreational drugs

g) Exposed tooth roots

h) Orthodontic appliances

In the risk assessment procedure any items on this list with a positive response are marked with a yes (Table 5.1) in the appropriate column. Each yes adds to the risk level. Items a and b can be modified by behavioural management. A yes to items c and d will normally indicate extreme risk if other risk factors and disease indicators suggest at least high risk. Deep pits and fissures suggest the use of preventive sealants. Item f indicates a lifestyle issue and most likely hyposalivation, depending on the drugs used. 'Meth mouth' is an extreme caries risk situation. Older people almost all have exposed tooth roots, indicating more attention is needed to fluoride and other preventive measures. Orthodontic brackets automatically places the patient at least into moderate risk because the appliances trap cariogenic bacteria, leading to their preferential growth during the time of the orthodontic treatment.

Add up the number of 'yes' checks and use this number to determine whether the patient is at low, moderate, or high risk, when balanced against the protective factors (below). Also use the yes indications to modify behaviour or determine additional therapy (see below).

Protective Factors

Protective factors are environmental or chemical therapy that helps to swing the caries balance to caries prevention or reversal. The most important factors that are proven effective are:

a) Lives, goes to school, or works in a fluoridated drinking water area

b) Uses a fluoride toothpaste once daily

c) Uses a fluoride toothpaste at least twice daily (it is well established that twice daily provides considerable added benefit. Therefore if the patient is a yes to question c they are also a yes to question b)
d) Uses a high concentration prescription (5,000 ppm F) fluoride toothpaste twice daily (a yes here is also a yes to questions b and c)
e) Has had fluoride varnish applied in the last 6 months
f) Uses 0.05% sodium fluoride mouthrinse daily
g) Uses 0.12% or 0.2% chlorhexidine gluconate mouthrinse daily for one week each month as prescribed for caries control
h) Has normal adequate salivary flow and function by inspection or measurement

Each of these items with a positive response receives a yes score and the number of 'protective factor' yes's are added up to offset the pathological score.

Determining the Caries Risk as Low, Moderate, High, or Extreme

1) **High and extreme risk.** One or more disease indicators signals at least high risk. If there is also hyposalivastion the patient is at extreme risk. With no hyposalivation the patient is at high risk. Even if there are no positive disease indicators the patient can still be at high risk if the pathological factors definitively outweigh the protective factors. Think of the caries balance.
2) **Low risk.** If there are no disease indicators, very few or no pathological factors and the protective factors prevail, the patient is at low risk. Usually this is obvious.
3) **Moderate risk.** If the patient is not obviously at high, or extreme risk and there is doubt about low risk, then the patient should be allocated to moderate risk and followed carefully, with additional chemical therapy added. An example would be a patient who had a root canal as a result of caries 4 years ago, and has no new clinical caries lesions, but has exposed tooth roots and only uses a fluoride toothpaste once a day.

Levels of Chemical Therapy Needed According to the Caries Risk Assessment

The following guidelines have been used and proven by two clinical trials and by outcomes assessment in thousands of patients (Featherstone et al. 2012; Featherstone and Chaffee 2018; Rechmann et al. 2018). Availability may vary by country, so these must be taken as guidelines and modified according to product availability. Chemical therapy must be included in the treatment plan for all patients, based upon the determined caries risk level. Restorative work, as needed will be included, in conjunction with the chemical therapy. The restorative work must be done according to the principles of minimal intervention dentistry (Featherstone and Doméjean 2012). The biggest issue is compliance. It is essential to work with the patient through motivational interviewing so that they use the home use regimens as prescribed, or the therapy will not be effective.

Low Caries Risk Chemical Therapy

The guideline is to 'keep it simple'. Whatever the patient is doing appears to be working. If the plaque levels are low, oral hygiene looks good, and the patient uses a fluoride toothpaste daily, then the recommendation is simple: 'keep doing what you are doing and use an over the counter fluoride toothpaste (1,000–1,450 ppm F) at least twice daily'. Recall for a follow-up visit at 12-month intervals.

Moderate Caries Risk Chemical Therapy

The moderate risk patient need additional therapy to keep them where they are, or better, to move them to low risk. Two alternatives are given, depending on the level of compliance.

1) Alternative 1: Over the counter fluoride toothpaste twice daily, plus 0.05% sodium fluoride mouthrinse daily at night. The patient should also be counselled to reduce between meal snacking, and to conscientiously follow this regimen.
2) Alternative 2: Prescription, high fluoride (5,000 ppm F) toothpaste, at least twice daily. Plus counselling on reducing between meal snacking of fermentable carbohydrates. This regimen is very simple and is recommended for those who may not comply with the toothpaste plus fluoride mouthrinse as in 1 above. The disadvantage is the prescription F toothpaste and the additional cost. Tha advantage is the simplicity of the protocol, and better likelihood of compliance.

Recall at 6 monthly intervals for follow-up visits.

High Caries Risk Chemical Therapy

The high risk patient **MUST** have antibacterial therapy to lower the bacterial challenge. Fluoride alone, at whatever concentration and frequency, will not be enough and the caries will continue to develop. The best proven antibacterial therapy that we currently have available is chlorhexidine mouthrinse (or gel). It is not ideal, as it is only partially effective. It is the best we currentlky have and was proven effective in a clinical trial, provided a specific regimen is used (Featherstone et al. 2012). New and better therapy will be available in the future. Silver diamine fluoride has recently gained popularity, and guidelines are being developed for its use. As of the time of writing, here is the proven chemical therapy for high caries risk patients (Featherstone et al. 2012; Featherstone and Chaffee 2018; Rechmann et al. 2018). There are three components:

a) Fluoride varnish applied in the clinic at the time of the clinical visit and reapplied every 4-6 months (for children and adults).
b) Brushing with a prescription, high fluoride (5,000 ppm F) toothpaste, at least twice daily. Plus counselling on reducing between meal snacking of fermentable carbohydrates.
c) Rinse for one minute once daily for one week each month with a chlorhexidine gluconate mouthrinse (0.12% or 0.2%). This should be done at least one hour apart from the fluoride toothbrushing, preferably last thing at night before bed. The regimen is to be continued for at least a year, until the disease is controlled and the risk level is lowered.

Recall at 4–6 month intervals for follow-up visits depending on the severity of the decay.

Extreme Caries Risk Chemical Therapy

The extreme risk patient must have antibacterial therapy to lower the bacterial challenge. Fluoride alone, at whatever concentration and frequency, will not be enough and the caries will continue to develop. This is even more so for the extreme risk patient. The therapy is the same as for high risk plus additional buffering and antibacterial therapy.

a) Fluoride varnish applied in the clinic at the time of the clinical visit and reapplied every 4–6 months (for children and adults).

b) Brushing with a prescription, high fluoride (5,000 ppm F) toothpaste, at least twice daily. Plus counselling on reducing between meal snacking of fermentable carbohydrates.

c) Rinse for one minute once daily for one week each month with a chlorhexidine gluconate mouthrinse (0.12% or 0.2%). This should be done at least one hour apart from the fluoride toothbrushing, preferably last thing at night before bed. The regimen is to be continued for at least a year, until the disease is controlled and the risk level is lowered to moderate or low.

d) Rinse ad libitum throughout the day every day with a baking soda solution, made fresh daily (2 teaspoons in 8 ounces (250 mL) of water).

e) In difficult cases consider adding at home use of fluoride trays with 5,000 ppm F gel for 5 minutes daily.

Recall at 3–4 month intervals for follow-up visits depending on the severity of the decay.

Anticaries Agents and Delivery Systems

- Fluoride in its various delivery forms has been well established to work through topical mechanisms via the plaque and the surface of the teeth to inhibit demineralisation and enhance remineralisation (Featherstone 2004). Numerous clinical trials have established the efficacy of fluoride-containing toothpastes in markedly reducing future dental caries. 'Over the counter' products contain 1,000–1,450 ppm F in one of its various forms. The use of fluoride toothpaste twice a day, rather than once a day or less, has been shown to even further reduce caries progression. High concentration fluoride toothpastes with 5,000 ppm F have been shown to be significantly more effective than 1,000 or 1,450 ppm F products against root caries and enamel caries. Fluoride varnish (22,000 ppm F) has been shown in several clinical trials to have additional benefit in reducing dental caries progression. Mouthrinse containing sodium fluoride at 0.05% has been shown very effective in reducing dental caries.

- Chlorhexidine gluconate (a cationic bis-biguanide) has been used for many years as an antiplaque agent and has been shown to suppress *Streptococcus mutans*, so it is potentially useful used for caries prevention. However, clinical results have been mixed. A number of chlorhexidine preparations are available, as rinses, toothpastes, gels, thymol-containing varnishes, chewing gums, and sprays. Especially relevant to this chapter are two clinical trials that showed the efficacy of 0.12% chlorhexidine gluconate mouthrinse, in conjunction with fluoride toothpaste, in altering the caries balance, and reducing caries in high caries risk adults (Featherstone et al. 2012; Rechmann et al. 2018). It is important to note that the successful regimen was developed based upon bacterial measures in humans over time, and consists of rinsing once a day with 10 mL for one week each month.

- Xylitol is a non-cariogenic sugar-alcohol that has similar sweetness to sucrose. It cannot be metabolised by cariogenic bacteria and is a very effective substitute for sucrose in reducing the frequency of fermentable carbohydrate snacking. Numerous studies indicated that xylitol gum or mints may reduce dental caries, but results have been mixed. In the clinical outcomes studies for caries management by risk assessment described above (Featherstone and Chaffee 2018), xylitol use was not significantly related to caries reduction or negatively related to caries risk assessment.
- Casein Phosphopeptide-Amorphous Calcium Phosphate (CPP-ACP): Considerable work has been done with this material. It is a casein phosphopeptide that contains soluble calcium phosphate that is readily available to enhance remineralisation in smooth surface lesions. It is valuable as additional therapy in hyposalivatory patients and when smooth surface lesions are progressing, such as in orthodontic patients. However, clinical results are mixed.
- Functionalised Tricalcium phosphate is used as an additive to fluoride-containing products such as 5,000 ppm F toothpaste and fluoride varnish. It has been shown in laboratory studies to enhance remineralisation beyond the effect of fluoride alone.

Bioactive Materials and the Future

Considerable research is being carried out around the world to develop materials that enhance remineralisation. We can expect such products to be proven and marketed in the near future. Further, considerable effort is being devoted to new antibacterial agents, especially those that can beneficially modify the biofilm without necessarily killing the cariogenic bacteria, but rather subduing their effect. Genetic modification of the microbiome (biofilm on the tooth) is also being pursued and shows promise. All of these approaches will take time and money before they are clinically available for use.

When to Consider Conventional Treatment in High Risk Patients?

High and extreme caries risk patients cannot be controlled by conventional fluoride therapy and conventional restorative work alone. All clinical studies on such subjects clearly show major caries progression in spite of combined fluoride and restorative therapy. Therefore, antibacterial therapy, dietary modification, fluoride therapy, and minimally invasive restorative procedures must all be used in combination to manage dental caries in high and extreme risk patients. In extreme risk patients pH control must also be added, as described above.

Summary

The most desirable treatment for dental caries is remineralisation since the ultimate aim is to preserve the tooth structure in an appropriate approach. Remineralisation is the natural repair process of non-cavitated lesions that can be arrested, or even reversed. However, if the bacterial challenge is high the amount of acid produced, when fermentable carbohydrates are ingested, can overcome the effects of remineralisation and lesions can progress to cavitation.

Minimally invasive strategies for the management of dental caries starts with identifying the caries risk, tailoring the prevention and treatment options for the patient's needs. There are widely researched anti-caries agents such as fluoride, chlorhexidine, thymol, CPP-ACP, and functionalised tricalcium phosphate in the literature. Nowadays, bioactive materials are being incorporated into dental products to enhance remineralisation and to prevent demineralisation. Their antimicrobial effects have not been fully investigated, although considerable research is in progress. Genetic modification of the microbiome (biofilm on the tooth) is also being pursued and shows promise. All these approaches ultimately aim to preserve tooth structure by the employment of minimally invasive strategies since being in a restorative cycle despite the degree of caries risk is less than ideal for the survival of teeth. Therefore, advances in research are still required.

Caries management by risk assessment has been clinically proven effective and should be employed with all patients as part of the minimal intervention approach. Improvements in chemical therapy appropriate to risk levels will be available in the future.

Further Reading

Chaffee, B.W., Featherstone, J.D., Gansky, S.A., Cheng, J., and Zhan, L. (2016). Caries risk assessment item importance: Risk designation and caries status in children under age 6. *JDR Clin. Trans. Res.* 1 (2): 131–142. PMID: 27403458. PMCID: PMC4937437.

Featherstone, J., Fontana, M., and Wolff, M. (2018). Novel anticaries and remineralization agents: Future research needs. *J. Dent. Res.* 97: 125–127. PMID: 29355470.

Rechmann, P., Bekmezian, S., Rechmann, B.M.T., Chaffee, B.W., and Featherstone, J.D.B. (2018). MI varnish and MI paste plus in a caries prevention and remineralization study: a randomized controlled trial. *Clin. Oral. Investig.* PMID: 29299732.

Rechmann, P., Chaffee, B.W., Rechmann, B.M., and Featherstone, J.D.B. (2018). Changes in caries risk in a practice based randomized controlled trial. *Adv. Dent. Res.* 29 (1), 15–23.

Rechmann, P., Rechmann, B.M.T., Kinsel, R., and Featherstone, J. (2018). Change of salivary fluoride level with intake of fluoride releasing lozenges: A pilot study. *J. Investig. Clin. Dent.* 30: e12336. PMID: 29603891.

References

Backer Dirks, O. (1966). Posteruptive changes in dental enamel. *J. Dent. Res.* 3: 503–511.

Baysan, A., and Lynch, E. (2001). Management of primary root caries with a high fluoride dentifrice. *Quintenssence Book, Chapter* 2: 37–48.

Featherstone, J.D., and Chaffee, B.W. (2018). The evidence for caries management by risk assessment (CAMBRA®). *Adv. Dent. Res.* 29: 9–14.

Featherstone, J.D., and Doméjean, S. (2012). Minimal intervention dentistry: Part 1. From "compulsive" restorative dentistry to rational therapeutic strategies. *Br. Dent. J.* 9 (213): 41–445.

Featherstone, J.D., White, J.M., Hoover, C.I., Rapozo-Hilo, M., Weintraub, J.A., Wilson, R.S., Zhan, L., and Gansky, S.A. (2012). A randomized clinical trial of anticaries therapies targeted according to risk assessment (Caries Management by Risk Assessment). *Caries Res.* 46: 118–129.

Featherstone, J.D.B. (2000). The science and practice of caries prevention. *J. Am. Dent. Assoc.* 131: 887–899.

Featherstone, J.D.B. (2004). The continuum of dental caries – evidence for a dynamic process. *J. Dent. Res.* 83 (Special issue C): C39–42.

Featherstone, J.D.B., Crystal, Y.O., Alston, P., Chaffee, B.W., Doméjean, S., Rechmann, P., Zhan, L., and Ramos-Gomez, F. (2021a). A comparison of four caries risk assessment methods. *Front. Oral. Health.* https://doi.org/10.3389/froh.2021.656558

Featherstone, J.D.B., Crystal, Y.O., Alston, P., Chaffee, B.W., Doméjean, S., Rechmann, P., Zhan, L., and Ramos-Gomez, F. (2021b). Evidence-based caries management for all ages-practical guidelines. *Front. Oral. Health.* https://doi.org/10.3389/froh.2021.657518

Featherstone, J.D.B., Young, D.A., Domejean-Orliaguet, S., Jenson, L., and Wolff, M. (2007). Caries risk assessment appropriate for age 6 through adult. *CDA Journal* 35: 703–713.

Petersen, P.E. (2003). The world oral health report 2003: Continuous improvement of oral health in the 21st century–The approach of the WHO Global Oral Health Programme. *Community Dent. Oral Epidemiol.* 31 (Suppl 1): 3–24.

Ramos-Gomez, F., Crall, J., Slayton, R., and Featherstone, J.D. (2007). Caries risk assessment appropriate for the age one visit. *CDA J.* 35: 689–702.

Rechmann, P., Chaffee, B.W., Rechmann, B.M.T., and Featherstone, J.D.B. (2018). Changes in caries risk in a practice-based randomized controlled trial. *Adv. Dent. Res.* 29(1): 15–a23.

6

Intraoral Vaccine and Their Potential Clinical Use

Lesley Ann Bergmeier

Key Topics

- History of vaccination
- Definitions of immune functions
- Defining vaccination terminology
- Potential of iIntraoral vaccination

Learning Objectives

- To understand the concepts of vaccination and immune protection
- To understand the functions of the immune system in the oral cavity
- To be able to appreciate the potential for intraoral vaccination in oral health care
- To be able to appreciate the role of the immune system in oral health

Introduction

The concept of intraoral vaccination is relatively new and contrasts with conventional vaccination by directly targeting the oral cavity to induce local immune responses or to modulate already established immune functions or disease presentations. Methods such as the passive application of antibodies or the induction of tolerance have been successful in both animal models and in human clinical trials for a variety of oral conditions and systemic diseases with oral presentations.

The purpose of this chapter is to introduce the concept of **intraoral** vaccination and to review the current knowledge of the capacity of the oral cavity as an inductive site for immune responses.

Minimally Invasive Dentistry: Interdisciplinary Clinical and Scientific Approaches, First Edition.
Edited by Aylin Baysan and Paul Anderson.
© 2026 John Wiley & Sons Ltd. Published 2026 by John Wiley & Sons Ltd.
Companion website: www.wiley.com/go/baysan/minimally_invasive_dentistry

A Brief History of Vaccination

Vaccination has a long and important history in public health which precedes the most well-known discovery of Edward Jenner in the 18th century. The process of 'inoculation' is thought to have been used against smallpox as early as the 10th century in China, while the earliest recorded examples of vaccination date from the 17th century when powdered scabs from individuals infected with smallpox were used to protect against the disease. Edward Jenner observed that individuals who had recovered from the much less serious disease, cowpox, seemed to be immune from smallpox. His pioneering work in the field of the smallpox vaccination led eventually to the complete eradication of the disease in 1980 (Figure 6.1). The toll of infectious diseases, in terms of both mortality and morbidity, have been vastly decreased by the development and world-wide adoption of vaccination strategies. Many once common diseases are now rare and some, like polio are very close to eradication, while vaccination against diphtheria and measles have been highly successful. The World Health Organisation Global Action plan for vaccination 2011–2020 currently lists 26 available vaccines with 23 in pipeline development (http://www.who.int/immunization/global_vaccine_action_plan/GVAP_doc_2011_2020/en/). (Pre-SARS-CoV-2 vaccine roll out).

Principals of Vaccination

The aims of vaccination are to induce specific immune responses in the B- and T-cell compartments through administration of a 'non-virulent' antigen preparation (Box 6.1). In broad terms, the induction of B cells producing specific antibodies is the key

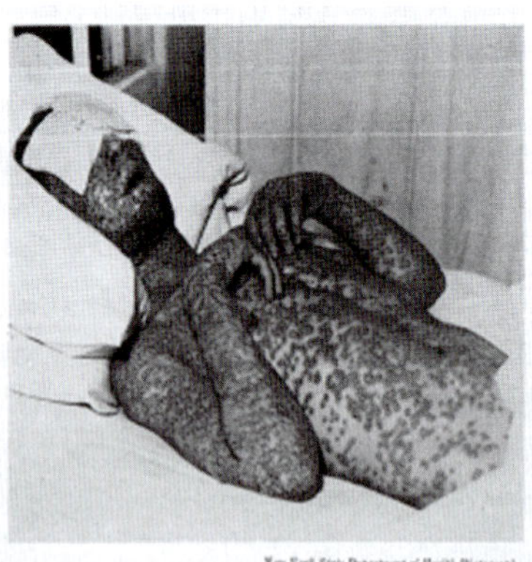

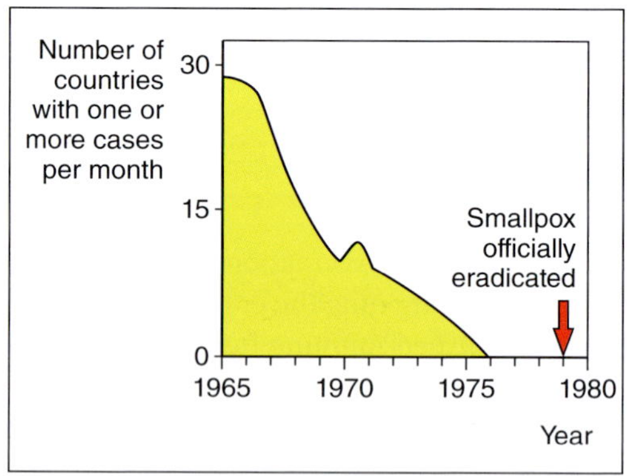

Figure 6.1 Smallpox: Eradication and the power of vaccination. This photograph of a smallpox victim appeared in the Baltimore Health News in 1939 as a warning to people who had not been vaccinated. ('This Man Was Never Vaccinated Against Smallpox', Baltimore Health News 16, no. 2 (Nov. 1939). Source: Chapin Library of Rare Books, Williams College, reproduced under Creative Commons.

Box 6.1   Key protective immune responses following vaccination

Antibody mediated protection (B-cell compartment)

Antibodies produced following immunisation can be very effective against extracellular organisms and their products (toxins). Antibodies can block viruses and bacteria from entering and infecting host cells and can also mediate killing of pathogens. The ability of antibodies to neutralise toxins can prevent the damaging effects of infections such as *diphtheria* or *clostridium*. The type of antibody induced is important as IgG is primarily effective in blood whereas secretory IgA (SIgA) is the principal antibody associated with mucosal surfaces.

Cell-mediated immune protection (T-cell compartment)

The cell-mediated immune response is characterised by two distinct activities: **Cytotoxic T cells** (CD8$^+$), able to kill cells infected with viruses or other intracellular pathogens including some bacterial, fungal, and protozoa and **CD4$^+$ T helper cells** which are important activators of other T cells but also activate polymorphonuclear leukocytes (PMNs), natural killer cells (NKT) cells by their ability to secrete a wide range of cytokines, chemokines, and growth factors.

  CD4$^+$ T helper cells are also key to the induction and maturation of antibody secreting cells and their ability to generate memory cells which migrate back to the draining lymph nodes where they wait in readiness for the next exposure to the antigen (infection) for which they are specific.

---

protective response to bacterial infections, while the induction of cytotoxic T cells induces protection against intracellular infections such as viruses and some bacteria and parasites. The immune response will become re-activated when an individual is exposed to the disease-causing organism (or its toxins) due to the induction of *memory cells* which rapidly expand into **effector cells** to eliminate the disease-causing pathogen or to neutralise its toxins. The use of vaccination is recognised as one of the most effective interventions in the control of infectious diseases. When a significant proportion of any population has been vaccinated against a given organism the result is **herd immunity** where the potential for the spread or transmission of infectious organisms is disrupted and any non-vaccinated individuals are much less likely to be exposed to infection.

The standard set of vaccines in use today are given to all individuals and some are only given to those at high risk of infection (Table 6.1). The timing of vaccination depends on the group of individuals to be vaccinated. Vaccines against common infections are given as early as possible. Some vaccines do not work well in very young infants. This may be due to the presence of maternal antibodies which have crossed the placenta and provide protection to the infant in the first few months of life until the child's own immune system begins to become active and responsive to vaccination and/or infection.

Table 6.1 Current vaccines in use in UKNHS.

2 months: 5-in-1 vaccine Pneumococcal vaccine Rotavirus vaccine Men B vaccine	2, 3, and 4 years plus school years one and two: Children's annual flu vaccine	65 and over: Pneumococcal vaccine Annual flu vaccine
3 months: Men C vaccine 5-in-1 vaccine (2nd dose) Rotavirus vaccine (2nd dose)	3 years and 4 months: 4-in-1 pre-school booster MMR vaccine (2nd dose)	70 years: Shingles vaccine
4 months: 5-in-1 vaccine (3rd dose) Pneumococcal vaccine (2nd dose) Men B vaccine (2nd dose)	12–13 years: HPV vaccine 13–18 years: 3-in-1 teenage booster vaccine Men ACWY vaccine	Vaccines only for at-risk groups: BCG (TB) vaccine (birth to age 35) Chickenpox vaccine (any age) Flu vaccine (adults) Flu vaccine (children) Pneumococcal vaccine (2 years to 65 years)
12–13 months: MMR vaccine Hib/Men C booster vaccine Pneumococcal vaccine (3rd dose) Men B vaccine (3rd dose)	Travel vaccines: Hep A Typhoid Cholera Yellow fever Rabies (post exposure + antibody)	Hepatitis B vaccine (birth onwards)

(http://www.nhs.uk/Conditions/vaccinations/Pages/vaccination-schedule-age-checklist.aspx?tabname=NHS%20vaccination%20schedule).

Types of Vaccine Preparations

The milestones achieved in vaccination in the past have relied on whole-killed or *attenuated* pathogen preparations but more recent research has investigated *subunit* vaccines where fragments of pathogens or specific proteins or peptides are used as the vaccine antigen (Figure 6.2). These vaccines are more pure, safer, and easier to produce, especially if they are recombinant proteins. However, these subunit vaccines are often poorly immunogenic and are dependent on highly efficient enhancers of immune responses known as **adjuvants** (Box 6.2) (Matzinger 1994; Moser and Leo 2010).

Adjuvants are substances that enhance the immune response to an antigen with which it is mixed. Non-living vaccines (especially small molecule-peptide vaccines) require the addition of adjuvants to boost the response to these antigens. These adjuvants are frequently microbial in origin, however can be synthetic and some are endogenous materials. At present only calcium and aluminium salts are used in human vaccine preparations. These salts function by producing a 'depot' effect that allows for slow release of the antigen. Adjuvants must preserve the integrity of the antigen with which they are used and the slow release of the antigen helps in effective targeting of antigen presenting

- Antigens
  - Whole inactivated or attenuated organisms or a mixture of various strains
  - Isolated and purified proteins, glycoproteins or carbohydrates
  - Recombinant proteins and glycoproteins
- Immune potentiators (adjuvants)
  - Bacterial products
  - Toxins and lipids
  - Nucleic acids
  - Peptidoglycans
  - Carbohydrates, peptides
  - Cytokines and hormones
  - Small molecules
- Delivery systems
  - Mineral salts (e.g. Alum)
  - Surface active agents
  - Synthetic microparticles (ISCOMS, VLPs)
  - Oli-in water emulsions
  - Liposomes

Type of antigen	Viruses	Bacteria
Normal Organism	Vaccinia (cowpox)	
Live attenuated	Measles Mumps Rubella Polio (Sabin) Yellow Fever Varicella zoster	BCG Typhoid
Whole killed organisms	Rabies Polio (Salk) Influenza	Pertussis Typhoid Cholera
Subcellular fragments		Diphtheria Tetanus Cholera
Capsular polysaccharides		Meningococcus Pneumococcus Haemophilus Typhoid
Surface antigens	Hep B	

Figure 6.2 The key components of vaccines. Examples of the types of antigen used in different vaccines currently in use are shown in the inset box.

Box 6.2 Enhancing the immune response: Adjuvants

substance that enhance the immune response to an antigen with which it is mixed. Non-living vaccines (especially small molecule peptide vaccines) require the addition of adjuvants to boost the responses to these antigens.

- Adjuvants are frequently microbial in origin, but can be synthetic and some are endogenous materials. At present only calcium and aluminium salts are the permitted adjuvants for use in humans.
- Adjuvants must preserve the integrity of the antigen that they are used with and allow for the slow release of the antigen and effective targeting of antigen presenting cells.
- These substances frequently engage with innate immune cell receptors such as the toll-like receptors (TLRs) (Allan 2008; Gutjahr et al. 2016). New preparations in clinical development were recently reviewed by Correia-Pinto et al. (2013).
- Adjuvants can also act as delivery systems (Wack and Rappuoli 2015), which can increase the immune responses depending on their particular characteristics (Basith et al. 2011).
- For mucosal applications, different adjuvants are required (Lycke 2012; Correia-Pinto et al. 2013; Holmgren and Czerkinsky 2005; Holmgren and Svennerholm 2012), see Table 6.2.

Table 6.2 Mucosal adjuvants showing the induction of mucosal IgA and the activation of different T helper cells: + or – indicates the strength of induced immune response.

Mucosal adjuvants

Composition	Target	Th1	Th2	Th17	CTL	Mucosal IgA
		T cell mediated immune response				
MDP	TLR2	+	+	–	–	+
MPL	TLR4	+	–	–	+	+
Flagellin	TLR5	+	–	–	+	++
Cholera toxin	GM1	–	+	+	+	++++++
CTA1-DD	Ig heavy chain	+	+	+	+	+++++
Quillaja saponins	DCs	+	+	–	+	++
Cationic DNA	Not known	+	–	–	+	++
Chitosan	Tight junctions	–	+	–	–	++
IL-1	IL-1 R	+	+	–	–	+++
IL-12	IL-12 R	+	–	–	+	+

+ or – in this table means the strength of induced immune response.
CTL, cytotoxic T lymphocytes; MDP, muramyl dipeptide; TLR, Toll-like receptor; MPL, monophosphoryl lipid A; CT, cholera toxin; DC, dendritic cell; DDA, dimethyldioctadecylammonium; ND, not determined; IL, interleukin.
Source: Adapted from Lycke (2012), Kim and Jang (2017), and Novak et al. (2008).

cells (APCs). Adjuvants are usually categorised as immunostimulants (Reed et al. 2009) and they frequently engage the innate immune cells receptors such as the tll-like receptors (Allan 2008; Gutjahr et al. 2016) (TLRs) or delivery systems (Wack and Rappuoli 2015) They can increase the immune responses depending on their particular characteristics (Basith et al. 2011).

The type of materials that have been used in mucosal vaccination are different from those used in parenteral immunisation. The most effective are the enterotoxins cholera toxin and *E.coli* heat labile toxin (Lycke 2012). The choice of mucosal adjuvant is very important as it will dictate the type and quality of immune response which is induced. Many of the adjuvants will act through

TLRs either on the cell surface or in the cytoplasm of antigen presenting cells such as dendritic cells (DCs). The different T-helper cells, which are induced, will have a profound effect on the immune effector cells that are activated. For example Muramyl dipeptide acts through TLR 2 and induces both Th1 and Th2 cells and gives rise to some mucosal IgA, but cholera toxin binds to GM1 ganglioside and induces Th2, Th17, and Cytotoxic T cells as well as high levels of mucosal IgA (Lycke 2012; Apostolico et al. 2016; Kim and Jang 2017).

Immunisation

Vaccines that provoke immune responses, induce protection in the individual who has been vaccinated. This immune response may induce high levels of antibodies that can be transferred to other individuals in a passive manner. This has given rise to the concepts of active and passive immunisation defined below:

Active immunisation: The administration of a vaccine containing microbial products with or without adjuvants to obtain long-lasting immunological protection against the infective organism. There are two routes of immunisation; systemic (intramuscular or subcutaneous) or mucosal (oral or intranasal). Mucosal immunisation is the route of choice for polio (oral) and intranasal immunisation is frequently used for flu vaccines, especially in children or the needle-phobic.

Most of the vaccines in current use are delivered by either subcutaneous or intramuscular injection, which does not give rise to good mucosal immunity. To induce immunity in mucosal tissues it is important to use a route of immunisation which will induce good mucosal immunity. However, some vaccines are delivered by mucosal immunisation such as o-ral polio vaccination and there are preparations of flu vaccine which are delivered by nasal spray, especially formulated for children (Table 6.3).

Table 6.3 Mucosal vaccines in use in humans. At present, there are no vaccines for oral diseases.

Mucosal vaccine currently in use in humans

Infection	Vaccine	Route	Comments
Polio	Oral Polio (Sabin)	Oral	3 Attenuated serotypes
Salmonella Typhi	Ty21a (Vivotyl*)	Oral	Live attenuated S. typhi
Cholera	Dukoral*	Oral	Killed Vibrio cholera plus CTB
	CVD103HgR	Oral	Live attenuated V.cholreae
Influenza	HA + LT	Intranasal	Withdrawn: Attenuated virus
	Flumist*	Intranasal	
Rotavirus	Rotashield*	Oral	Withdrawn
	Rotarix*		Attenuated virus, monovalent
	Rota Teq*		Attenuated virus, pentavalent
Adenovirus	Adenovirus	Oral	Live Adenovirus types 4 and 7: Military use only

OPV, oral polio vaccine; CTL, cytotoxic T lymphocytes; CTB, cholera toxin B subunit; LPS, lipopolysaccharide; CTB, Cholera toxin B subunit; HA, hemagglutinin; LT, *E.colt* heat labile enterotoxin.
Source: Adapted from Russell and Mestecky: Mucosal vaccines: An Overview. Chapter 55: Mucosal Immunology 2015.

Passive immunisation: The administration of preformed antibodies either intravenously or intramuscularly. This method can be used to provide protection against certain infections such as diphtheria or tetanus or in the event of accidental exposure to pathogens such as hepatitis B. It can also be used to protect immunocompromised individuals. The use of so called 'biologics,' namely monoclonal antibodies for the treatment of disease is now very common (see below).

There are also examples of so called *natural antibodies* present in serum, which are able to cross the gingival margin and protect against dental caries (Challacombe et al. 1984b). The observation that this occurs gave rise to the notion that antibodies might be used in the dental clinic particularly for dental caries and periodontal disease.

Antibodies have the potential to protect against oral disease, but how does the immune system operate in the oral cavity?

The Structure and Function of the Oral Cavity

In addition to the functions associated with nutrition (masticatory, sensory, pain, and temperature perception) the oral cavity has a barrier function that defends against infection with pathogenic organisms. The oral cavity is also host to more than 700 species of commensal bacteria of which about 60% are cultivatable (www.homd.org). In normal healthy individuals the oral mucosa is regarded as a tolerogenic environment (Novak et al. 2008).

The oral cavity can be divided into two regions—the outer oral vestibule found between the lips and cheeks on the outside and the maxillary and mandibular arches on the inside and the oral cavity proper situated within the dental arches (Figure 6.3).

The main structural features of the oral mucosa are the oral epithelium, lamina propria, and submucosa. The oral epithelium is described as a stratified squamous epithelium and

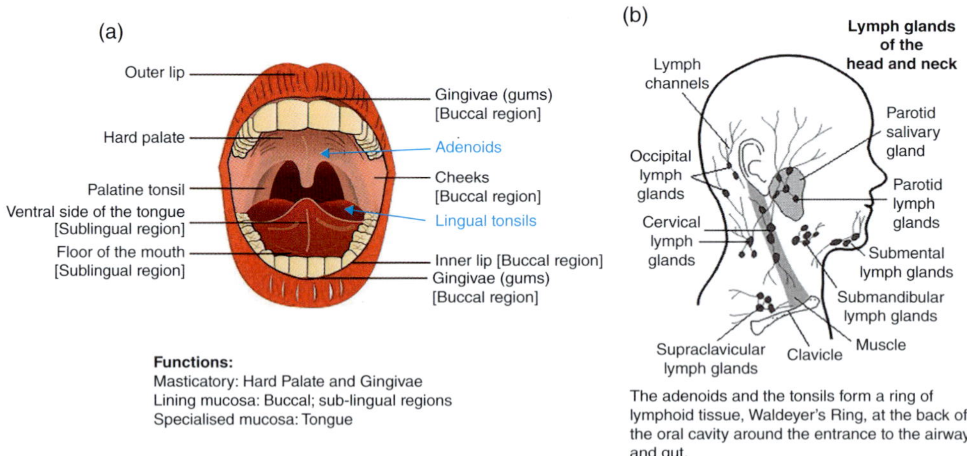

Figure 6.3 The anatomy of the oral cavity showing the main structures and the lymphoid tissues of the tonsils and adenoids plus the draining lymph nodes of the head and neck. Source: (a) Adapted from Kraan et al. (2014); (b) https://patient.info/signs-symptoms/neck-lumps-and-bumps-leaflet/swollen-lymph-glands. Reprinted with permission.

contains multiple layers of cells with different morphologies arranged into discrete layers. The main elements of the immune response are to be found within the epithlium and the lamina propria.

Immune Responses in the Oral Cavity

Inflammation and the Immune Response: Defending the Barricades

Mammals have evolved a sophisticated innate and adaptive immune system that integrates a network of tissues, cells, and effector molecules and protects the body from disease by recognition of potential pathogens or diseased tissues (discriminating between self, 'non-self', and altered-self: Figure 6.4).

The immune system is further divided into the **systemic immune response,** an enclosed system protecting the systemic tissues, which includes the circulation through which cells migrate to areas of inflammation and/or injury to effect destruction of invading organisms or to initiate repair mechanisms.

The oral cavity is part of the mucosal immune system with the total surface area of the oral mucosa estimated at about 0.8 M^2 and is continuous, but distinct from, the gut with a total surface area of about 400 M^2 compared to about 2 M^2 of skin.

The **mucosal immune system,**is open to the environment and is constantly bathed in fluid (saliva and gastric juices), from the mouth through the gut. Material entering the oral cavity by air or in food will be partially broken down by the masticatory process and by salivary enzymes.

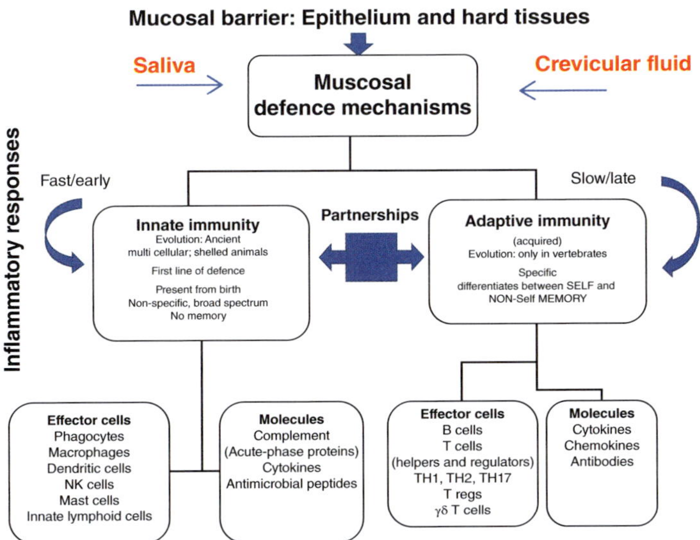

Figure 6.4 Partnerships at the mucosal surfaces. Cells and molecules in innate and adaptive immune responses interact with the epithelial tissues providing cells and molecules that contribute to protection but can also contribute to disease when the systems become dysregulated.

The presence of antigenic material in the oral cavity has the potential of inducing immune responses and early work on the development of vaccines against dental caries showed that ingestion of *step. mutans* gave rise to the induction of IgA antibodies not only in the saliva but also in tears and introduced the concept of a common **mucosal immune system** where induction of immune responses at one mucosal surface gave rise to a widely disseminated immune response into other mucosal tissues (Mestecky et al. 1978a, 1978b). Later the compartmentalisation of the common mucosal immune system was redefined in the context of vaccine development (Holmgren and Czerkinsky 2005).

Innate responses are present from birth, are a first line of defence and are the rapid response force; innate cells protect against invading pathogens by the recognition of pathogen associated molecular patterns (PAMPS) or damage associated molecular patterns (DAMPS) in diseased or damaged cells and induce an inflammatory response to which cells of the immune response are recruited. Polymorphisms in these molecules (TLRs, NLRs, and RIGI receptors) are known to be associated with inflammatory mucosal disease (Lavelle et al. 2010). These genetically encoded **pattern recognition receptors** (PRRs) activate the innate immune system which in turn 'educates' adaptive cells which migrate to the draining lymph nodes where the induction of a robust immune response is initiated. PRRs include the toll-like receptors which recognise a wide range of bacterial and viral antigens and have been shown to exhibit splice variants in disease such as Behçet's syndrome which might result in aberrant signalling and the induction of chronic inflammation characteristic of this disease (Seoudi et al. 2014).

Following activation, clones of antigen specific cells migrate from the lymph node to the site of infection/inflammation and carry out effector functions such as secretion of specific antibody (B cells) for the clearance of bacterial (and some viral) infections; induction of cytotoxic $CD8^+T$ cells which will kill viral (or intracellular bacteria) infected cells or damaged or dying cells; cytotoxicity occurs either directly or with the help of antibodies (NK cells/Antibody Dependent Cellular Cytotoxicity-ADCC). **Memory cells** are induced which recirculate back to the draining lymph nodes where they will wait, 'armed' for the next exposure to their 'cognate' antigen. The most important of these educators, acting at the interface of the innate and adaptive responses are **antigen presenting cells** (APCs) and include Langerhans' cells (LCs) and DCs, macrophages, and other phagocytic cells such as neutrophils. DCs and LCs can penetrate the epithelial junctions to sample luminal antigens (Hussain and Lehner 1995). DCs were shown to polarise effector responses toward TH1 (inflammatory) or TH2 (anti-inflammatory) depending on the type of endotoxin encountered (Pulendran et al. 1997, 1999, 2001). In investigating the effect of *P. gingivalis* LPS on DCs it was apparent that sub-optimal maturation occurs with the result that IL-10 (an immunosuppressive/TH2 cytokine) tends to be induced (reviewed by Cutler and Jotwani 2006). A cartoon of the main events of immune activation is shown in Figure 6.5.

It is becoming increasingly clear that these PRR bearing cells can control the adaptive immune response and in turn feed back into the maintenance of homeostasis (Palm and Medzhitov 2009; Hovav 2014).

Epithelial cells, macrophages, and DCs all secrete a variety of cytokines that have profound effects on the recruitemt of T cells to the oral mucosa and their ultimate effector function (Wu et al. 2014).

The cytokines secreted by T helper cells are grouped according to the effector cells which they induce (Figure 6.6). The T helper 1 (Th1) cytokines (IL-2, IFNγ, TNFα) activate

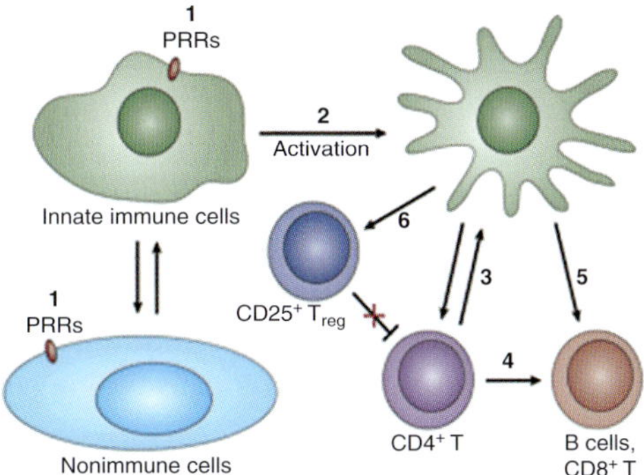

Figure 6.5 The initiation of an immune response: Upon interaction with PAMPs (1), resting innate immune cells and certain nonimmune cells, such as tissue epithelial cells, secrete cytokines and chemokines. Double arrows indicate cross-talk between cells. Key features of this early activation are an increase in APC function characterised by increased costimulatory capacity and upregulation of surface major histocompatibility complex molecules (2). Cells of the adaptive immune system, such as CD4$^+$ and CD8$^+$ T cells, then recognise presented antigen and undergo clonal expansion (3). Cognate interaction between T and B cells leads to B-cell activation, expansion and conversion to plasma cells that secrete specific antibodies (4). Activated DCs can also act directly on CD8$^+$ T cells to license them to become effector CTLs (5) and may also secrete soluble factors that block the immunosuppressive effects of CD25$^+$ T$_{reg}$ (6). A proportion of adaptive immune cells also differentiate into memory cells that will be ready for a secondary encounter with the specific pathogen. Thus, complete elimination of pathogens is achieved by effector cells and soluble factors of both the innate and adaptive immune systems.

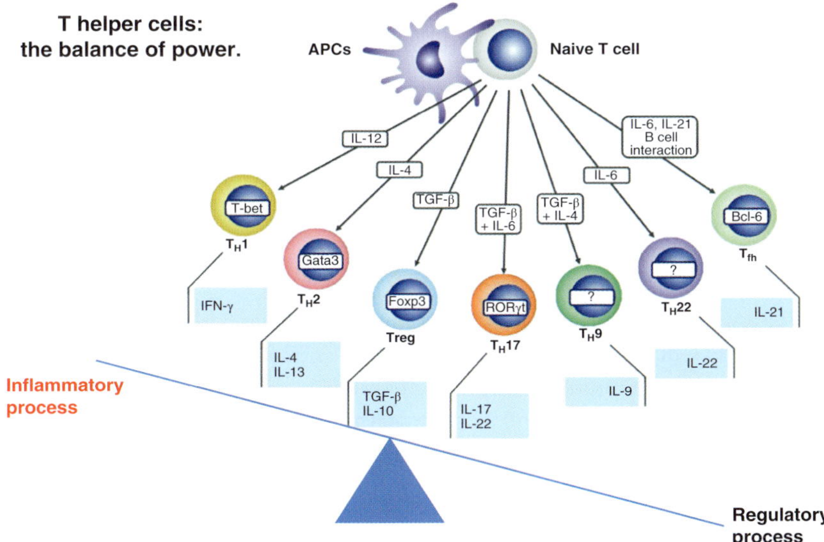

Figure 6.6 Signalling pathways induced by APC/T cell interactions dictate T helper cell effector functions and downstream pathogenesis or regulation. Cytokines and chemokines are important effector molecules in the oral mucosa influencing recruitment of other cells into the tissue and orchestrating the balance between inflammation and regulation as well as tissue breakdown and repair. Source: Adapted from Wu et al. (2014).

macrophages, induce B cells to class switch to IgG1 or IgG3 and supress Th2 responses, while Th2 cytokines (IL-4, 5, 6, 10, and 13) activate B cells, induce class switching to IgG2, IgA, or IgE and supress the Th1 response. In recent years, more subsets of T-helper cells have been identified and Th17 cells have been recognised as important contributors to the host response to periodontal pathogens and are characterised by the secretion of IL-17. This subset is related to Th1 but its induction is dependent on IL-21 and TGFβ. Another subset of CD4 helper cells are the T regulatory cells (T_{regs}) which play an important role in maintaining self-tolerance. They are also important in contributing to the limitation of immune responses in other words when to shut the response down when it is no longer required (Wu et al. 2014) (Figure 6.3).

Destructive effector mechanisms require powerful regulation, and the immune system has evolved intricate feedback loops that limit the duration of responses thus avoiding the potential for bystander damage resulting from prolonged inflammatory responses. This balance between inflammation and regulation is dictated by the induction of specific effector T cells responding to unique signalling and transcription pathways resulting in the production of cytokines able to either regulate the inflammation or drive specific functions (Figure 6.6); for example production of IL-4 and IL-13 by Th2 cells supports antibody production while Th17 cells secrete IL-17, which has been associated with autoimmune diseases and also the exacerbation of periodontal disease once homeostasis of the oral microbiome has been disrupted and dysbiosis has been established. Regulatory molecules such as the Suppressor of Cytokine Signalling family (SOCS) have also been shown to be upregulated in conditions such as Behçet's and Sjögren's syndromes (Hamedi et al. 2014; Vartoukian et al. 2014).

A recent systematic characterisation of the immune cell network at the gingival barrier in a large cohort of healthy individuals indicated a predominant number of T cells, minimal B cells and large numbers of granulocytes/neutrophils and a sophisticated network of antigen presenting cells. A small number of innate lymphoid cells were also present (Dutzan et al. 2016). However, in six untreated periodontitis patients, displaying severe bone loss and visible inflammation, there was a significant increase in IL-17 producing CD4$^+$ T helper cells.

Inductive and Effector Sites in the Oral Cavity

Mucosal **inductive sites** include the Nasal Associated Lymphoid Tissues (NALT) and the Payers patches of the Gut (GALT), for the induction of mucosal secretory IgA (SIgA) antibody responses. Homing of memory and/or activated T and B cells from NALT to nasal passages and oral cavity occurs and is part of the compartmentalisation of the immune system (Holmgren and Czerkinsky 2005). In the oral cavity, inductive sites consist of the buccal mucosa, salivary glands and Waldeyer's ring consisting of the adenoids (unpaired naso-pharyngeal tonsils) and the paired palatine and lingual tonsils (Figure 6.3). Human tonsils have deep branched antigen retaining crypts with a reticular endothelium which contains M cells—a highly developed antigen capture cell which is vital for the induction of B-cell diversity and memory. About 50% of the cells are B cells that are present in lymphoid follicles containing germinal centres, where immune responses are induced. Palatine tonsils contain a significant sub-epithelial population that may be crucial in the production of antibody specific for inhaled antigens taken up by M cells. These cells act as a portal to the outside environment delivering antigens to the lymphoid cells in the lamina propria for the induction of antigen specific immune responses.

Inductive sites in the oral mucosa have been investigated in the context of active immunisation and also tolerisation (Kraan et al. 2014). The buccal mucosa has been shown to have a distinct set of APCs which are potential targets for the induction of immune responses while the sublingual mucosa appears to be more tolerogenic and has the potential for use as a site for desensitisation rather than active immunisation.

Effector sites for oral mucosal immune responses include the epithelium, lamina propria and the salivary glands. There are also scattered intraepithelial lymphoid cells throughout the mucosa (Novak et al. 2008).

Mucosal Immunisation and Oral Tolerance

The concept of oral tolerance is based on the observations that feeding an animal with an antigen followed by a booster vaccination via subcutaneous or intramuscular immunisation resulted in the dissemination of IgA antibodies (mucosal) to the saliva (through the common mucosal immune system) but no systemic antibody response (IgG in the serum). Tolerance is defined as a state of specific immunological unresponsiveness to food and bacterial antigens in the gut and is B and T cell mediated. The mechanism of oral tolerance includes the induction of various populations of T regulatory cells and suppressive cytokines and is well established in several animal models including mice, rats, and guinea pigs. There have been many studies in which animal models have been used to mimic human disease such as multiple sclerosis, where myelin basic protein was fed to animals and lesions were resolved. However, this occurs through the tolerogenic mechanisms in the gut and are not strictly 'oral'.

Nevertheless, this has led to speculation that this method might be used to 'de-sensitise' individuals who have mounted an inappropriate immune response as in autoimmune disease.

Oral Diseases and Vaccination

Diseases of the oral cavity can be divided into those directly caused by infective agents such as the relationship between dental caries and *Streptococcus mutans;* candida infection and the host response to periodontal organisms that drive the progression from gingivitis to periodontal disease and oral mucosal diseases such as those listed in Figure 6.7 and systemic diseases with significant oral manifestations.

Dental Caries

Vaccine strategies against dental caries have a long history with the *S. mutans* antigen I/II demonstrably affected in animal studies (Russell et al. 1980a, 1980b). Natural IgG antibodies to *S. mutans* were shown in serum and were associated with low or no caries (Challacombe et al. 1984a) (Figure 6.8) while passage of immunoglobulins from the serum to the gingival crevicular fluid had previously been demonstrated in the rhesus macaque (Challacombe et al. 1978a, 1978b).

Passive application of monoclonal antibodies specific for antigen I/II were successfully used in preventing re- colonisation by *S. mutans* in the 1990s Ma et al. 1990; Ma and Lehner 1990; Lehner et al. 1992).

- **Infection in the oral cavity**
  - Dental caries
  - Periodontal disease
  - Candidiasis
- **Oral mucosal diseases**
  - Pemphigus and pemphigoid
  - Recurrent aphthous stomatitis
  - Behçet's disease
  - Lichen planus
- **Oral manifestations of systemic diseases**
  - Celiac disease
  - Crohn's disease
  - Ulcerative colitis
  - Food allergy and oral tolerance
  - Sjögrens
  - HIV

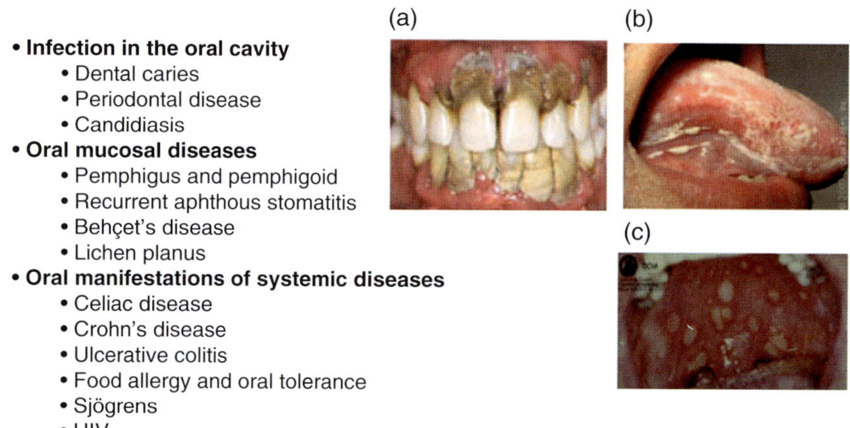

Figure 6.7 Immunology in the Dental Clinic: A role for vaccines. Source: (a,b) Bergmeier 2018, Springer Nature; (c) Mendes et al. 2009, Elsevier.

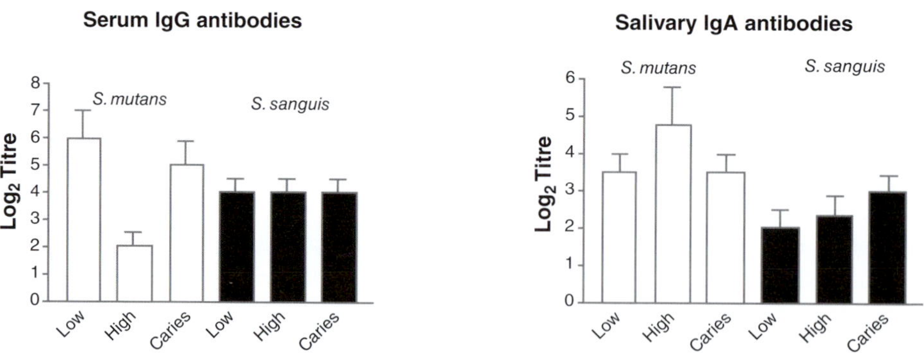

Figure 6.8 Natural antibodies to SAI/II. These observations along with protection studies in non-human primates demonstrated that immune responses to *S. mutans* antigens could protect against dental caries. Source: Challacombe et al. (1984a).

Periodontal Disease

Active immunisation against periodontal disease has also been investigated in animal models and the response to gingipains of *P. gingivalis* has been shown to induce specific responses (O'Brien-Simpson et al. 2016). However, the complex interplay between the immune response to *P. gingivalis* and the contribution of the host response to the chronic inflammatory response that results in the loss of attachment of the periodontal ligament and bone loss. The beneficial effects of vaccination are to induce a specific IgG response that will result in the phagocytosis of bacteria, while IgA antibodies in the saliva prevent bacterial adherence. The induction of the complement cascade by bacterial endotoxin and the release of cytokines such as IL-12 will recruit immune cells to the site of inflammation, including phagocytic cells. T helper cells will induce class switching in B cells producing specific antibodies to periodontal organisms (Table 6.4). However, the antigen/antibody immune complexes (and complement) are capable of inducing hypersensitivity, while cytokines can induce and prolong the inflammatory process and contribute to tissue damage by inducing the secretion of osteoclast-activating factors. High levels of IL-17 are associated with periodontal disease (Abusleme and Moutsopoulos 2016) and phagocytes release proteases further contributing to tissue damage (Cheng et al. 2016, 2017).

Monoclonal antibodies specific to periodontal pathogens have also been used in passive vaccination strategies but have had limited success. *P. gingivalis* was greatly reduced or absent in patients for up to 9 months (Booth et al. 1996; Booth and Lehner 1997; Kelly et al. 1997).

Table 6.4 Complex interplay between immune responses for resolution and pathogenesis in periodontal disease.

Periodontal disease

Complex interplay between bacterial species and host defences

Beneficial effects	Harmful effects
● IgG phagocytosis of bacteria	● Ag/Ab complexes-hypersensitivity-attract leucocytes-release proteases-tissue damage
● IgA bacterial adherence	
● Complement-activated by endotoxin-initiates inflammatory process-recruits neutrophils	● Complement could induce hypersensitivity
● Cytokines IL-12 recruits immune cells	
● Phagocytes destroy bacteria	● Cytokines-too much pro-inflammatory cytokine secretion contributes to tissue damage-e.g., osteoclast-activating factor
● T cells produce antibody	
● B cells produce antibodies against perio- organisms	● Phagocytes-release protease-tissue damage

Behçet's Disease (BD)

BD is a chronic auto inflammatory disease where high levels of Th1 cytokines drive a vasculitis in many organs of the body. Patients frequently present with oral ulceration and uveitis is also very common. Immune responses to self-antigens such as HSP (which cross react with oral microbial antigens) have been observed to induce a shift to a TH1 cytokine profile. A rat model of the uveitis observed in BD has been exploited in the context of down regulation of immune responses. Oral immunisation with HSP65 peptides conjugated to the mucosal adjuvant, cholera toxin B subunit (CTB) were shown to down regulate Th1 responses (Lehner et al. 2003; Stanford et al. 1994, 2004) and in a small clinical trial patients with uveitis were tolerised to the peptide and experienced remission in their uveitis over a period of about 18 months (Stanford et al. 2004). This is a classical oral tolerisation where induction of immune responses in the gut has resulted in down regulation of peripheral pathological responses.

Sublingual and Buccal Vaccine Delivery

Sublingual Immunotherapy (SLIT) is the only *truly* intraoral vaccination strategy currently available and to date has been used extensively for the immunomodulation of allergy.

Allergy has a profound effect on suffers and is frequently life threatening, especially due to food allergies inducing anaphylaxis. The potential for desensitisation using the SLIT is considerable and several clinical trials with hypersensitive individuals have taken place with extremely promising results, for example for peanut allergy (Gomez et al. 2017). Other allergens that have shown regulatory responses following SLIT include; birch pollen, grass pollen, house dust mite allergens, cow's milk, and peanuts (Kraan et al. 2014; Jay and Nadeau 2014). However, this very powerful method of harnessing the regulatory power of the immune system has great potential for the development of other oral vaccine strategies.

Particular subsets of DCs (CD103$^-$CD11b$^+$ cells) have been shown to present sublingual antigens and to induce regulatory T cells in the draining lymph nodes of mice (Tanaka et al. 2017) (Figure 6.9).

SLIT has recently been used in non-human primates with gp41 subunit vaccines against HIV (Hervouet et al. 2010; Bekri et al. 2017).

S. mutans colonisation was reduced following sublingual immunisation with a phosphate-binding-protein (PstS) in a mouse model of dental caries (Ferreira et al. 2016).

A subunit influenza vaccine administered (in mice) by this route induced systemic immunity which compared very well with intramuscular immunisation, but additionally induced local IgA and Th17 responses (Gallorini et al. 2014).

The sublingual mucosa has been used for many years as fast delivery routes for small drugs such as those required in acute angina pectoris attacks. However, it seems clear that vaccine antigens do not enter the blood stream through sublingual or buccal mucosa but are dependent on specific uptake by dendritic cells (mainly Langerhans cells). This allows for an effective adaptive immune response to be induced. These cells have been shown to 'sample' antigens in the lumen and to migrate to draining lymph nodes where they are able to prime both naïve CD4 and CD8 T lymphocytes. The buccal epithelium has been shown to be a very good site for the priming of CD8 T cells. After activation in the lymph nodes the

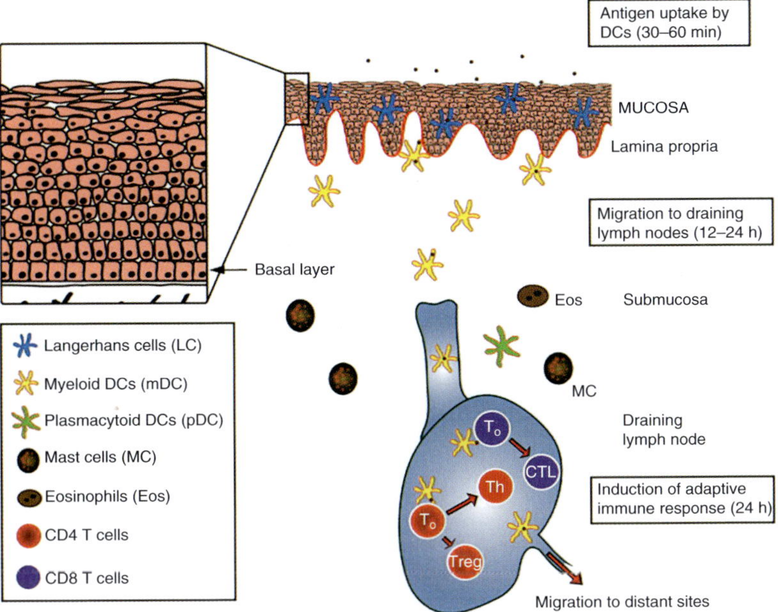

Figure 6.9 Antigen delivery through DCs or LCs and homing to distant sites following buccal or sublingual immunisation. Source: From Kraan et al. (2014) with permission from the publisher.

cells will migrate to other mucosal sites where they will differentiate in to memory or effector cells. If CD4 T cells are induced then, helper cells and /or T regulatory cells will be able to mediate immune responses.

The lack of keratinisation makes antigen uptake in the buccal and sublingual mucosa superior to that of skin. There is no risk of breakdown of the vaccine antigen through gastric acid action as would happen in the stomach, although there is some enzymatic activity in the oral cavity. There is now an extensive literature charting the progress of a variety of vaccine formulations that have been used in buccal or sublingual vaccinations (Kraan et al. 2014). These include; live attenuated flu vaccine; live vaccine carriers for infections such as HIV and Ebola virus; inactivated viruses (Flu, HPV, RSV, HIV). To date all these studies have been carried out as pre-clinical proof of principle models.

'Biologics'-passive Immunotherapy with Monoclonal Antibodies

Immunotherapy using monoclonal antibodies is a more recent addition to the clinicians' armamentarium. Here, monoclonal antibodies are used that target immune functions such as B cells producing antibodies. Anti CD20 antibodies (Rituximab) have been used to deplete the pathogen clones of B cells producing antibodies specific for desmoglein in Pemphigus vulgaris (Eming et al. 2008). Depletion lasted from 6 to 12 months resulting in dramatic decline in the serum autoantibodies. Remission of the skin blistering is seen following 4 weekly rounds of passive immunisation of the biologic. In the example shown here the skin shows a tremendous improvement following use of this monoclonal antibody which is directed against B cells and therefore eliminates the cells that are producing the anti-DSG3 antibodies that are causing pathology. This would also be effective in patients with oral manifestations of pemphigus (Figure 6.10).

Monoclonal antibodies are also used in many diseases where high levels of proinflammatory cytokines are produced. In Behçet's disease there are high levels of TNF-α which can be controlled by infusions of a monoclonal antibody which is able to 'mop-up' excess cytokine (Table 6.5).

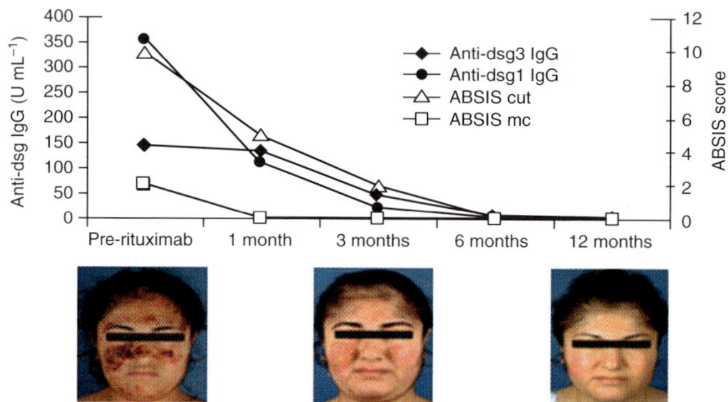

Figure 6.10 Resolution of skin blistering in pemphigus vulgaris following treatment with a monoclonal antibody specific for CD20⁺ B cell (Rituximab). Clinical response to rituximab in recalcitrant pemphigus vulgaris (PV). Clinical course of a representative patient with chronic erosions of the face and scalp (partly shown) before rituximab treatment and 3 and 12 months afterward, respectively. Complete clinical remission as illustrated by reduction of the disease scores for cutaneous (ABSIS cut) and mucosal (ABSIS mc) involvement was paralleled by a decrease of desmoglein1 (dsg1)- and dsg3-reactive IgG autoantibodies. Source: Eming et al. (2008)/Reproduced with permission from Elsevier.

Table 6.5 A selection of monoclonal antibodies in use in Behçet's disease to control the over production of pro-inflammatory cytokines.

'Biologics' in Behçet's	Infliximab: binds to TNF-α and TNF-β and lyses TNF-producing cells which neutralises their activity.	Reduces inflammation by specifically inhibiting different molecules
	Etanercept: a recombinant dimer of human TNF receptor proteins fused and bound to human IgG1, preventing the binding of TNF to its cell surface receptor.	
	Adalimumab: a monoclonal fully human anti-TNF-α antibody which binds to TNF-α with high affinity; *reviewed by* Nash and Florin (2005) and Silva et al. (2010).	
	Rituximab: anti-CD20. Anakinra: anti-IL-1.	
	Daclizumab: anti IL-2. Tocilizumab: anti-IL-6. Secukinumab: anti-IL-17	
	Anti-IFN-α therapy which acts by targeting various immune cells that produce Type I interferons. *reviewed by* Nava et al. (2014) and Saleh and Arayssi (2014).	

Cancer

Head and neck cancers particularly oropharynx squamous cell carcinoma have been increasing of late. These cancers have been associated with human papilloma virus 16 (HPV-16) infection. It has therefore been suggested that vaccination might be a cost-effective measure to reduce the numbers of individuals with this disease (Marur et al. 2010).

Active vaccination using peptides from an apoptosis molecule (survivin) have been shown to reduce metastatic tumours by up to 70% following the 5th vaccination as seen in Figure 6.11 (Miyazaki et al. 2011).

Summary

Vaccination to protect mucosal surfaces is an important area of clinical and basic sciences discovery, since the majority of infective disease cross mucosal barriers.

Vaccination has also been used therapeutically to treat a variety of conditions including allergy, autoimmune diseases, and in cancer therapy (Lake and Robinson 2005; Larché and Wraith 2005; Neninger et al. 2009).

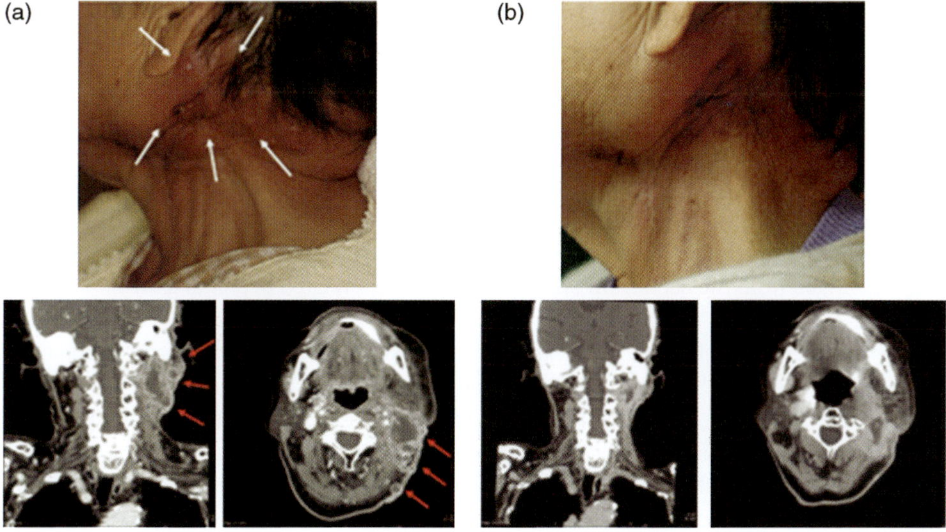

Figure 6.11 Vaccination in oral cancer. Photograph of skin on the neck and computed tomography (CT) scan image of the neck showing metastatic tumours of case 10. (a) Photograph of skin on the neck and CT scan image of the neck before vaccination. Axial contrast-enhanced CT image shows multiple metastatic tumors (arrows). (b) Photograph of skin on the neck and CT scan image of the neck after the fifth vaccination. The metastatic tumours show significant remission after the fifth vaccination compared with before vaccination (70% reduction). Source: Miyazaki et al. (2011)/ Reproduced with permission from Wiley.

The purpose of this chapter was two-fold:

1) To revise and show the importance of the immune response in the oral cavity,
2) To illustrate the dynamic potential of the immune responses in the control of a variety of both oral mucosal disease and systemic disease with oral manifestations and to illustrate how the 'immunology toolbox' has enormous potential in minimal invasive dentistry

References

Abusleme, L., and Moutsopoulos, N.M. (2016). IL-17: overview and role in oral immunity and microbiome. *Oral Dis.* 23: 854–865.

Allan, S. (2008). Vaccines: Explaining alum: Immunologists' dirty little secret. *Nat. Rev. Immunol.* 8: 320–320.

Apostolico Jde, S., Lunardelli, V.A., Coirada, F.C., Boscardin, S.B., and Rosa, D.S. (2016). Adjuvants: Classification, modus operandi, and licensing. *J. Immunol. Res.*: 1459394.

Basith, S., Manavalan, B., Lee, G., Kim, S.G., and Choi, S. (2011). Toll-like receptor modulators: A patent review (2006–2010). *Expert Opin. Ther. Pat.* 21: 927–944.

Bekri, S., Bourdely, P., Luci, C., Dereuddre-Bosquet, N., Su, B., Martinon, F., Braud, V.M., Luque, I., Mateo, P.L., Crespillo, S., Conejero-Lara, F., Moog, C., Le Grand, R., and Anjuere, F. (2017). Sublingual priming with a HIV gp41-based subunit vaccine elicits mucosal antibodies and persistent B memory responses in non-human primates. *Front. Immunol.* 8: 63.

Bergmeier, L.A. (2018). Infections of the oral mucosa and immune responses. In: *Oral Mucosa in Health and Disease* (ed. L. Bergmeier). Cham: Springer.

Booth, V., and Lehner, T. (1997). Characterization of the Porphyromonas gingivalis antigen recognized by a monoclonal antibody which prevents colonization by the organism. *J. Periodontal. Res.* 32: 54–60.

Booth, V., Ashley, F.P., and Lehner, T. (1996). Passive immunization with monoclonal antibodies against Porphyromonas gingivalis in patients with periodontitis. *Infect Immun.* 64: 422–427.

Challacombe, S.J., Bergmeier, L.A., and Rees, A.S. (1984a). Natural antibodies in man to a protein antigen from the bacterium Streptococcus mutans related to dental caries experience. *Arch. Oral Biol.* 29: 179–184.

Challacombe, S.J., Bergmeier, L.A., Czerkinsky, C., and Rees, A.S. (1984b). Natural antibodies in man to Streptococcus mutans: Specificity and quantification. *Immunology* 52: 143–150.

Challacombe, S.J., Russell, M.W., and Hawkes, J. (1978a). Passage of intact IgG from plasma to the oral cavity via crevicular fluid. *Clin. Exp. Immunol.* 34: 417–422.

Challacombe, S.J., Russell, M.W., Hawkes, J., Bergmeier, L.A., and Lehner, T. (1978b). Passage of immunoglobulins from plasma to the oral cavity in rhesus monkeys. *Immunology* 35: 923–931.

Cheng, W.C., Hughes, F.J., and Taams, L.S. (2017). The presence, function and regulation of IL-17 and Th17 cells in periodontitis. *J. Clin. Periodontol.* 41: 541–549.

Cheng, W.C., van Asten, S.D., Burns, L.A., Evans, H.G., Walter, G.J., Hashim, A., Hughes, F.J., and Taams, L.S. (2016). Periodontitis-associated pathogens *P. gingivalis* and A. actinomycetemcomitans activate human CD14(+) monocytes leading to enhanced Th17/IL-17 responses. *Eur. J. Immunol.* 46: 2211–2221.

Correia-Pinto, J.F., Csaba, N., and Alonso, M.J. (2013). Vaccine delivery carriers: Insights and future perspectives. *Int. J. Pharm.* 440: 27–38.

Cutler, C.W., and Jotwani, R. (2006). Dendritic cells at the oral mucosal interface. *J. Dent. Res.* 85: 678–689.

Dutzan, N.J., Konkel, E., Greenwell-Wild, T., and Moutsopoulos, N.M. (2016). Characterization of the human immune cell network at the gingival barrier. *Mucosal Immunol.* 9: 1163–1172.

Eming, R., Nagel, A., Wolff-Franke, S., Podstawa, E., Debus, D., and Hertl, M. (2008). Rituximab exerts a dual effect in pemphigus vulgaris. *J. Invest Dermatol.* 128: 2850–2858.

Ferreira, E.L., Batista, M.T., Cavalcante, R.C., Pegos, V.R., Passos, H.M., Silva, D.A., Balan, A., Ferreira, L.C., and Ferreira, R.C. (2016). Sublingual immunization with the phosphatebinding-protein (PstS) reduces oral colonization by Streptococcus mutans. *Mol. Oral Microbiol.* 31: 410–422.

Gallorini, S., Taccone, M., Bonci, A., Nardelli, F., Casini, D., Bonificio, A., Kommareddy, S., Bertholet, S., O'Hagan, D.T., and Baudner, B.C. (2014). Sublingual immunization with a subunit influenza vaccine elicits comparable systemic immune response as intramuscular immunization, but also induces local IgA and TH17 responses. *Vaccine* 32: 2382–2388.

Gomcz, F., Bogas, G., Gonzalez, M., Campo, P., Salas, M., Diaz-Perales, A., Rodriguez, M.J., Prieto, A., Barber, D., Blanca, M., Torres, M.J., and Mayorga, C. (2017). The clinical and immunological effects of Pru p 3 sublingual immunotherapy on peach and peanut allergy in patients with systemic reactions. *Clin. Exp. Allergy* 47: 339–350.

Gutjahr, A., Tiraby, G., Perouzel, E., Verrier, B., and Paul, S. (2016). Triggering intracellular receptors for vaccine adjuvantation. *Trends Immunol.* 37: 573–587.

Hamedi, M., Bergmeier, L.A., Hagi-Pavli, E., Vartoukian, S.R., and Fortune, F. (2014). Differential expression of suppressor of cytokine signalling proteins in Behcet's disease. *Scand. J. Immunol.* 80: 369–376.

Hervouet, C., Luci, C., Cuburu, N., Cremel, M., Bekri, S., Vimeux, L., Maranon, C., Czerkinsky, C., Hosmalin, A., and Anjuere, F. (2010). Sublingual immunization with an HIV subunit vaccine induces antibodies and cytotoxic T cells in the mouse female genital tract. *Vaccine* 28: 5582–5590.

Holmgren, J., and Czerkinsky, C. (2005). Mucosal immunity and vaccines. *Nat. Med.* 11 (4 Suppl): S45–53.

Holmgren, J., and Svennerholm, A.M. (2012). Vaccines against mucosal infections. *Curr. Opin. Immunol.* 24: 343–353.

Hovav, A.H. (2014). Dendritic cells of the oral mucosa. *Mucosal Immunol.* 7: 27–37.

Hussain, L.A., and Lehner, T. (1995). Comparative investigation of Langerhans' cells and potential receptors for HIV in oral, genitourinary and rectal epithelia. *Immunology* 85: 475–484.

Jay, D.C., and Nadeau, K.C. (2014). Immune mechanisms of sublingual immunotherapy. *Curr. Allergy Asthma Rep.* 14: 473.

Kelly, C.G., Booth, V., Kendal, H., Slaney, J.M., Curtis, M.A., and Lehner, T. (1997). The relationship between colonization and haemagglutination inhibiting and B cell epitopes of Porphyromonas gingivalis. *Clin. Exp. Immunol.* 110: 285–291.

Kim, S.H., and Jang, Y.S. (2017). The development of mucosal vaccines for both mucosal and systemic immune induction and the roles played by adjuvants. *Clin. Exp. Vaccine Res.* 6: 15–21.

Kraan, H., Vrieling, H., Czerkinsky, C., Jiskoot, W., Kersten, G., and Amorij, J.P. (2014). Buccal and sublingual vaccine delivery. *J. Control Release* 190: 580–592.

Lake, R.A., and Robinson, B.W. (2005). Immunotherapy and chemotherapy–a practical partnership. *Nat. Rev. Cancer* 5: 397–405.

Larché, M., and Wraith, D.C. (2005). Peptide-based therapeutic vaccines for allergic and autoimmune diseases. *Nat. Med. 11* (4 Suppl): S69–76.

Lavelle, E.C., Murphy, C., O'Neill, L.A.J., and Creagh, E.M. (2010). The role of TLRs, NLRs, and RLRs in mucosal innate immunity and homeostasis. *Mucosal Immunol.* 3: 17–28.

Lehner, T., Ma, J.K., and Kelly, C.G. (1992). A mechanism of passive immunization with monoclonal antibodies to a 185,000 M(r) streptococcal antigen. *Adv. Exp. Med. Biol.* 327: 151–163.

Lehner, T., Stanford, M.R., Phipps, P.A., Sun, J.B., Xiao, B.G., Holmgren, J., Shinnick, T., Hasan, A., and Mizushima, Y. (2003). Immunopathogenesis and prevention of uveitis with the Behcet's disease-specific peptide linked to cholera toxin B. *Adv. Exp. Med. Biol.* 528: 173–180.

Lycke, N. (2012). Recent progress in mucosal vaccine development: Potential and limitations. *Nat. Rev. Immunol.* 12: 592–605.

Ma, J.K., and Lehner, T. (1990). Prevention of colonization of Streptococcus mutans by topical application of monoclonal antibodies in human subjects. *Arch. Oral Biol.* 35 (Suppl): 115S–122S.

Ma, J.K., Hunjan, M., Smith, R., Kelly, C., and Lehner, T. (1990). An investigation into the mechanism of protection by local passive immunization with monoclonal antibodies against Streptococcus mutans. *Infect Immun.* 58: 3407–3414.

Marur, S., D'Souza, G., Westra, W.H., and Forastiere, A.A. (2010). HPV-associated head and neck cancer: A virus-related cancer epidemic. *Lancet Oncol.* 11: 781–789.

Matzinger, P. (1994). Tolerance, danger, and the extended family. *Annu. Rev. Immunol.* 12: 991–1045.

Mestecky, J., McGhee, J.R., Arnold, R.R., Michalek, S.M., Prince, S.J., and Babb, J.L. (1978). Selective induction of an immune response in human external secretions by ingestion of bacterial antigen. *J. Clin. Invest.* 61: 731–737.

Mestecky, J., McGhee, J.R., Michalek, S.M., Arnold, R.R., Crago, S.S., and Babb, J.L. (1978). Concept of the local and common mucosal immune response. *Adv. Exp. Med. Biol.* 107: 185–192.

Mendes, D., Correia, M., Barbedo, M., Vaio, T., Mota, M., Gonçalves, O., and Valente, J. (2009). Behçet's disease – A contemporary review. *J. Autoimmun.* 32 (3–4). 178–188.

Miyazaki, A., Kobayashi, J., Torigoe, T., Hirohashi, Y., Yamamoto, T., Yamaguchi, A., Asanuma, H., Takahashi, A., Michifuri, Y., Nakamori, K., Nagai, I., Sato, N., and Hiratsuka, H. (2011). Phase I clinical trial of survivin-derived peptide vaccine therapy for patients with advanced or recurrent oral cancer. *Cancer Sci.* 102: 324–329.

Moser, M., and Leo, O. (2010). Key concepts in immunology. *Vaccine* 28 (Suppl 3): C2–13.

Nash, P.T., and Florin, T.H. (2005). Tumour necrosis factor inhibitors. *Med. J. Aust.* 183: 205–208.

Nava, F., Ghilotti, F., Maggi, L., Hatemi, G., Del Bianco, A., Merlo, C., Filippini, G., and Tramacere, I. (2014). Biologics, colchicine, corticosteroids, immunosuppressants and interferon-alpha for Neuro-Behcet's Syndrome. *Cochrane Database Syst. Rev.* 12: 18.

Neninger, E., Verdecia, B.G., Crombet, T., Viada, C., Pereda, S., Leonard, I., Mazorra, Z., Fleites, G., González, M., Wilkinson, B., González, G., and Lage, A. (2009). Combining an

EGFbased cancer vaccine with chemotherapy in advanced nonsmall cell lung cancer. *J. Immunother.* 32: 92–99.

Novak, N., Haberstok, J., Bieber, T., and Allam, J.P. (2008). The immune privilege of the oral mucosa. *Trends Mol. Med.* 14: 191–198.

O'Brien-Simpson, N.M., Holden, J.A., Lenzo, J.C., Tan, Y., Brammar, G.C., Walsh, K.A., Singleton, W., Orth, R.K.H., Slakeski, N., Cross, K.J., Darby, I.B., Becher, D., Rowe, T., Morelli, A.B., Hammet, A., Nash, A., Brown, A., Ma, B., Vingadassalom Mccluskey, J., Kleanthous, H., and Reynolds, E.C. (2016). A therapeutic Porphyromonas gingivalis gingipain vaccine induces neutralising IgG1 antibodies that protect against experimental periodontitis. *Npj Vaccines* 1: 16022.

Palm, N.W., and Medzhitov, R. (2009). Pattern recognition receptors and control of adaptive immunity. *Immunol. Rev.* 227: 221–233.

Pulendran, B., Lingappa, J., Kennedy, M.K., Smith, J., Teepe, M., Rudensky, A., Maliszewski, C.R., and Maraskovsky, E. (1997). Developmental pathways of dendritic cells in vivo: Distinct function, phenotype, and localization of dendritic cell subsets in FLT3 ligand-treated mice. *J. Immunol.* 159: 2222–2231.

Pulendran, B., Smith, J.L., Caspary, G., Brasel, K., Pettit, D., Maraskovsky, E., and Maliszewski, C.R. (1999). Distinct dendritic cell subsets differentially regulate the class of immune response *in vivo*. *Proc. Natl. Acad. Sci. U S A* 96: 1036–1041.

Pulendran, B.P., Kumar, C., Cutler, W., Mohamadzadeh, M., Van Dyke, T., and Banchereau, J. (2001). Lipopolysaccharides from distinct pathogens induce different classes of immune responses *in vivo*. *J. Immunol.* 167: 5067–5076.

Reed, S.G., Bertholet, S., Coler, R.N., and Friede, M. (2009). New horizons in adjuvants for vaccine development. *Trends Immunol.* 30: 23–32.

Russell, M.W., Bergmeier, L.A., Zanders, E.D., and Lehner, T. (1980a). Protein antigens of Streptococcus mutans: Purification and properties of a double antigen and its proteaseresistant component. *Infect Immun.* 28: 486–493.

Russell, M.W., Zanders, E.D., Bergmeier, L.A., and Lehner, T. (1980b). Affinity purification and characterization of protease-susceptible antigen I of Streptococcus mutans. *Infect Immun.* 29: 999–1006.

Saleh, Z., and Arayssi, T. (2014). Update on the therapy of Behcet disease. *Ther. Adv. Chronic Dis.* 5: 112–134.

Seoudi, N., Bergmeier, L.A., Hagi-Pavli, E., Bibby, D., Curtis, M.A., and Fortune, F. (2014). The role of TLR2 and 4 in Behcet's disease pathogenesis. *Innate Immun.* 20: 412–422.

Silva, L.C., Ortigosa, L.C., and Benard, G. (2010). Anti-TNF-alpha agents in the treatment of immune-mediated inflammatory diseases: mechanisms of action and pitfalls. *Immunotherapy* 2: 817–833.

Stanford, M., Whittall, T., Bergmeier, L.A., Lindblad, M., Lundin, S., Shinnick, T., Mizushima, Y., Holmgren, J., and Lehner, T. (2004). Oral tolerization with peptide 336-351 linked to cholera toxin B subunit in preventing relapses of uveitis in Behcet's disease. *Clin. Exp. Immunol.* 137: 201–208.

Stanford, M.R., Kasp, E., Whiston, R., Hasan, A., Todryk, S., Shinnick, T., Mizushima, Y., Dumonde, D.C., van der Zee, R., and Lehner, T. (1994). Heat shock protein peptides reactive in patients with Behcet's disease are uveitogenic in Lewis rats. *Clin. Exp. Immunol.* 97: 226–231.

Tanaka, Y., Nagashima, H., Bando, K., Lu, L., Ozaki, A., Morita, Y., Fukumoto, S., Ishii, N., and Sugawara, S. (2017). Oral CD103-CD11b+ classical dendritic cells present sublingual antigen and induce Foxp3+ regulatory T cells in draining lymph nodes. *Mucosal Immunol.* 10: 79–90.

Vartoukian, S.R., Tilakaratne, V.M., Seoudi, N., Bombardieri, M., Bergmeier, L., Tappuni, A.R., and Fortune, F. (2014). Dysregulation of the suppressor of cytokine signalling 3-signal transducer and activator of transcription-3 pathway in the aetiopathogenesis of Sjogren's syndrome. *Clin. Exp. Immunol.* 177: 618–629.

Wack, A., and Rappuoli, R. (2015). Vaccinology at the beginning of the 21st century. *Curr. Opin. Immunol.* 17: 411–418.

Wu, R.Q., Zhang, D.F., Tu, E., Chen, Q.M., and Chen, W. (2014). The mucosal immune system in the oral cavity-an orchestra of T cell diversity. *Int. J. Oral Sci.* 6: 125–132.

7

Can Minimally Invasive Strategies Be Applicable in Restorative Dentistry?

Sevil Gurgan, Zeynep Bilge Kutuk, and Aylin Baysan

Key Topics

- Evolution of Minimally Invasive (MI) strategies in restorative dentistry
- MI operative management strategies in anterior and posterior dentition
- Management of tooth discoloration with MI approach
- Management of tooth wear with MI approaches
- MID strategies in tooth loss
- Repair of defective restorations

Learning Objectives

- Be able to define the MID principles in restorative dentistry
- Be able to know the restorative procedures in different stages of dental caries using MI strategies
- Be able to appreciate the MI restorative strategies in relation to tooth discolouration
- Be able to recognise the MID strategies for the management of tooth surface loss/tooth wear
- Be able to state the MID approaches for the management of tooth loss
- Be able to understand "repair concept" in MID philosophy

Introduction

In the 21st century, dental diseases still have an enormous social and financial impact for individuals and also to the governments. The World Health Organisation (WHO) recently stated that oral diseases are the fourth-most expensive diseases to treat [1]. There are also indirect costs involved with regards to loss of productivity due to absenteeism from school/ work. In this respect, Hayes et al. [2] reported that oral diseases accounted for productivity loss of >$1 billion yearly in Canada.

Minimally Invasive Dentistry: Interdisciplinary Clinical and Scientific Approaches, First Edition.
Edited by Aylin Baysan and Paul Anderson.
© 2026 John Wiley & Sons Ltd. Published 2026 by John Wiley & Sons Ltd.
Companion website: www.wiley.com/go/baysan/minimally_invasive_dentistry

The concept of Minimally Invasive Dentistry (MID) in restorative dentistry is referred as a conservative, biologically acceptable/biomimetic and tooth-structure-saving approach with an optimum aesthetic outcome when carrying out dental procedures such as for dental caries, enamel discoloration, tooth wear, and tooth loss.

MID is the delivery of patient care that deals with the causes of dental disease and not just the symptoms. The field of MID is wide, including the detection of diseases as early as possible, identification of risk factors (risk assessment) and the implementation of preventive strategies with health education for patients. The ultimate aim of MI approach is to preserve the tooth structure. Therefore, restorative treatment when required is carried out with tailored and personalised approaches to provide optimum benefit to the oral health of patients in long-term.

Evolution of Minimally Invasive (MI) Strategies in Restorative Dentistry

MID in restorative dentistry evolved with the development of adhesive dentistry and scientific progress in understanding the nature of dental diseases. Clinicians began to consider holistic approaches instead of removing and replacing diseased tissue(s) since historically, applied knowledge in preservation of tooth structure was unclear in addition to lack of understanding with regards to the disease process and deficiencies in the available restorative materials.

The ability to detect the earliest signs of dental diseases is still a concern in clinical practice. The accuracy of special investigations such as dental radiographs and further assessment using variety of tests and detection systems for dental diseases i.e., dental caries, tooth wear, tooth loss is not completely sufficient. Clinicians need to acknowledge that neither fluoride nor the prevention of microbial microleakage between the tooth and restoration would be adequate to prevent further disease activity. Engagement by involving patients in the management of their disease would be the key for the successful treatment outcomes. Therefore, restorative procedures need to be carried out in conjunction with a holistic approach to diagnose early and manage dental diseases with well-understood preventive techniques and by providing an optimum patient education.

MID is a response to the traditional, surgical manner of managing dental caries that is based on the operative concepts of G.V. Black of more than a century ago. In 1955, Buonocore described a technique for etching enamel surfaces to make them retentive for a restoration and Bowen in 1962 invented adhesive materials, which led to the invention of MI preparations. Mount and Hume [3] suggested key changes in the principles of operative dentistry on the basis of three factors:

1) Demineralisation–remineralisation cycle
2) Adhesion in restorative dentistry
3) Biomimetic restorative materials

In this respect, "extension for prevention" concept has been moved away to a new paradigm of MI approaches in restorative dentistry. The development of adhesive dentistry as part of the MI approach in understanding the nature of dental disease has enabled clinicians to consider a holistic and tailored strategy rather than restoring or replacing missing teeth with a conventional approach. The rationale behind a minimalist approach is ultimately to curtail the restoration/re-restoration cycle for the patient benefit. The ultimate aim is to conserve as much healthy tooth structure as possible through clinical procedures that first assess the risk, detect the disease early prior to lesion cavitation, restore caries with maximum retention of sound tooth structure, and seal unaffected areas [4, 5].

In the middle of the 1980s, the enamel microabrasion technique was successfully used for removing superficial enamel stains of any colour and correction of surface irregularities and imperfect enamel acquired after the removal of orthodontic appliances [4, 5]. The application was under rubber dam isolation using a mixture of 18% hydrochloric acid and fine pumice on the stained areas of enamel using wooden stick. Interestingly, a total of 15 applications were required [4]. The current practice of microabrasion follows the minimally invasive strategy by using a mixture of phosphoric acid with pumice or other "ready-to-use" products available in the market, which are typically comprised of up to 6.6% hydrochloric acid associated with fine-grit silicon carbide abrasive particles, such as Opalustre (Ultradent Inc., South Jordan, UT, USA) [4–8]. In some circumstances, teeth may become darker or yellow after enamel microabrasion since the remaining enamel surface becomes thin, allowing the dentine to show more evidently [5]. This situation might then be overcome by the application of carbamide peroxide (dental bleaching) in acetate trays, which has demonstrated considerable clinical success [4, 6–9].

MI Operative Management Strategies in Anterior and Posterior Dentition

MI Management of Early Carious Lesions

Assessing the patient's caries risk and assigning individualised preventive, non-operative care measures based upon the disease risk factors and indicators led to need for less invasive operative treatments [3, 10–15].

Classifying carious lesions at a non-cavitated stage could allow clinicians to evaluate if noninvasive measures would be successful [15, 16]. Non-cavitated carious lesions in enamel and dentine can be managed by means of remineralisation without restorative intervention [15, 16]. Remineralisation of incipient carious lesions might be possible with a variety of currently available agents containing fluoride either with or without bioactive glasses, bioavailable calcium and phosphate, and casein phosphoprotein amorphous calcium phosphate. To arrest caries progression by the employment of minimally invasive strategies, tooth surface needs to be sufficiently accessible to cleaning. This is influenced by the cavitation extent, severity of carious lesions, and pathological activity within the lesion. In this respect, the application of pit-and-fissure sealants could be considered as a treatment modality for non-cavitated carious lesions [17–19].

Fissure Sealants

The use of fissure sealants is a beneficial MI procedure for the management of non-cavitated occlusal caries. The initiation of dental caries occurs in the stagnant biofilm, which accumulates at the opening of a fissure. Traditionally, resin-based sealants have been the material of choice, with superior retention rates in comparison to glass ionomer cement (GIC) fissure sealants [19]. However, when the different types of sealers are compared with respect to prevention of occlusal caries on permanent teeth, GIC appears to be as effective as resin-based sealants. It should be noted that a key aspect of caries prevention by the employment of fissure sealants is the need for monitoring and maintaining this prescribed MI treatment.

Preventive Resin Restoration (PRR)

Resin composites might be considered to be the material of choice for ultra-conservative restoration of discrete carious lesions in the fissures of posterior teeth, where it is impossible to facilitate effective plaque removal and when fissure sealing alone is inappropriate. Depending on the size of the lesion (and the possible need to seal adjacent, unaffected, fissures), various guidelines have been proposed for preventive resin restorations (PRR) [20, 21]. These incipient lesions might be treated with an aim of remineralising the demineralised enamel. It has been clear for many years that G.V. Black's outline form for the restoration of occlusal cavity preparations is an anachronism in MI dentistry.

The outline of the cavity preparation is solely determined by the extent of dental caries. The PRR technique that encompasses carious lesion into dentine, where carious lesion removal can be achieved as conservatively as possible with the smallest possible burs, and restoration using the acid-etch technique with the most up-to-date restorative (resin composite/GIC) materials. Remineralisation would be considered for incipient lesions, particularly those entirely in enamel before any invasive restorative care is attempted [21].

Resin Infiltration Technique

Resin infiltration has been proposed as an alternative MID treatment for the management of non-cavitated enamel carious lesions on approximal and buccal surfaces [22–26]. The infiltration concept is based on the penetration of a low-viscosity resin material in the subsurface enamel porosities of the lesion, which is previously etched using hydrochloric acid. The infiltrant apparently creates a diffusion barrier for hydrogen ions to prevent lesion progression [25]. Laboratory-based and *in situ* studies reported that infiltrants are capable of inhibiting the progression of natural carious lesions [22–26], and subsequently, this has been confirmed by clinical studies [27, 28].

Interestingly, resin infiltration combined with fluoride varnish application was superior in arresting superficial carious lesions in proximal surfaces of primary molars when compared to dental varnish containing fluoride alone for a period of 3 years [27]. The progression of enamel and dentine carious lesions on distal surfaces of first primary molars in young children after 2.5 years was low for resin infiltration (46.4%) than for interdental flossing of these surfaces (71.4%) [29]. However, comparing the infiltration technique with sealing carious lesions in proximal surfaces of permanent teeth with a resin-bonding material failed to show any significant differences in carious lesion progression after 3 years [29].

Molar-Incisor Hypomineralisation (MIH) affects mechanical properties of hard dental tissues due to the disorganised prismatic structures with low mineral density and high protein content which leads to increased porosity and discolouration, i.e., especially in yellow and brown lesions. The affected enamel is likely to develop post-eruptive enamel breakdown (PEB) that would potentially facilitate plaque accumulation and development of carious lesions in high caries risk individuals [30]. Nogueira et al. [31] recently reported that resin infiltration treatment positively influenced the structural integrity maintenance of MIH-affected teeth in 223 children aged from 6 to 12 years by decreasing the risk of enamel breakdown when compared to the application of dental varnish containing fluoride (5% NaF; Duraphat; Colgate Palmolive, Germany) for a period of 18 months. This clinical study was the first to report the resin infiltration effect on MIH-affected teeth. However, management of MIH is challenging and the clinical effects of treatments for MIH-affected teeth to improve the physical characteristics of these lesions remain unknown. Therefore, further clinical data is required in relation to minimally invasive strategies for the management of these lesions.

In summary, the evidence currently available indicates that resin infiltration of enamel lesions is a promising micro-invasive method for reducing the progress of enamel lesions [31]. Further evidence is required for the management of enamel lesions.

MI Restorations in Non-Carious Cervical Lesions

Dental caries in anterior teeth would preferably be restored using resin composite due to its optimum aesthetic performance. According to a systematic review regarding effectiveness of adhesive materials (three-step etch and rinse adhesives, two-step etch and rinse adhesives, two-step self-etch adhesives, one-step self-etch adhesives, glass-ionomers, and self-adhesive composite resins) bonded to enamel and dentine in non-carious cervical lesions [32], glass-ionomers, and two-step self-etch adhesives showed the most favourable and durable bonding performance. However, despite the excellent clinical performance in terms of retention, glass-ionomers commonly present with lower aesthetic features, high surface roughness, low colour stability, and wear resistance with inferior mechanical properties when compared to resin-based restorative materials.

MI Management for Deep Carious Lesions

Despite the plea made by World Health Organisation (WHO), the FDI World Dental Federation and International Association for Dental Research (IADR) to reduce the use of restorative materials, especially dental amalgam, through placing much greater emphasis on caries preventive measures, the need for treating cavitated teeth would remain into the foreseeable future [13].

Remineralisation of Demineralised Dentine

The key strategy for managing a cavitated tooth is to remove decomposed (or "infected") dentine, to leave demineralised (or "affected") dentine behind and to provide an adequate seal with innovative restorative materials that have optimum biological and physical properties [33–39].

Remineralisation of demineralised dentine occurs through: the function of the odontoblast process, providing calcium and phosphate from the vital pulp [33], diffusion of ions (fluoride, calcium, and phosphate) from bioactive dental materials placed on the floor of restored cavities [34, 38, 39], and contact of saliva with carious lesions, providing calcium and phosphate in conjunction with oral hygiene measures [40].

In this respect, systematic reviews reported that micro-organisms left underneath the well-sealed restorations have no further ability to drive the caries process. Depriving micro-organisms from the source of metabolic nutrition would be required to discourage their survival and production of acid that demineralises tooth surfaces. This situation leads to a change in the environment of cariogenic microorganisms and inhibits their metabolic ability [41–43].

The adage of "the seal is the deal" should be adopted if oral healthcare professionals aim to provide the optimum patient care to the growing number of people with a functional natural dentition and keep their teeth healthy from youth into old age to achieve "teeth for life for all".

Cavity Design and Principles for MID

Conservation of tooth structure using minimally invasive cavity preparations could be possible since adhesive materials do not require the incorporation of mechanical retentive features. Biomimetic potential including the release of fluoride, calcium, and phosphate ions can be of value in enhancing remineralisation potential of carious lesions. Majority of restorative dental materials that can currently be used for this purpose are resin-based composites and GICs [39, 44].

The principles are:

- Gaining access to the body of the lesion without being destructive (shape of cavity is dictated by dental caries and unique for each carious lesion-conservative cavity preparation-macro mechanical retention is not required);
- Removal of tooth structure that is infected and soft, which is incapable of regeneration;
- Retaining the affected leathery type of dentine;
- Retaining and reinforcing sound, however undermined enamel needs to be removed;
- Reducing perimeter of the restoration;
- Keeping the margins of the restoration away from the gingiva; and
- Reducing occlusal stress on the final restoration [23].

Appropriate Excavation Methods

According to the concept of MID, only the infected dentine needs to be removed from within the cavity. However, the extent and type of carious dentine to be removed to achieve a mechanically and biologically successful restoration is still a matter of debate.

Deep caries has been defined radiographically as a condition where the teeth are damaged to 1/3 or 1/4 of the dentine near the dental pulp or at risk of dental pulp exposure. The traditional management involved the removal of all demineralised tissues and microbiologically contaminated dental tissues and restoration with various dental materials. However, there have been significant challenges for the management of deep caries lesions due to the risk of dental pulp exposure. Currently, there are three treatment options especially for deep carious lesions: total carious lesion excavation/complete caries excavation (TCLE), stepwise excavation (SWE), and incomplete carious lesion removal (ICLR). Nowadays, TCLE for deep carious lesions is not recommended due to the potential indirect dental pulp damage in permanent and primary teeth. This could be from the irritation going through the residual demineralised dentine and/or from the unnecessary weakening of tooth structure integrity. However, the aim of the ICRL technique, especially for the deep carious lesions, is to arrest the progression of dental caries and to maximise the remineralisation of the demineralised residual dentine in order to maintaining the dental pulp vitality [39].

In aiding this process, several techniques have been introduced, i.e., the use of caries detecting dyes (CDDs), chemo-mechanical excavation, excavation by sono-abrasion, air-abrasion excavation, fluorescence-aided caries excavation (FACE), excavation aided by laser-induced fluorescence, or laser excavation [45–49]. There is still lack of evidence on the detection systems to clinically define the severity of carious lesions, enabling complete removal of infected tissue without overextending cavity preparation. It should also be noted that restorations might be replaced prematurely since dentists do not have a consistent method to diagnose some lesions. Therefore, these lesions might be treated when the intervention is unnecessary.

The time involvement in cleaning the cavity is an issue and most likely will, among others, depend on the operators' experience. This then leaves hand excavation with an excavator and the use of conventional excavation with tungsten-carbide or carbon-steel burs still considered as effective methods for removing decomposed carious dentin prior to restoration. Irrespective of the caries excavation method chosen, it is recommended to finish the cavity margins in clean/sound tooth tissue to achieve the best performance of adhesive, while being at the same time least invasive with regard to caries excavation and most conservative with regard to sound-tissue preservation.

MI Restorations in Posterior Teeth

Resin composites may also be considered as the material of choice for the treatment of extensive primary carious lesions, where minimally invasive techniques can still be applied (Figure 7.1) [50–53]. However, some promising data of highly viscous GIs were also shown successfully retained in the treatment of posterior teeth (Figure 7.2) [51].

MI Restorations in The "Aesthetic Zone"

The use of ceramics in the form of veneers or crowns was considered as the only satisfactory and durable solution to address the optimum aesthetic demands in young as well as adult patients. This hegemony of ceramics, which for that matter tends to linger, is favoured

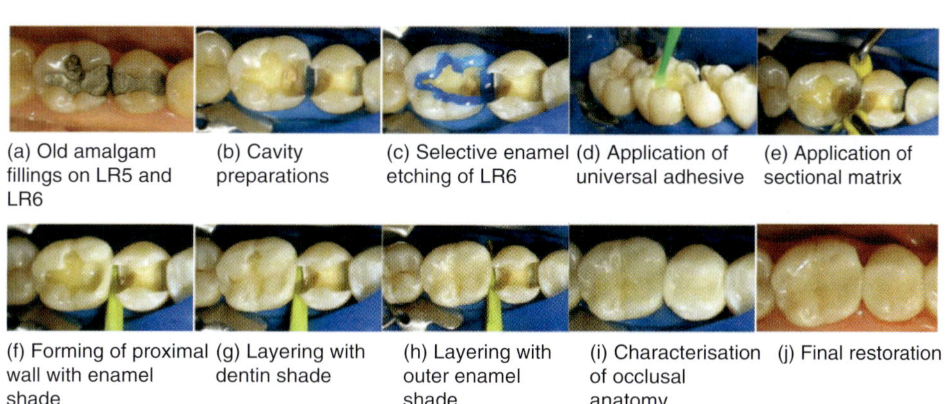

(a) Old amalgam fillings on LR5 and LR6

(b) Cavity preparations

(c) Selective enamel etching of LR6

(d) Application of universal adhesive

(e) Application of sectional matrix

(f) Forming of proximal wall with enamel shade

(g) Layering with dentin shade

(h) Layering with outer enamel shade

(i) Characterisation of occlusal anatomy

(j) Final restoration

Figure 7.1 Application of posterior composite resin restorations.

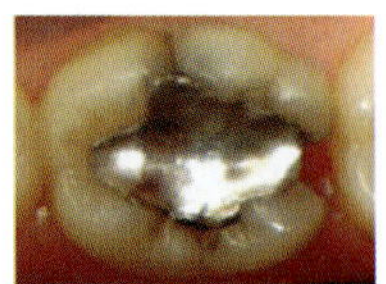 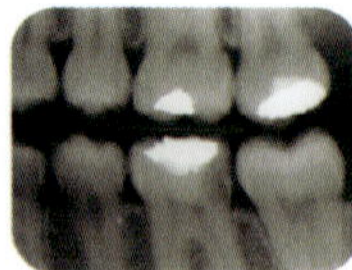 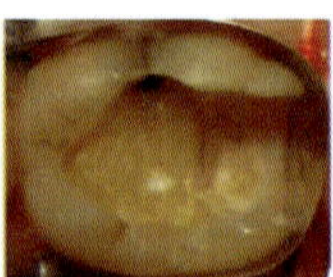 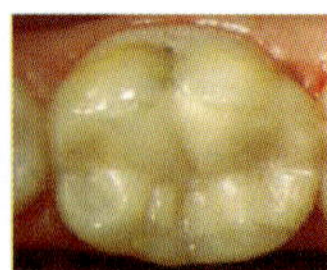 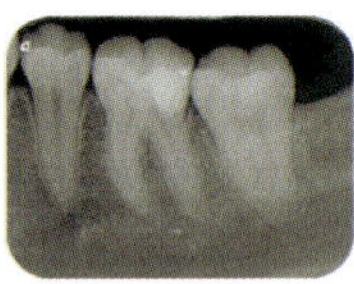

(a) Old amalgam filling at the LL6

(b) Pre-operative radiographic view (Left bitewing)

(c) Cavity preparation

(d) Restoration with permanent restorative GI

(e) Post-op radiographic view

Figure 7.2 The use of GI as a permanent restorative material in the treatment of extended size cavity in posterior region. (Please note. The tooth was assessed for tooth vitality and responded positive to the tooth sensibility tests using cold test-50 degrees and Electrical Pulp Tester).

by the dental industry that invests significant amounts of money to promote these materials and new technologies, without demonstrating any consideration for the biomechanics of the healthy tooth structures.

The sheer aesthetic criteria need to be weighed against the biological and mechanical fundamental principles of the natural tooth not only to ensure the longevity of the restorations, but also to preserve the vitality and the integrity of the dental hard tissues.

In this respect, these considerations have been encouraging clinicians to consider direct bonding techniques as a first-choice alternative to destructive preparations for the placement of ceramic restorations [52–56]. Direct resin composites have the advantages of combining reasonable cost, optimum aesthetics, encouraging patient satisfaction, and proven longevity [57–63]. In addition, these materials can be used effectively to conserve tooth tissue [63], avoiding the need for further tooth preparation, which may ultimately involve core build-up and crown preparation (Figure 7.3). The motivation should also be to perfect the least invasive methods for the preservation and repair of teeth for life [7].

"No-Prep" Adhesive Restorations: Another Way to Deal with Problems Related to Aesthetics

The improvement of the aesthetic properties of composite resin materials [52–60], also permitted to make direct restorations available to everyone, since they are not anymore only for the prerogative of gifted clinicians trained to complex stratification techniques, which are inaccessible to the general dental practitioners/general dentists.

Indeed, several systems have been developed during the past 10 years building on the "Concept of Natural Stratification", consisting of only two basic layers (enamel and dentine) and an appropriate shade guide. In addition, clinical results in the medium and long-term with regards to the use of direct composite resins have been proved to be reliable [53].

Clinical cases that illustrate the direct approach and aesthetic potential of composite resin systems based on the concept of natural stratification are presented in Figures 7.4 and 7.5.

Management of Tooth Discoloration with MI Approach

Tooth Whitening/Bleaching

In recent years, the focus of dentistry has shifted from "functional demand", where routine dental treatment is repairing the destructive effects of dental caries, to "*aesthetic dentistry*", where patients are concerned about the appearance of their teeth [64].

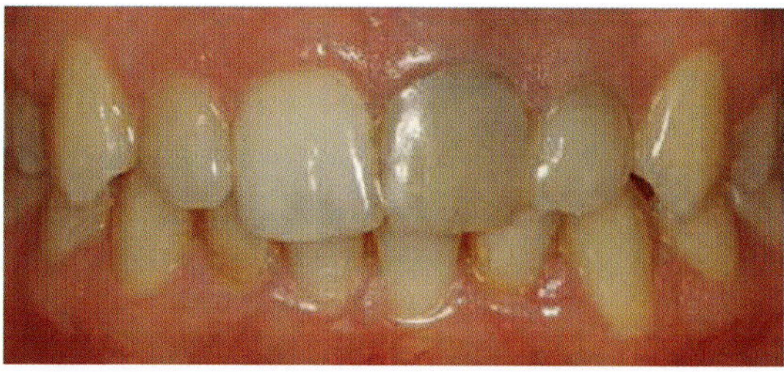
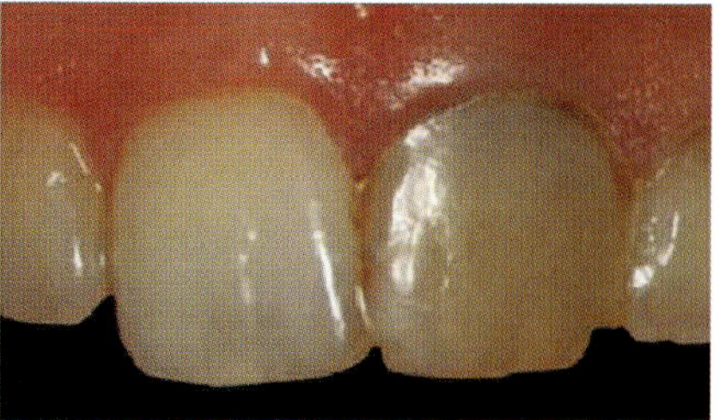

Preoperative view of the discoloured and old composite resin restoration at the tooth (UL1)

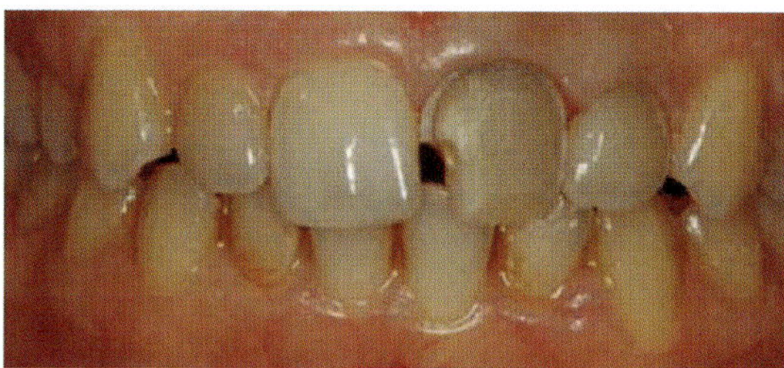
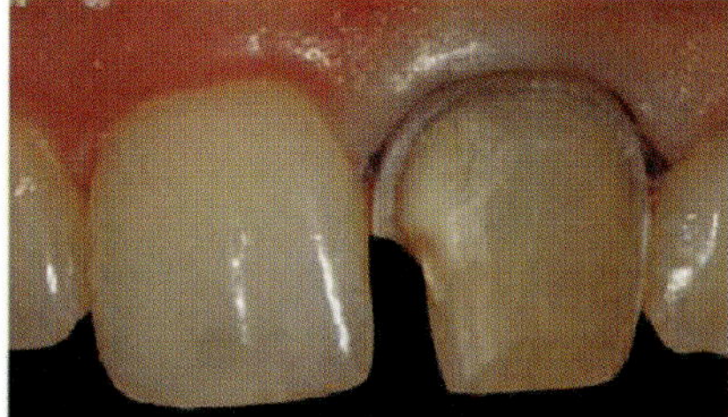

Removing old composite resin restoration and preparation of the UL1

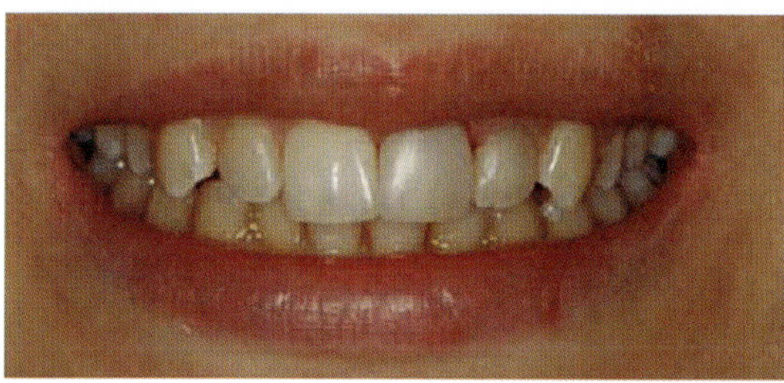
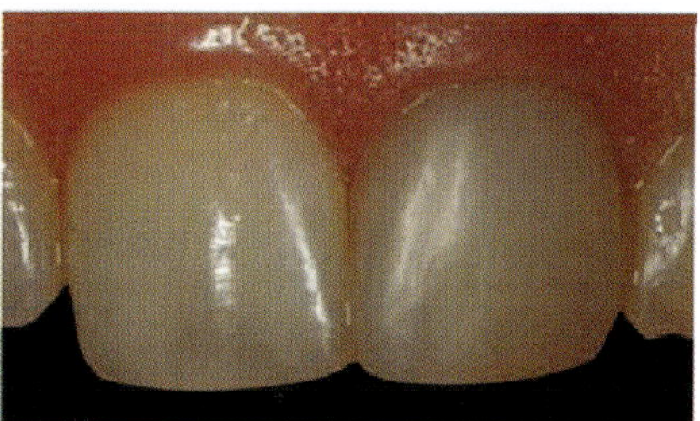

Post-operative view of the new direct composite resin restoration at the UL1

Figure 7.3　MI treatment of a discoloured anterior tooth. A 33-year-old female patient referred to the restorative dentistry clinic complaining of her unaesthetic smile due to the discoloured UL1. There was no relevant medical history and no medication. There were no reported known allergies.
What is the first step you would consider?
A thorough history taking, clinical examination including risk assessment analysis, then special investigations with radiographic examinations. In a brief note, Subjective, Objective, Assessment, and Plan (SOAP) could be followed.
What is your approach to your patient with regards to treatment options?
There were different treatment modalities with cost implications. These techniques might need further removal of the patient's sound tooth structure and require two or more sessions due to laboratory procedures.
What treatment option would you consider?
One option would be to restore the tooth in one session with the use of direct composite resin.

The importance of tooth whitening for patients and consumers has seen a dramatic rise in the number of tooth whitening products and procedures. There are a number of methods and approaches that have been described in the literature for the bleaching of vital and non-vital teeth utilizing different bleaching agents, concentrations, times of application, product format, application mode [64–67]. However, three fundamental bleaching approaches exist today, namely dentist-supervised night guard bleaching (NGVB), in office or power bleaching (Figure 7.6), and mass market bleaching products called as OTC (over

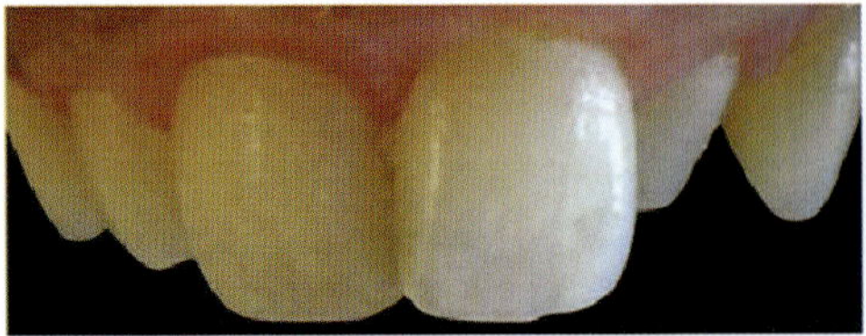

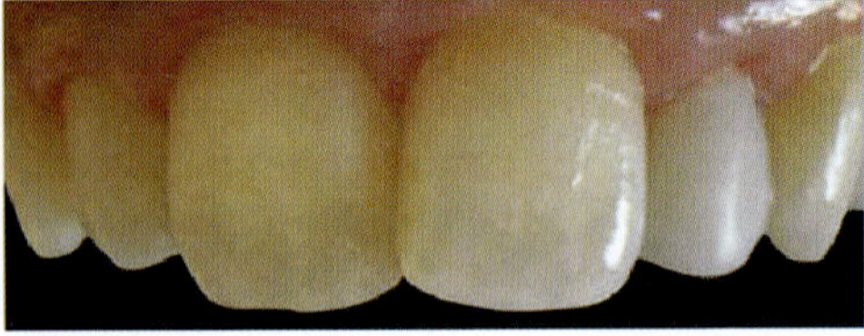

(a) Pre-operative upper anterior teeth view   (b) Post-operative upper anterior teeth view

Figure 7.4   This case is about a 24-year-old patient presented with hypodontia and peg-shaped UL2. There was no relevant medical history and no medication. There were also no reported known allergies.

What is the first step you would consider?
A thorough history taking, clinical examination including risk assessment analysis, then special investigations with radiographic examinations. In a brief note, Subjective, Objective, Assessment, and Plan (SOAP) could be followed.

What is your approach to your patient with regards to treatment options?
There were different treatment modalities with cost implications. These techniques might need further removal of the patient's sound tooth structure and require two or more sessions due to laboratory procedures.

What treatment option would you consider?
Patient indicated that that she could not afford an orthodontic treatment. The tooth could be reshaped without any reduction from the tooth structure in one session by using direct composite resin.

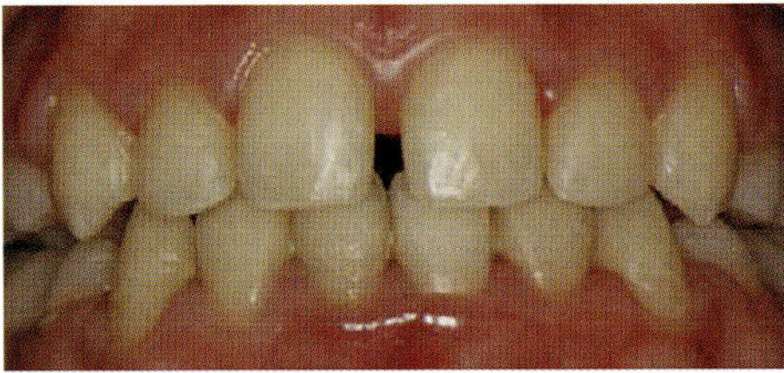

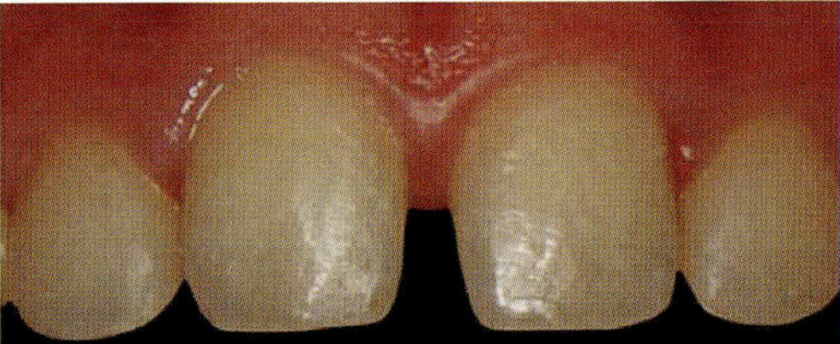

Pre-operative view of the patient with midline diastema

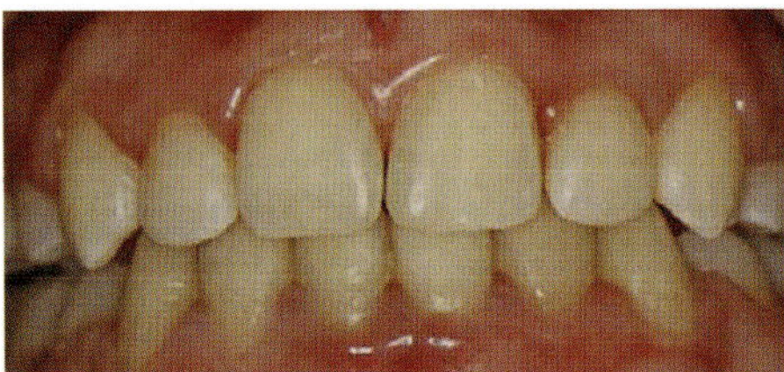

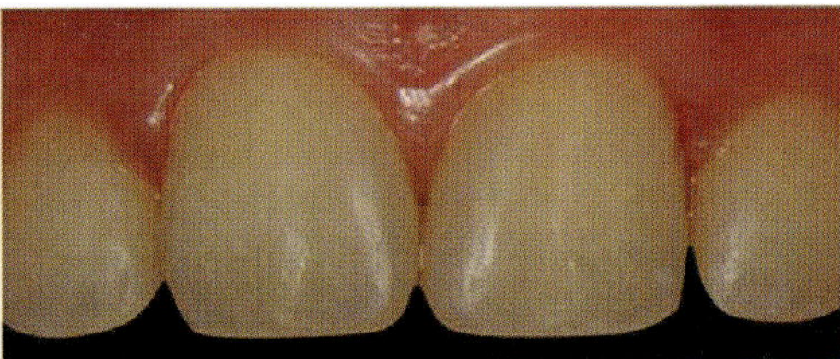

Post-operative view, a direct approach has naturally been followed in this case. Final view showing the optimum integration of the restorations. The aesthetics have been facilitated by the application of a single shade concept, easy to implement and predictable, ideal for the treatment of aesthetic deficiencies of a young smile

Figure 7.5   A diastema closure using direct composite resin without preparation. This case presents an application of direct bonding for diastema closure in a 17-year-old patient. There was no relevant medical history and no medication. There were no reported known allergies.

the counter) products [64]. Although home-based bleaching methods have a prominent place in the dental market, in office bleaching for vital teeth recently presented a steady increase in popularity.

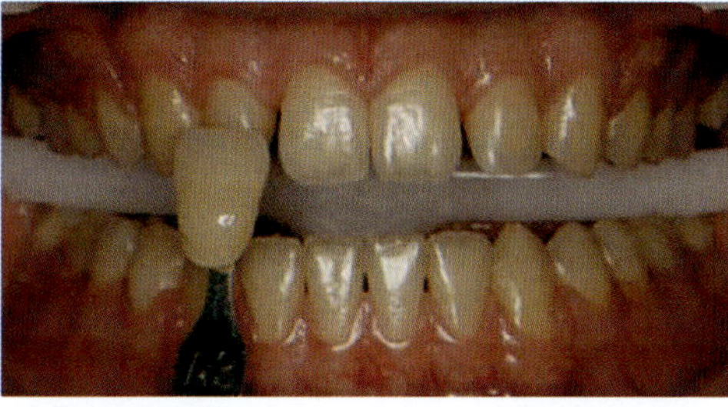

(a) Preoperative view and colour determination

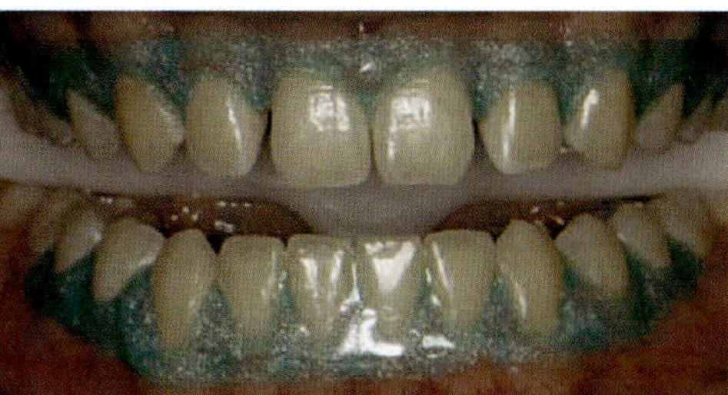

(b) Application of gingival barrier

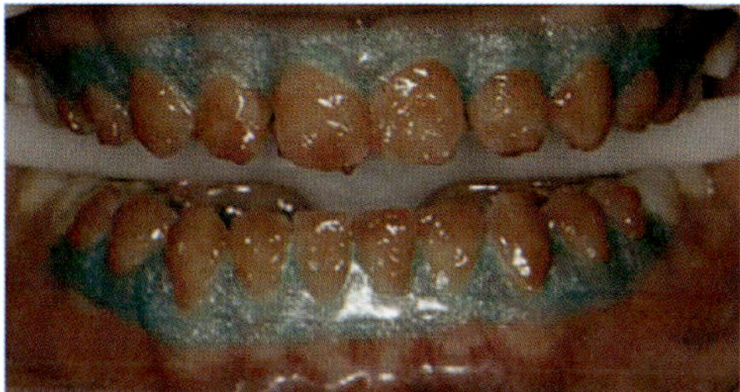

(c) Application of bleaching agent

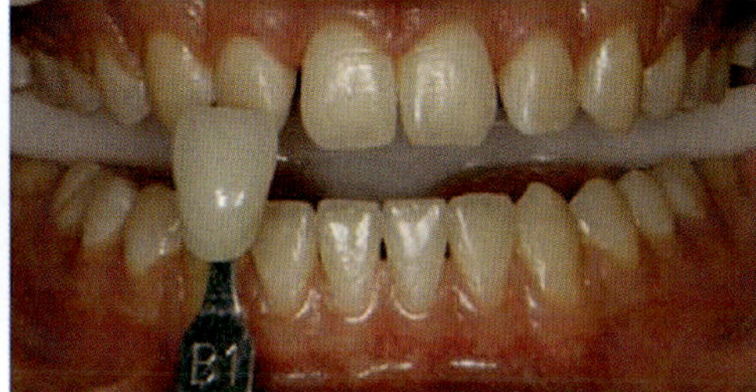

(d) Post-operative view after one week with no reported symptoms such as hypersensitivity

Figure 7.6   Vital tooth bleaching. Twenty-three-year-old male patient referred to the clinic as he was unhappy with the colour of his teeth after the orthodontic treatment. There was no relevant medical history and no medication. There were also no reported known allergies.
What is the first step you would consider?
A thorough history taking, clinical examination including risk assessment analysis, and then special investigations with radiographic examinations. In a brief note, Subjective, Objective, Assessment, and Plan (SOAP) could be followed. Clinical examination revealed a well-maintained dentition with shade A3 in Vita Shade Guide.
What is your approach to your patient with regards to treatment options?
One option is that the satisfactory aesthetical outcome could be achieved without any harm to his teeth by the employment of tooth whitening or bleaching.
What treatment can you offer him?
An office bleaching with 40% hydrogen peroxide could be applied for a period of 20 min/3 sessions.

Current tooth bleaching materials are based primarily on either hydrogen peroxide or carbamide peroxide [64–67]. Hydrogen peroxide is the active agent in most whitening products. This agent acts as a strong oxidising agent, producing reactive oxygen molecules and hydrogen peroxide anions. Hydrogen peroxide diffuses into enamel and dentine due its small molecule where it decomposes into different active oxygen species under specific temperature, pH, and light conditions. The free radicals created could oxidise the conjugated structure of the chromophores, and this oxidation would promote morphological changes on enamel surfaces [64]. Therefore, the bleaching process has the potential to provide satisfactory aesthetic outcome, however the effect of peroxides on hard tissues is still in question.

Management of Tooth Wear with MI Approaches

The incidence of tooth wear is increasing and oral rehabilitation of patients with non-carious tooth loss requires strategies that address all factors relevant to the aetiology and pathogenesis of this condition. The multifactorial nature of tooth wear and variability in its clinical presentation provide treatment challenges for the clinician. Management must include an appropriate mix of preventive and restorative strategies and an understanding that long-term restorative success is affected by the general and patient related factors, i.e., oral and general health, diet, plaque control, and lifestyle can modify the outcome [68].

MID philosophy is ideally suited to tooth wear cases and an overall MID strategy involving diagnosis, recognition and control of predisposing factors, stabilisation of the oral environment, remineralisation, and restoration of the tooth structure with maintenance can be implemented. When restorative treatment is required, contemporary materials and techniques are available that can provide cost-effective and conservative restorative alternatives for patients who are especially unable to undergo complex indirect restorative techniques that are both costly and time consuming to implement. These MI approaches are not only an economically viable solution, but also can provide aesthetic and functional rehabilitation by maintaining tooth structure as a precursor to more complex restorative options when/if required. Direct composite resins have been shown to be successful (Figure 7.7)

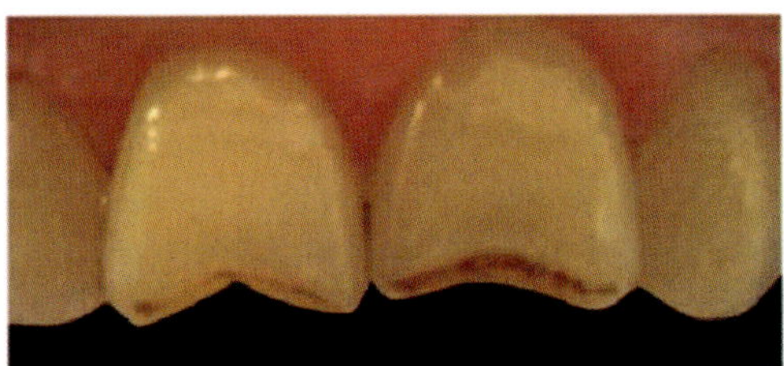

(a) Pre-operative view of the UL1 and UR1

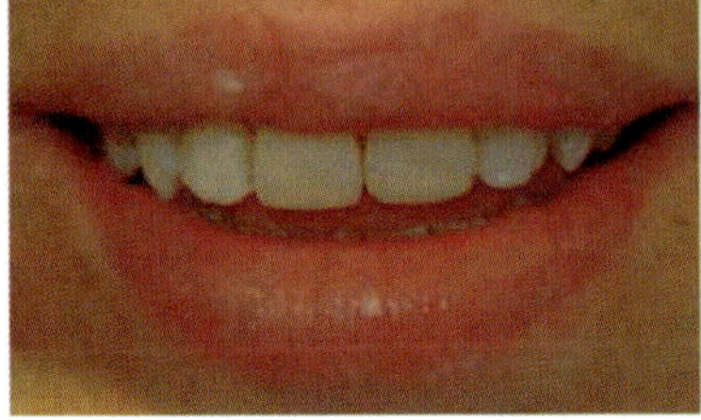

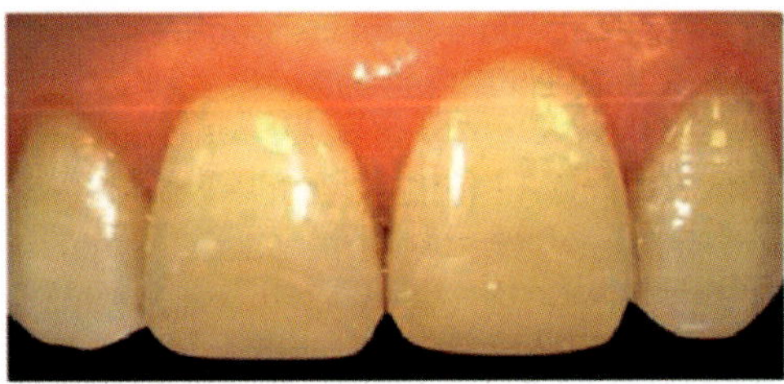

(b) Direct composite resin restorations at the UL1 and UR1

Figure 7.7 Direct composite restorations of wear on teeth at the UL1 and UR1. Forty-five-year-old female patient who was not satisfied with the appearance of her worn anterior teeth referred to the restorative clinic. A thorough history taking, clinical examination including risk assessment analysis, then special investigations with radiographic examinations. In a brief note, Subjective, Objective, Assessment, and Plan (SOAP) could also be followed. Diagnosis was tooth wear due to attrition and an element of erosion. Both teeth were restored with the direct composite resins.
What would the next step be?
Identification of aetiologic factors and checking the occlusion.
What would you discuss with your patient?
The long-term success of rehabilitation was depended on the identification of aetiological factors, lifestyle, diet, plaque control, consideration of occlusion, parafunctional habits, and regular maintenance.
What treatment would you offer to your patient?
The teeth could be restored by direct resin composite in order to restore what has been lost, improve aesthetics, and prevent further damage.

[68–71] in the rehabilitation of worn dentitions on a medium to long term (5–10 years) and sometimes even preferred over indirect full-ceramic restorations [68, 72].

In this respect, Milosevic et al. [73] reported the survival rate of 1010 direct composites placed in 164 patients due to suboptimal appearances of teeth. Mean follow-up time was 33.8 months. Seventy-one of 1010 restorations failed during follow-up. The estimated failure rate in the first year was 5.4% (95% CI 3.7–7.0%). In older patients presented with significantly high failure rates ($p = 0.005$) when there was a lack of posterior support ($p = 0.003$). Interestingly parafunctional habits such as bruxism and increase in the occlusal vertical dimension were not the associated factors for failure of these restorations. The proportion of failures was high in patients with Class 3 or edge-to-edge incisal relationship in comparison to the Class 1 and Class 2 cases, however this was statistically insignificant. In addition, failures were mainly in the lower arch (9.6%) when compared to the upper arch (6%) with the large number of composite resins on the maxillary incisors ($n = 519$). In conclusion, the repairability of composite resins and the ability to replace completely debonded build-ups improved the success rather than survival. Interestingly, it should be noted that 15.5% of 161 zirconia (Lava™) crowns used to restore severe anterior tooth wear for a period of 7 years. The main reasons were mainly due to attrition, which presented catastrophic failures and were unrepairable [73, 74].

Tooth Loss and MI Restorative Approaches

Replacing single missing teeth in posterior dentition encompasses a broad spectrum of treatment options. When neither functional nor aesthetic limitations are present, abandonment of a restorative therapy and monitoring of single tooth gaps could be an option. Alternatively, orthodontic interventions, tooth transplantations, or fixed/removable prosthesis can be considered as management options [75–77].

A mostly unknown treatment option for the posterior dentition is interdental closure by direct composite build-ups. In selected cases, MID would be implemented in order to reshape and widen teeth through adhesively applied resin composite materials thereby avoiding fixed dental prostheses and single-tooth implants [76, 77]. MID treatment guidelines and extended indications for resin composite as "restorative material of choice" in the posterior region are recommended also by the European Section of the Academy of Operative Dentistry (AODES) [78].

An Alternative Replacement Approach to Tooth Loss: Resin Bonded Bridges

The evolution of resin bonded or resin retained bridges (RBBs/RRBs) for the replacement of a short span or single tooth has been significant since the first description in the 1970s. The first type of RBB was called "Rochette Bridge". The retention of this type bridge depended on the perforated metal retainer and resin cement tags [79]. However, the compromised longevity of this type of bridges led the alteration of the metal retainer surface to improve the micromechanical retention [80]. Subsequently "Maryland Bridge" was introduced at the University of Maryland with a view of electrochemical etching process for the retainer. Following these developments, the retention of RBBs improved further by the development of resin cements that bond chemically to both tooth surface and the retainer (Figure 7.8a–c) [81].

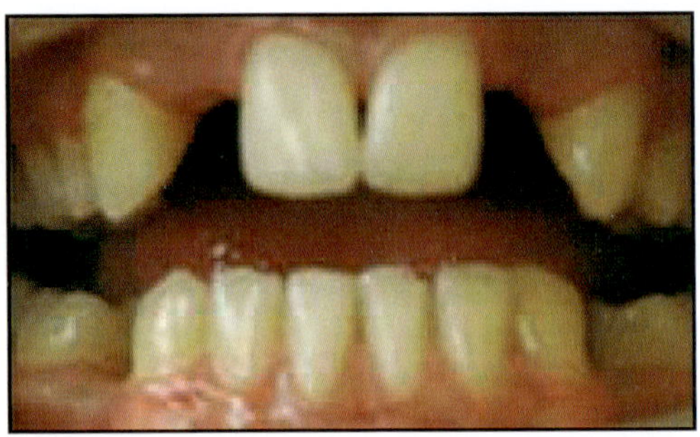

Figure 7.8(a) Young patient with hypodontia at the UR2, UL2, LR5, and LL5. Source: Dr Baysan (Author).

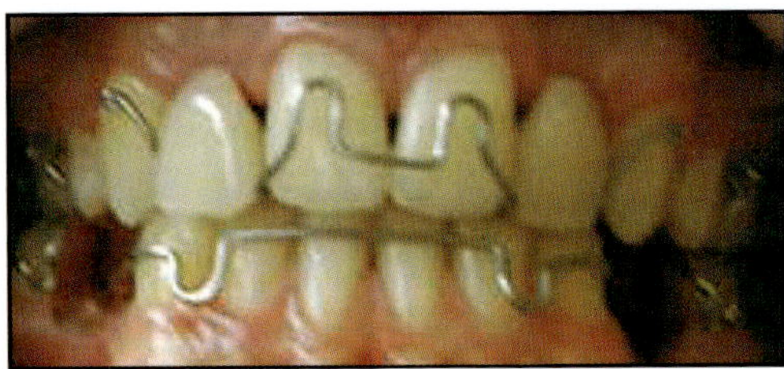

Figure 7.8(b) Upper and lower removable retainers following the orthodontic treatment to replace congenitally missing teeth and to prevent relapse of tooth movement

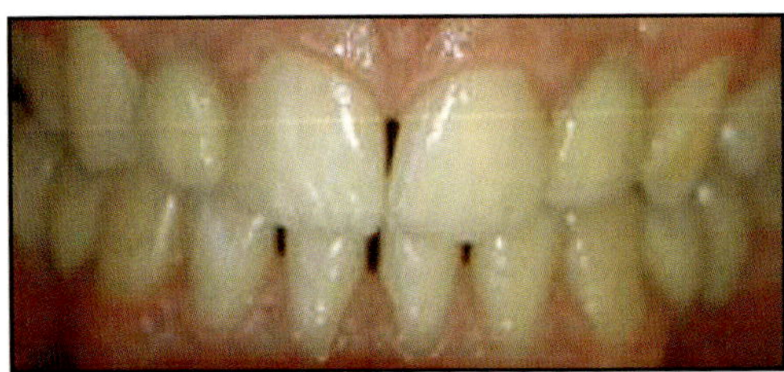

Figure 7.8(c) RBBs to replace upper lateral incisors and lower second premolars without any tooth preparation

With respect to MID strategies, the main advantage of RBBs is no preparation or minimal preparation without the need of local anaesthetics in comparison to the conventional fixed prosthesis. In addition, Djemal et al. [82] reported the clinical performance of 832 resin-retained bridges and splints provided in post-graduate teaching hospital. The recall data was available for 58.4% of cases and the median survival was 7 years and 10 months. The survival of these bridges was significantly affected by their design and retainer coverage. Interestingly, the experience of the operator presented a remarkable effect, however the reasons of this finding was unclear. Resin-retained restorations with minimal tooth preparation were shown to be capable of extended clinical service and their failure rarely resulted in adverse consequences for the patient. In addition, patient satisfaction was found to be high [82].

Subsequently, the systematic review indicated the five-year survival rates for bridgework as 87.7% for RBBs and over 90% for conventional bridges depending on the design [83]. It should be noted that these rates were low in comparison to the success of implant retained single crowns, which is 94.5% [84], however RBBs have the advantages of being less invasive, requiring a short total treatment time and less financial commitment with less catastrophic failure outcomes in comparison to the conventional bridges (loss of tooth vitality) and implant retained single crowns (peri-mucositis/implantitis). In addition, it was reported that the annual debonding rate for RBBs placed on posterior teeth (5.03%), whilst for the anterior-placed RBBs, this was 3.05% and the failure difference according to the location was insignificant ($p = 0.157$). With respect to biological complications, 1.5% RBBs debonded due to dental caries on abutments (1.5%), whilst 2.1% RBBs were lost due to periodontitis.

One of the main disadvantages of metal based-RBBs is the greying effect of the metal wing showing through abutment teeth, known as "shine through". In addition, the rare disadvantage could be corrosion and potential allergy to the nonprecious alloys used. Therefore, fiber-reinforced composite RBBs has recently been introduced and reported to provide optimum aesthetic outcome, however these types of RBBs were perceived as temporary [85]. Therefore, all-ceramic RBBs (glass-infiltrated alumina ceramic or zirconia ceramic) were suggested during early 1990s due to the growing demand on aesthetics [86]. However, limited evidence is available on the survival and design of these types of RBBs.

Despite the reported benefits of RBBs, this treatment modality is not widely implemented in clinical practice due to potential repeated debonding, available materials for retainers, and limitations of resin-based cements despite recent innovations. The outcome could be related to various factors such as patient-related factors, plaque control, compliance, abutment tooth selection, design, retainer coverage, occlusion, and technique sensitive cementation of RBB. It should be noted that the outcome of this treatment could be shaped with applied knowledge and careful planning [82, 87].

In conclusion, there is still limited evidence with regards to survival and clinical performance of RBBs. The impact of different levels of skill and experience of clinicians in addition to the RBB design and materials used such as nickel-chromium/ceramic require further investigation.

Repair of Defective Restorations

MID strategies aim to limit unnecessary removal of healthy tooth structure, and repair of defective restorations. The diagnostic finding "defective" for an existing restoration is a critical step in treatment planning and invariably affects the longevity of the restored tooth.

Secondary caries and staining of the margins of existing restorations are the most common reasons for restoration replacement [88–90]. Although the criteria for the diagnosis of a defective restoration may solely be based on visual and tactile examination, the subsequent management plan could take the holistic approach into account by including through patient assessment with risk analysis and professional's judgment of benefit versus risk since the replacement of restorations could lead to [4]:

- Weakening of tooth structure due to the increased surface area of the cavity,
- The increased surface area tends to make more complex form of restoration,
- Large restorations, which usually have a shorter life span than their predecessors, and
- Possible damage to adjacent teeth.

In this respect, Wilson et al. [10] reviewed the criteria for the replacement of restorations and reported that further research in the area is required (i.e., establishment of risk assessment of defective and failing restorations). Innovative diagnostic tools to assess functionality and suitability of existing restorations are still required. This research could run in parallel with regenerative endodontic advancements.

When the clinician is evaluating an existing restoration with one or more localised clinical features that deviate from ideal and the restoration is considered defective, the clinician should assess whether the tooth in question will truly benefit from a new restoration. When a clinician faces with a borderline situation, the patient's past dental history and current caries risk status, and the optimum treatment for the tooth in question need to be considered. If the clinician is unsure whether the defective area can be removed by polishing or by sealing the affected area, another conservative and predictable approach would be to repair the restoration by removing the deteriorated area and re-restoring this area only.

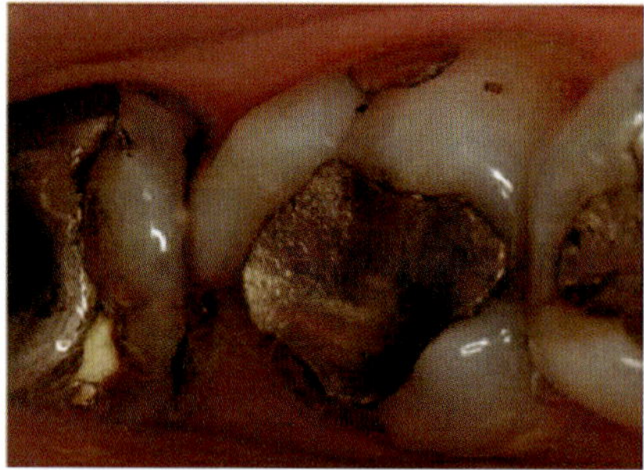

(a) Preoperative view

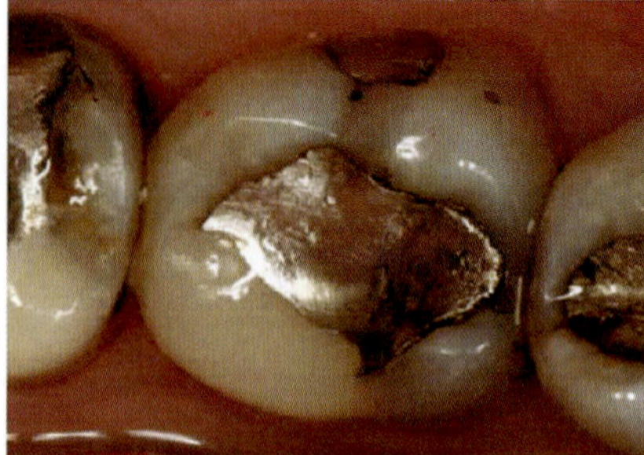

(b) Post-operative view

Figure 7.9 Repair of fractured amalgam restoration. Fifty-five-year-old male patient referred to the restorative clinic complaining sensitivity on his right lower posterior region. A fracture at lingual cusp of an amalgam restoration on tooth LR7 was observed at the oral examination. The old amalgam, which was over 20 years old, repaired with direct composite resin instead of removing the old restoration.
What are the available options for this patient?
To restore with a new restoration (intra or extracoronal) or repair of fractured cusp using direct resin composite.
What would you discuss with the patient?
Treatment options with advantages and disadvantages need to be explained such as in correctly selected cases, repairing the restoration could be conservative by preserving the remaining sound tooth structures, less financial impact, and time-saver.

During recent years, new strategies such as repair and refinishing or sealing of localised defects have shown an overall improvement in the clinical properties of defective restorations, thereby increasing their longevity through minimal intervention [91–96]. In addition, repair of restorations with correct case selection can be more cost-effective and acceptable to patients than restoration replacement. Since this MI procedure preserves tooth structure, the "repair" approach when carried out at the right case would have the potential to allow patients to retain most of their teeth during their lifetime.

Prospective studies have shown that repaired restorations in permanent teeth have the same or increased longevity as restorations that were replaced completely [91, 93–95]. In addition, it should be noted that repaired restorations could present a reduction in-patient and/or the third-party payers' expenses, which would potentially increase the number of individuals who could afford dental care instead of ignoring the treatment due to various reasons such as financial implications (Figure 7.9) [96].

Summary

MID is a philosophy that attempts to ensure that teeth are kept functional for life. The main goal of MID in relation to restorative dentistry is to increase the life of the teeth, which was restored with less intervention. Therefore, MID concept is not only restricted to the management of dental caries but is also applicable in restorative dentistry.

Further Reading

General

General Dental Council, Tooth whitening position statement. https://www.gdc-uk.org/docs/default-source/what-is-the-legal-position/tooth-whitening-position-statement.pdf.

Loomans, B., Opdam, N., Attin, T., Bartlett, D., Edelhoff, D., Frankenberger, R., Benic, G., Ramseyer, S., Wetselaar, P., Sterenborg, B., Hickel, R., Pallesen, U., Mehta, S., Banerji, S., Lussi, A., and Wilson, N. (2017). Severe tooth wear: European Consensus Statement on management guidelines. *J Adhes. Dent.* 19(2):111–119. doi: 10.3290/j.jad.a38102. PMID: 28439579.

The British Society of Restorative Dentistry is building a resource for dentists by providing guidelines on managing challenging clinical situations. https://www.bsrd.org.uk/Guidelines.aspx

References

1   Petersen, E. (2013). http://www.who.int/oral_health/media/en/orh_report03_en.pdf.

2   Hayes, A., Azarpazhooh, A., Dempster, L., Ravaghi, V., and Quinonez, C. (2013). Time loss due to dental problems and treatment in the Canadian population: Analysis of a nationwide cross-sectional survey. *BMC Oral Health* 13: 17.

3   Mount, G.J., and Hume, W.R. (1997 May). A revised classification of carious lesions by site and size. *Quintessence Int.* 28 (5): 301–303. PMID: 9452692.

4   Bhatiya, P., and Thosar, N. (2015). Minimal invasive dentistry – An emerging trend in pediatric dentistry: A review. *Int. J. Contemp. Dent. Med. Rev.* 2015. Article ID: 320115. doi: 10.15713/ins.ijcdmr. 514.

5   White, J.M., and Eakle, W.S. (2000). Rationale and treatment approach in minimally invasive dentistry. *J. Am. Dent. Assoc.* 131 (Suppl): 13S–9S.

6   Neena, I., Edagunji, G., Poornima, P., Nagaveni, N., Roopa, K., and Bharath, K. (2015). Minimal invasive dentistry. *Int. J. Contemp. Dent. Med. Rev.* 2015: 1–4.

7   Mackenzie, L., Parmar, D., Shortall, A.C., and Burke, F.J. (2013). Direct anterior composites: A practical guide. *Dent. Update* 40 (4): 297–299, 301–302, 5–8 passim.

8   Brostek, A.M., Bochenek, A.J., and Walsh, L.J. (2006). Minimally invasive dentistry: A review and update. *Shanghai Kou Qiang Yi Xue* 15 (3): 225–249.

9   Mertz-Fairhurst, E.J., Adair, S.M., Sams, D.R., Curtis, J.W., Jr., Ergle, J.W., Hawkins, K.I., Mackert, J.R. Jr., O'Dell, N.L., Richards, E.E., and Rueggeberg, F. (1995). Cariostatic and ultraconservative sealed restorations: Nine-year results among children and adults. *ASDC J. Dent. Child.* 62 (2): 97–107.

10 Wilson, N., Lynch, C.D., Brunton, P.A., Hickel, R., Meyer-Lueckel, H., Gurgan, S., Pallesen, U., Shearer, A.C., Tarle, Z., Cotti, E., Vanherle, G., and Opdam, N. (2016 September). Criteria for the replacement of restorations: Academy of operative dentistry European Section. *Oper. Dent.* 41 (S7): S48–S57. doi: 10.2341/15-058-O. PMID: 27689930.

11 Mertz-Fairhurst, E.J., Curtis, J.W., Jr., Ergle, J.W., Rueggeberg, F.A., and Adair, S.M. (1998). Ultraconservative and cariostatic sealed restorations: Results at year 10. *J. Am. Dent. Assoc.* 129 (1): 55–66.

12 Vidnes-Kopperud, S., Tveit, A.B., and Espelid, I. (2011). Changes in the treatment concept for approximal caries from 1983 to 2009 in Norway. *Caries Res.* 45 (2): 113–120.

13 Frencken, J.E., Peters, M.C., Manton, D.J., Leal, S.C., Gordan, V.V., and Eden, E. (2012). Minimal intervention dentistry for managing dental caries – a review: Report of a FDI task group. *Int. Dent. J.* 62 (5): 223–243.

14 Hausen, H. (2004). How to improve the effectiveness of caries-preventive programs based on fluoride. *Caries Res.* 38 (3): 263–267.

15 Featherstone, J.D., White, J.M., Hoover, C.I., Rapozo-Hilo, M., Weintraub, J.A., and Wilson, R.S. (2012). A randomized clinical trial of anticaries therapies targeted according to risk assessment (caries management by risk assessment). *Caries Res.* 46 (2): 118–129.

16 Featherstone, J.D. (1999). Prevention and reversal of dental caries: Role of low level fluoride. *Community Dent. Oral Epidemiol.* 27 (1): 31–40.

17 Holmgren, C., Gaucher, C., Decerle, N., and Domejean, S. (2014). Minimal intervention dentistry II: Part 3. Management of non-cavitated (initial) occlusal caries lesions–non-invasive approaches through remineralisation and therapeutic sealants. *BDJ* 216 (5): 237–243.

18 Beauchamp, J., Caufield, P.W., Crall, J.J., Donly, K., Feigal, R., Gooch, B., Ismail, A., Kohn, W., Siegal, M., Simonsen, R., and American Dental Association Council on Scientific Affairs. (2008). Evidence-based clinical recommendations for the use of pit-and-fissure sealants: A report of the American Dental Association Council on Scientific Affairs. *J. Am. Dent. Assoc.* 139 (3): 257–268.

19 Wright, J.T., Tampi, M.P., Graham, L., Estrich, C., Crall, J.J., Fontana, M., Gillette, E.J., Nový, B.B., Dhar, V., Donly, K., Hewlett, E.R., Quinonez, R.B., Chaffin, J., Crespin, M., Iafolla, T., Siegal, M.D., and Carrasco-Labra, A. (2016). Sealants for preventing and arresting pit-and-fissure occlusal caries in primary and permanent molars: A systematic review of randomized controlled trials-a report of the American Dental Association and the American Academy of Pediatric Dentistry. *J. Am. Dent. Assoc.* 147 (8): 631–45 e18.

20 Mackenzie, L., Shortall, A.C., and Burke, F.J. (2009). Direct posterior composites: A practical guide. *Dent. Update* 36 (2): 71–2, 4–6, 9–80 passim.

21 Simonsen, R.J. (2011). From prevention to therapy: Minimal intervention with sealants and resin restorative materials. *J. Dent.* 39 (Suppl 2): S27–33.

22 Paris, S., Meyer-Lueckel, H., and Kielbassa, A.M. (2007). Resin infiltration of natural caries lesions. *J. Dent. Res.* 86 (7): 662–666.

23 Meyer-Lueckel, H., Paris, S., and Kielbassa, A.M. (2007). Surface layer erosion of natural caries lesions with phosphoric and hydrochloric acid gels in preparation for resin infiltration. *Caries Res.* 41 (3): 223–230.

24 Paris, S., and Meyer-Lueckel, H. (2010). Infiltrants inhibit progression of natural caries lesions in vitro. *J. Dent. Res.* 89 (11): 1276–1280.

25 Paris, S., and Meyer-Lueckel, H. (2010). Inhibition of caries progression by resin infiltration in situ. *Caries Res.* 44 (1): 47–54.

26 Ekstrand, K.R., Luna, L.E., Promisiero, L., Cortes, A., Cuevas, S., Reyes, J.F., Torres, C.E., and Martignon, S. (2011). The reliability and accuracy of two methods for proximal caries detection and depth on directly visible proximal surfaces: An *in vitro* study. *Caries Res.* 45 (2): 93–99.

27 Martignon, S., Ekstrand, K.R., Gomez, J., Lara, J.S., and Cortes, A. (2012). Infiltrating/sealing proximal caries lesions: A 3-year randomized clinical trial. *J. Dent. Res.* 91 (3): 288–292.

28 Kielbassa, A.M., Muller, J., and Gernhardt, C.R. (2009). Closing the gap between oral hygiene and minimally invasive dentistry: A review on the resin infiltration technique of incipient (proximal) enamel lesions. *Quintessence Int.* 40 (8): 663–681.

29 Martignon, S., Tellez, M., Santamaría, R.M., Gomez, J., and Ekstrand, K.R. (2010). Sealing distal proximal caries lesions in first primary molars: Efficacy after 2.5 years. *Caries Res.* 44 (6): 562–570. doi: 10.1159/000321986. Epub 2010 Nov 19. PMID: 21088401. .

30 Da Costa-Silva, C.M., Ambrosano, G.M., Jeremias, F., De Souza, J.F., and Mialhe, F.L. (2011). Increase in severity of molar-incisor hypomineralization and its relationship with the colour of enamel opacity: A prospective cohort study. *Int. J. Paediatr. Dent.* 25: 333–341. doi: 10.1111/j.1365-263x.2011.01128.

31 Nogueira, V.K.C., Soares, I.P.M., Fragelli, C.M.B., Boldieri, T., Manton, D.J., Bussaneli, D.G., and Cordeiro, R.C.L. (2021). Structural integrity of MIH-affected teeth after treatment with fluoride varnish or resin infiltration: An 18-Month randomized clinical trial. *J. Dent.* 105: 103570. ISSN 0300-5712. doi: 10.1016/j.jdent.2020.103570.

32 Peumans, M., De Munck, J., Mine, A., and Van Meerbeek, B. (2014). Clinical effectiveness of contemporary adhesives for the restoration of non-carious cervical lesions. A systematic review. *Dent. Mater.* 30: 1089–1103. doi: 10.1016/j.dental.2014.07.007. Epub 2014 Aug 3. PMID: 25091726.

33 Peters, M.C., Bresciani, E., Barata, T.J., Fagundes, T.C., Navarro, R.L., Navarro, M.F., and Dickens, S.H. (2010). In vivo dentin remineralization by calcium-phosphate cement. *J. Dent. Res.* 89: 286–291.

34 Bjorndal, L., Larsen, T., and Thylstrup, A. (1997). A clinical and microbiological study of deep carious lesions during stepwise excavation using long treatment intervals. *Caries Res.* 31: 411–417.

35 Ribeiro, C.C., Baratieri, L.N., Perdigao, J., Baratieri, N.M., and Ritter, A.V. (1999). A clinical, radiographic, and scanning electron microscopic evaluation of adhesive restorations on carious dentin in primary teeth. *Quintessence Int.* 30: 591–599.

36 Massara, M.L., Alves, J.B., and Brandao, P.R. (2002). Atraumatic restorative treatment: Clinical, ultrastructural and chemical analysis. *Caries Res.* 36: 430–436.

37 Santiago, B.M., Ventin, D.A., Primo, L.G., and Barcelos, R. (2005). Microhardness of dentine underlying ART restorations in primary molars: An in vivo pilot study. *BDJ* 199: 103–106.

38 Ngo, H.C., Mount, G., Mc Intyre, J., Tuisuva, J., and Von Doussa, R.J. (2006). Chemical exchange between glass-ionomer restorations and residual carious dentine in permanent molars: An *in vivo* study. *J. Dent.* 34: 608–613.

39 Zain, S., Davis, G.R., Hill, R., Anderson, P., and Baysan, A. (2020). Mineral exchange within restorative materials following incomplete carious lesion removal using 3D non-destructive XMT subtraction methodology. *J. Dent.* 99: 103389. doi: 10.1016/j.jdent. 2020.103389. Epub 2020 May 31. PMID: 32492503.

40 van Loveren, C., and Duggal, M.S. (2001). The role of diet in caries prevention. *Int. Dent. J.* 51 (6 Suppl 1): 399–406.

41 Oong, E.M., Griffin, S.O., Kohn, W.G., Gooch, B.F., and Caufield, P.W. (2008). The effect of dental sealants on bacteria levels in caries lesions: A review of the evidence. *J. Am. Dent. Assoc.* 139: 271–278, quiz 357–8.

42 Peumans, M., Kanumilli, P., De Munck, J., Van Landuyt, K., Lambrechts, P., and Van Meerbeek, B. (2005). Clinical effectiveness of contemporary adhesives: A systematic review of current clinical trials. *Dent. Mater.* 21: 864–881.

43 Mickenautsch, S., Yengopal, V., and Banerjee, A. (2010). Atraumatic restorative treatment versus amalgam restoration longevity: A systematic review. *Clin. Oral Investig.* 14: 233–240.

44 Ritter, A.V. (2008). Posterior composites revisited. *J. Esthet. Restor. Dent.* 20: 57–67.

45 Bennett, A. (2009). Emerging technologies for diagnosis of dental caries: The road so far. *J. Appl. Phys.* 105: 102047, 0021-8979/2009/10510/102047/9.

46 Foros, P., Oikonomou, E., Koletsi, D., and Rahiotis, C. (2021). Detection methods for early caries diagnosis: A systematic review and meta-analysis. *Caries Res.* 55 (4): 247–259. doi: 10.1159/000516084. Epub 2021 Jun 15. PMID: 34130279.

47 de Souza, L.A., Cancio, V., and Tostes, M.A. (2018 July). Accuracy of pen-type laser fluorescence device and radiographic methods in detecting approximal carious lesions in primary teeth – an *in vivo* study. *Int. J. Paediatr. Dent.* 28: 472–480.

48 Peskersoy, C., Turkun, M., and Onal, B. (2015). Comparative clinical evaluation of the efficacy of a new method for caries diagnosis and excavation. *J. Conserv. Dent.* 18: 364–368. doi: 10.4103/0972-0707.164032. PMID: 26430298; PMCID: PMC4578179.

49 Tassery, H., Levallois, B., Terrer, E., Manton, D., Otsuki, M., Koubi, S., Gugnani, N., Panayotov, I., Jacquot, B., Cuisinier, F., and Rechmann, P. (2013). Use of new minimum intervention dentistry technologies in caries management. *Aust. Dent. J.* 58: 40–59. doi: 10.1111/adj.12049.

50 Lopes, G.C., Vieira, L.C., and Araujo, E. (2004). Direct composite resin restorations: A review of some clinical procedures to achieve predictable results in posterior teeth. *J. Esthet. Restor. Dent.* 16 (1): 19–31, discussion 2.

51 Gurgan, S., Kutuk, Z.B., Ergin, E., Oztas, S.S., and Cakir, F.Y. (2015). Four-year randomized clinical trial to evaluate the clinical performance of a glass ionomer restorative system. *Oper. Dent.* 40 (2): 134–143.

52 Macedo, G., Raj, V., and Ritter, A.V. (2006). Longevity of anterior composite restorations. *J. Esthet. Restor. Dent.* 18 (6): 310–311.

53 Peumans, M., Van Meerbeek, B., Lambrechts, P., and Vanherle, G. (1997). The 5-year clinical performance of direct composite additions to correct tooth form and position. I. Esthetic qualities. *Clin. Oral Investig.* 1 (1): 12–18.

54 Dietschi, D., Ardu, S., and Krejci, I. (2006). A new shading concept based on natural tooth color applied to direct composite restorations. *Quintessence Int.* 37 (2): 91–102.

55 Magne, P., and So, W.S. (2008). Optical integration of incisoproximal restorations using the natural layering concept. *Quintessence Int.* 39 (8): 633–643.

56 Dietschi, D. (2008). Optimizing smile composition and esthetics with resin composites and other conservative esthetic procedures. *Eur. J. Esthet. Dent.* 3 (1): 14–29.

57 Wolff, D., Kraus, T., Schach, C., Pritsch, M., Mente, J., Staehle, H.J., and Ding, P. (2010). Recontouring teeth and closing diastemas with direct composite buildups: A clinical evaluation of survival and quality parameters. *J. Dent.* 38 (12): 1001–1009.

58 Summitt, J., Robbins, J., Hilton, T., Schwartz, R., and Santos, J. (2006). *Fundamentals of Operative Dentistry: A Contemporary Approach.* Illinois, USA: Quintessence Books.

59 Dietschi, D., Ardu, S., and Krejci, I. (2000). *Exploring the Layering Concepts for Anterior Teeth.* JF IR, M D, editors. Berlin: Quintessence Publishing.

60 Dietschi, D. (1997). Free-hand bonding in the esthetic treatment of anterior teeth: Creating the illusion. *J. Esthet. Dent.* 9 (4): 156–164.

61 Dietschi, D. (1995). Free-hand composite resin restorations: A key to anterior aesthetics. *Pract. Periodontics Aesthet. Dent.* 7 (7): 15–25, quiz 7.

62 Dietschi, D. (2001). Layering concepts in anterior composite restorations. *J. Adhes. Dent.* 3 (1): 71–80.

63 Samorodnitzky-Naveh, G.R., Geiger, S.B., and Levin, L. (2007). Patients' satisfaction with dental esthetics. *J. Am. Dent. Assoc.* 138 (6): 805–808.

64 Joiner, A. (2006). The bleaching of teeth: A review of the literature. *J. Dent.* 34 (7): 412–419.

65 Patil, A.G., Hiremath, V., Kumar, R.S., Sheetal, A., and Nagaral, S. (2014). Bleaching of a non-vital anterior tooth to remove the intrinsic discoloration. *J. Nat. Sci. Biol. Med.* 5 (2): 476–479.

66 Kugel, G., and Ferreira, S. (2005). The art and science of tooth whitening. *J. Mass Dent. Soc.* 53 (4): 34–37.

67 Kihn, P.W. (2007). Vital tooth whitening. *Dent. Clin. N. Am.* 51 (2): 319–331, viii.

68 Burke, F.J., Kelleher, M.G., Wilson, N., and Bishop, K. (2011). Introducing the concept of pragmatic esthetics, with special reference to the treatment of tooth wear. *J. Esthet. Restor. Dent.* 23 (5): 277–293.

69 Meyers, I.A. (2008). Diagnosis and management of the worn dentition: Conservative restorative options. *Ann. R. Australas Coll. Dent. Surg.* 19: 31–34.

70 Dietschi, D., and Argente, A. (2011). A comprehensive and conservative approach for the restoration of abrasion and erosion. part II: Clinical procedures and case report. *Eur. J. Esthet. Dent.* 6 (2): 142–159.

71 Dietschi, D., and Argente, A. (2011). A comprehensive and conservative approach for the restoration of abrasion and erosion. Part I: Concepts and clinical rationale for early intervention using adhesive techniques. *Eur. J. Esthet. Dent.* 6 (1): 20–33.

72 Zero, D.T., and Lussi, A. (2005). Erosion–chemical and biological factors of importance to the dental practitioner. *Int. Dent. J.* 55 (4 Suppl 1): 285–290.

73 Milosevic, A., and Burnside, G. (2016 January). The survival of direct composite restorations in the management of severe tooth wear including attrition and erosion: A prospective 8-year study. *J. Dent.* 44: 13–19. doi: 10.1016/j.jdent.2015.10.015. Epub 2015 Nov 2. PMID: 26542166.

74 Milosevic, A. (2014). The survival of zirconia based crowns (Lava™) in the management of severe anterior tooth wear up to 7-years follow-up. *Oral Biol. Dent.* 2: 9. doi: 10.7243/2053-5775-2-9.

75 Thiebot, N., Hamdani, A., Blanchet, F., Dame, M., Tawfik, S., Mbapou, E., Ali Kaddouh, A., and Alantar, A. (2022). Implant failure rate and the prevalence of associated risk factors: A 6-year retrospective observational survey. *J. Oral Med. Oral Surg.* 28 (2): 19. doi: 10.1051/mbcb/2021045.

76 Setzer, F.C., and Kim, S. (2014). Comparison of long-term survival of implants and endodontically treated teeth. *J. Dent. Res.* 93: 19–26. doi: 10.1177/0022034513504782. Epub 2013 Sep 24. PMID: 24065635; PMCID: PMC3872851.

77 Burke, F.J., and Shortall, A.C. (2001). Successful restoration of load-bearing cavities in posterior teeth with direct-replacement resin-based composite. *Dent. Update* 28: 388–398.

78 Lynch, C.D., Opdam, N.J., Hickel, R., Brunton, P.A., Gurgan, S., Kakaboura, A., Shearer, A.C., Vanherle, G., and Wilson, N. (2014). Guidance on posterior resin composites: Academy of operative dentistry – European Section. *J. Dent.* 42 (4): 377–383. ISSN 0300-5712. doi: 10.1016/j.jdent.2014.01.009.

79 Howe, D.F., and Denehy, G.E. (1977). Anterior fixed partial dentures utilizing the acid-etch technique and a cast metal framework. *J. Prosthet. Dent.* 37: 28–31.

80 St George, G., Hemmings, K., and Patel, K. (2002). Resin-retained bridges re-visited. Part 1. History and indications. *Prim. Dent. Care* 9: 87–91.

81 Durey, K., Nixon, P., Robinson, S., and Chan, M.F. (2011). Resin bonded bridges: Techniques for success. *Br. Dent. J.* 211: 113–118. doi: 10.1038/sj.bdj.2011.619.

82 Djemal, S., Setchell, D., King, P., and Wickens, J. (1999 April). Long-term survival characteristics of 832 resin-retained bridges and splints provided in a post-graduate teaching hospital between 1978 and 1993. *J. Oral Rehabil.* 26 (4): 302–320. doi: 10.1046/j.1365-2842.1999.00374.x. PMID: 10232858.

83 Pjetursson, B.E., Tan, W.C., Tan, K., Bragger, U., Zwahlen, M., and Lang, N.P. (2008). A systematic review of the survival and complication rates of resin-bonded bridges after an observation period of at least 5 years. *Clin. Oral Implants Res.* 19: 131–141.

84 Pjetursson, B.E., Bragger, U., Lang, N.P., and Zwahlen, M. (2007). Comparison of survival and complication rates of tooth-supported fixed dental prostheses (FDPs) and implant-supported FDPs and single crowns (SCs). *Clin. Oral Implants Res.* 18 (Suppl 3): 97–113.

85 Burke, T. (2008). Resin-retained bridges: Fibre reinforced versus metal. *Dent. Update* 35: 521–526.

86 Pospiech, P., Rammelsberg, P., Goldhofer, G., and Gernet, W. (1996). All-ceramic resin-bonded bridges. A 3-dimensional finite-element analysis study. *Eur. J. Oral Sci.* 104: 390–395.

87 Patsiatzi, E., and Grey, N.J. (2004). An investigation of aspects of design of resin-bonded bridges in general dental practice and hospital services. *Prim. Dent. Care* 11: 87–89.

88 Mjor, I.A., Moorhead, J.E., and Dahl, J.E. (2000). Reasons for replacement of restorations in permanent teeth in general dental practice. *Int. Dent. J.* 50 (6): 361–366.

89 Deligeorgi, V., Wilson, N.H., Fouzas, D., Kouklaki, E., Burke, F.J., and Mjor, I.A. (2000). Reasons for placement and replacement of restorations in student clinics in Manchester and Athens. *Eur. J. Dent. Educ.* 4 (4): 153–159.

90 Gordan, V.V., Garvan, C.W., Blaser, P.K., Mondragon, E., and Mjor, I.A. (2009). A long-term evaluation of alternative treatments to replacement of resin-based composite restorations: Results of a seven-year study. *J. Am. Dent. Assoc.* 140 (12): 1476–1484.

91 Fernandez, E.M., Martin, J.A., Angel, P.A., Mjor, I.A., Gordan, V.V., and Moncada, G.A. (2011). Survival rate of sealed, refurbished and repaired defective restorations: 4-year follow-up. *Braz. Dent. J.* 22 (2): 134–139.

92 Moncada, G., Martin, J., Fernandez, E., Hempel, M.C., Mjor, I.A., and Gordan, V.V. (2009). Sealing, refurbishment and repair of Class I and Class II defective restorations: A three-year clinical trial. *J. Am. Dent. Assoc.* 140 (4): 425–432.

93 Mjor, I.A. (1993). Repair versus replacement of failed restorations. *Int. Dent. J.* 43: 466–472.

94 Setcos, J.C., Khosravi, R., Wilson, N.H., Shen, C., Yang, M., and Mjor, I.A. (2004). Repair or replacement of amalgam restorations: Decisions at a USA and a UK dental school. *Oper. Dent.* 29: 392–397.

95 Gordan, V.V., Riley, J.L., 3rd, Blaser, P.K., Mondragon, E., Garvan, C.W., and Mjor, I.A. (2011). Alternative treatments to replacement of defective amalgam restorations: Results of a seven-year clinical study. *J. Am. Dent. Assoc.* 142: 842–849.

96 Gordan, V.V., Garvan, C.W., Richman, J.S., Fellows, J.L., Rindal, D.B., Qvist, V., Heft, M.W., Williams, O.D., Gilbert, G.H., and DPBRN Collaborative Group. (2009). How dentists diagnose and treat defective restorations: Evidence from the dental practice-based research network. *Oper. Dent.* 34: 664–673.

8

Dental Materials and Their Clinical Implications in Minimally Invasive Dentistry

Saroash Shahid and Robert Hill

Key Topics

- Concept of remineralization
- Role of remineralization in minimally invasive dentistry
- Concept of bioactive glasses for dental applications

Learning Objectives

- Be able to critically analyse the remineralizing properties of currently available restorative materials
- Be able to understand the concept behind bioactive glasses
- Be able to understand the concept behind the development of fluoride containing bioactive glasses
- Be able to understand the clinical advantages of using fluoride-containing bioactive glasses

Introduction

The minimally invasive approach in treating dental caries incorporates the dental science of detecting, diagnosing, intercepting and treating dental caries at the microscopic level. This approach has evolved from an increased understanding of the caries process and the development of adhesive and biomimetic restorative materials. With minimally invasive dentistry, dental caries is treated as an infectious condition rather than an end product of it. Now no longer radical 'extension for prevention' is practiced but has changed to 'constriction with conviction'.

Minimally Invasive Dentistry: Interdisciplinary Clinical and Scientific Approaches, First Edition.
Edited by Aylin Baysan and Paul Anderson.
© 2026 John Wiley & Sons Ltd. Published 2026 by John Wiley & Sons Ltd.
Companion website: www.wiley.com/go/baysan/minimally_invasive_dentistry

In order to develop a dental restorative for minimally invasive dentistry, it must fulfil the following criteria:

- Control the disease through the reduction of cariogenic flora.
- Remineralize early lesions.
- Perform minimal intervention surgical procedures, as/when required.

Glass Ionomer Cements and the Atraumatic Restorative Treatment (ART)

Frenken and co-workers pioneered the atraumatic restorative treatment (ART). Glass ionomer cements (GICs) are the material of choice for ART for a number of reasons including they set by an acid-base reaction and no polymerization is involved, there is no polymerization shrinkage and providing there is no shrinkage to water loss, they exhibit good marginal adaptation and no marginal gaps. High-viscosity GICs are recommended for ART to give improved mechanical properties. If the concentration and molar mass of the polyacid in a GIC are increased, their viscosity increases and more importantly their strength and fracture toughness. In addition, GICs release fluoride, which has a well-documented anticaries role. The fluoride can be exchanged for hydroxyl ions in hydroxyapatite in the adjacent enamel and dentine forming much more acid-durable fluorapatite.

Table 8.1 gives the chemical composition of five commercial glasses used in GICs. Whilst GICs release fluoride they contain very little phosphorus as can be seen from Table 8.1 and they are thus not capable of releasing much orthophosphate.

An ideal GIC for ART would not only release fluoride but also release calcium and orthophosphate ions, form fluorapatite, and have the potential to remineralize any hard carious dentine left after ART restoration. In the vicinity of carious lesions, calcium and phosphate are not likely to be readily available since tertiary/reparative dentine is likely to form, and this has a random orientation of dentinal tubules. Consequently, dentinal fluid containing calcium and phosphate required for remineralization is unlikely to be able to diffuse through the dentinal tubules to the carious lesion. This means that in order for a GIC to have a remineralization effect, the calcium and phosphate must come from the GIC. It might seem that a simple solution to this would be to increase the amount of phosphate

Table 8.1 Chemical composition of typical ionomer glasses in atomic percent.

Glass	Al	Si	P	Ca	O	F	Sr	La	Na
Fuji IX	0.129	0.115	0.017	0.000	0.547	0.126	0.056	0	0.010
G2	0.140	0.158	0.011	0.038	0.528	0.192	0.000	0	0.058
G338	0.131	0.098	0.030	0.041	0.536	0.143	0	0	0.055
G2SR	0.168	0.106	0.027	0.031	0.567	0.061	0.061	0	0.007
Molar	0.104	0.104	0.015	0.060	0.515	0.163	0	0.043	0.021

in the ionomer glass composition. Dupree et al. showed that phosphate in alumino-silicates systems exists as $AlPO_7$ species (Dupree et al. 1989). High phosphate content may give rise to more metastable Al—O—P linkages within the glass network, which makes Al(IV) unavailable for PAA crosslinking (Zainuddin et al. 2012).

It was believed by Griffin and Hill (2000) that phosphate content in fluoro-alumino-silicate glasses will influence GIC setting properties because P5+ competes with Al^{3+} and Ca^{2+} for COO− groups. However, it is now understood that Al—O—P linkages within the network are not hydrolysable, and as such aluminium charge balanced by phosphorus does not take part in the GIC setting reaction. Griffin and Hill (2000) found that low phosphate content is beneficial in that it extends working and setting times of the cements and also observed small improvements in compressive strength with low phosphate glasses. Griffin and Hill (2000) also concluded that glasses higher in phosphate excessively disrupt the crosslinking process in the cement by competing with metal ions for carboxylate groups and also observed significant reduction of compressive strength and Young's moduli and increase in working and setting times of the cement pastes.

Many research groups have focused on enhancing the remineralization potential of GICs through the incorporation of various remineralizing agents such apatite, amorphous calcium phosphate and bioactive glasses. However, the addition of various agents to promote the remineralization potential has always come at the expense of sustaining clinically acceptable physical and mechanical properties (Ana et al. 2003; Choi et al. 2008; De Caluwe et al. 2016).

Moshaverinia is a modified commercial GIC by the addition of nanoparticles of HAp and FAp. This resulted in an improved compressive strength (Moshaverinia et al. 2008). Lucas et al. (2001) also reported an increase in fracture toughness of the tested GICs upon the incorporation of HAp.

Another model was examined by Zainuddin et al. (2012), who looked at the commercial product Glass Carbomer® (produced by GCP, Netherlands), that was deliberately designed to promote remineralization to FAp in the mouth. The production of this material has discontinued. Glass Carbomer contained nanocrystals of calcium hydroxyfluoroapatite, which was claimed to act as a nucleus for the remineralization process. The study suggested that the apatite present in the Glass Carbomer is a mixture of HAp and FAp. 31P MAS-NMR spectra showed that the peak intensity of crystalline calcium orthophosphate (apatite) gradually decreased after 10 months; this indicates HAp was consumed in the setting reaction. Thus, less apatite is available to promote remineralization.

ACP has been incorporated into ionomer cements as a filler. Taking the advantage of ACP to release calcium and phosphate. This release was observed to be more in an acidic environment. CPP-ACP has been investigated as a highly promising anticariogenic agent. CPP is a group of peptides that have been shown to stabilize calcium and phosphate preserving them in amorphous calcium phosphate. In a study that modified GIC through the incorporation of CPP-ACP and tested the effect on shear bond strength to demineralized dentine, the results revealed that CPP-ACP did not negatively affect adhesion (Zhao et al. 2017). It is critical to note that these results were obtained under controlled laboratory conditions that do not exactly mimic clinical situations.

Hill et al. (2004) have highlighted the synergistic role of strontium in aiding the remineralization process. Strontium was found to substitute for calcium ions and form strontium fluorapatite Sr (FAp).

It can be seen that some of them including Fuji IX contain strontium, which is largely added to confer radio-opacity. In the case of Fuji IX, there is no significant calcium. However Sr^{2+} exhibits complete solid solution phase behaviour in apatites and replaces Ca^{2+} ions in the apatite lattice. In addition, strontium has an antibacterial effect (Huang et al. 2016) and can also upregulate odontoblasts to produce tertiary dentine (Sriranganathan et al. 2016). Other glasses used to form GICs have lanthanum or barium to confer radio-opacity; however, these have no potent.

Bioactive Dental Composites

Two composites, Cention N (by Ivoclar) and Activa Restorative (by PulpDent), have been launched that claim remineralization. In addition, this a growing and active area of research.

Cention N

Cention N is a self-cure composite resin. The organic, monomer part of Cention N consists of four different dimethacrylates, which comprise approximately 20% by weight of the final mixed material. A combination of UDMA, DCP, an aromatic aliphatic-UDMA and PEG-400 DMA which cross-links during polymerization results in strong mechanical properties and good long-term stability. Cention N does not contain Bis-GMA, HEMA or TEGDMA. The remaining 80% by weight consists of three glasses plus Yterbium fluoride and a stress-relieving filler. The first glass is a chemically conventional inert barium boro-alumino-silicate glass, the second is an ionomer glass of the type used in GICs and the third is a degradable calcium fluorosilicate containing glass, which is similar to bioactive glasses discussed later but contains no phosphate. This third glass degrades by an ion-exchange process with H^+ ions from the external medium being exchanged for Ca^{2+} ions, which results in a reduction in the H^+ ion concentration and an increasing pH that is claimed to inhibit acidophyllic bacteria associated with caries. The alkaline calcium fluorosilicate glass accounts for 24.6% in weight of the final material and the manufacturer claims this glass releases substantial levels of fluoride (F−) ions —comparable to those released by traditional glass ionomers.

The manufacturers claim the release of ions from Cention N depends on the pH value in the oral cavity. When the pH value is low (acidic), due for example to an active plaque biofilm, Cention N releases a significantly larger amount of ions than when the pH value is neutral. Thus Cention N is a smart material that responds to its chemical environment. In this behaviour the calcium fluorosilicate glass behaves like bioactive glasses and bioactive glass composites.

Tiskaya et al. (2019) noted that Cention N released more therapeutic ions in artificial saliva and formed an apatite-like phase. The authors concluded that Cention N has bioactive properties that may explain the low incidence of secondary caries found clinically with this composite resin.

Activa Bioactive

The technical brochure on the Activa Bioactive materials provides little exact information on the composition and in particular the type or composition of the glass used in these products. Apatite formation is the essential requirement of bioactive materials. It is claimed ACTIVA stimulates mineral apatite formation and the natural remineralization process that knits the restoration and the tooth. The technical description of Activa and the one published paper leads us to believe the glass in Activa is a bioactive glass of the type first developed by Larry Hench. These glasses are based on the SiO_2–P_2O_5–CaO–Na_2O system and dissolve in body fluids and form apatite. However, we suspect the glass used is an ionomer glass. The Activa composite is claimed to form fluorapatite; however, work done by Tiskaya et al. (2019) demonstrated that Activa does not form apatite and thus its ability to remineralize is questionable.

Bioactive Glass as Remineralizing Agent

Hench and co-workers first developed bioactive glasses in the late 60s (Hench, 2006). A bioactive glass dissolves or degrades in physiological-like fluids and forms hydroxycarbonated apatite. They were originally developed as bone substitutes, but in the last fifteen years they have been increasingly used as an additive in remineralizing hypersensitivity toothpastes (Greenspan 2010; Earl et al. 2010, 2011a, 2011b; Gillam et al. 2002). The glass compositions are based on SiO_2–P_2O_5–CaO–Na_2O system. Some typical bioactive glass compositions are given in Table 8.2.

The mechanism of BAG degradation described by Hench (2006) starts with the hydrolysis of the glass with the subsequent rapid cation exchange of Na^+ and/or Ca^{2+} cations from BAG with the H^+ or H_3O^+ protons from the solution. Local pH rises consequently due to the accumulation of hydroxyl ions (OH−), resulting in the alkaline hydrolysis of Si—O—Si and the formation of silanol groups (SiOH) at the glass surface. Subsequently, a cation-depleted silica-rich layer forms on the glass surface because of rearrangement by polycondensation of adjacent silanols. Phosphate is also leached from the glass. The Ca^{2+} and PO_4^{3-} migrate back from the solution to the silica-rich layer forming an amorphous calcium phosphate CaO–P_2O_5 (CaP) film. This film of CaP begins to crystallize through the incorporation of hydroxide (OH−) and carbonate (CO_3^{2-}) groups to form HAp (Hench et al. 2004; Jones 2013).

Table 8.2 Bioactive glass compositions in mole percent.

Glass	SiO$_2$	P$_2$O$_5$	CaO	Na$_2$O	K$_2$O	MgO	CaF$_2$	SrF$_2$	NC
45S5	46.1	2.6	26.9	24.4			0		2.11
53P4	54	2.0	22	23			0		2.56
BioMinF	40.2	5.25	29.5	23.25			1.8		2.16
45S5F	46.1	2.6	16.9	24.4			10		2.55

Hill questioned this mechanism and developed a network connectivity NC model for predicting the dissolution and apatite-forming ability of bioactive glasses (Hill 1996).

This model treats bioactive glasses as polymers based on silicon. In a pure SiO_2 glass, each silicon is linked via a bridging oxygen (an Si—O—Si) to four other silicons and the network connectivity is four. In a calcium metasilicate glass containing equimolar ratios of CaO and SiO_2, each CaO introduces two non-bridging oxygens (Si—O$^-$) breaking up the three-dimensional network. Each silicon is now linked to only two other silicons and the NC = 2. The glass corresponds to a linear silicate chain and may be considered a silicate polymer of $[SiO_3^{2-}]_n$. Crystalline calcium metasilicate known as Wollastonite in fact consists of such linear silicate chains. Reducing the CaO content results in the NC increasing beyond 2 and the polymeric chains become increasingly cross-linked. Based on this concept, dissolution and bioactivity would be expected to be highly dependent on the NC and a sharp cut off in bioactivity would be expected at an NC of 2.0. Practically dissolution and bioactivity often extend above an NC of 2.0 towards a cut-off value of 2.4.

The NC model predicted the bioactivity and apatite-forming ability quite well but did not work well for glasses with higher phosphate contents than the 45S5 glass or compositions containing MgO or ZnO. One of the problems in calculating NC is structural assumptions about the role of the various oxides that have to be made. In the original model it was assumed that the phosphate formed Si—O—P bonds; however, O'Donnell et al. (2008a, 2008b, 2009) showed the phosphorus formed orthophosphate (PO_4^{3-}) locally charge balanced by Ca^{2+} and Na^+ ions and was thus not part of the silicate network.

In such glasses, the modified NC' is given by (Hill and Brauer 2011):

$$NC' = \left(\left[SiO_2 \right] \times 4 - 2 \times \text{sum of} \left[NMO \right] + 6 \times \left[P_2O_5 \right] \right) / \left[SiO_2 \right]$$

Eden developed his split network model the values which correspond exactly to those for the modified NC' (Edén, 2011).

O'Donnell et al. (2008a, 2008b, 2009) investigated the structural role of phosphate in bioactive glasses and the influence of phosphate on the physical properties dissolution behaviour and ability of the glasses to form an apatite in simulated body fluid (SBF). Phosphorus was shown to exist as orthophosphate and when the phosphate content was increased, whilst maintaining a fixed network connectivity by adding additional CaO and Na_2O, the time to form an apatite-like phase decreased and the amount of apatite increased. Eden (2011) also demonstrated the importance of phosphate content and stated 'as long as phosphorus remains predominantly as orthophosphate and the average silicate network-polymerization is favorable, the bioactivity enhances monotonically for increasing phosphorus content of the Bioactive Glass'.

Hill and co-workers developed strontium-containing bioactive glasses by replacing Ca by Sr (Fredholm et al. 2010, 2012; Gentlemen et al. 2010; Lotfibakhshaiesh et al. 2011). The initial glasses developed had a low phosphate content and it was found that strontium expanded the glass network resulting in faster degradation and dissolution of the glass as well as faster apatite formation. Structural neutron scattering studies (Martin et al. 2012) later confirmed this as well as molecular dynamics simulations (Xiang and Du 2011). Strontium lies below Ca in Group II of the periodic table and exhibits complete solid substitution for calcium in all apatites (O'Donnell et al. 2008c) Strontium up-regulates osteoblasts down-regulates osteoclasts and being of high atomic number confers radio-opacity. Strontium has a mild anticaries role and is thought to have a synergistic action with fluoride in preventing caries (Curzon et al. 1978; Thuy et al. 2008; Liu et al. 2016a). Strontium is also bacteriocidal and recent studies indicate it inhibits the growth of the microbes involved in periodontal disease (Huang et al. 2016).

Recently it has also been shown that strontium up-regulates odontoblasts (Sriranganathan et al. 2016). High strontium contents in high phosphate bioactive glasses however inhibit apatite formation, probably because the hydroxyapatite forms below pH 9 via an octacalcium phosphate precursor phase (Brown et al. 1987; Chow and Eanes 2001) and only small amounts of strontium can replace Ca and be incorporated in OCP. However, in the presence of fluoride, apatite forms directly without going via OCP, and where fluoride is present in bioactive glasses, strontium does not suppress apatite formation (Sriranganathan et al. 2017).

Original Studies by Hench and Spilman on Incorporating Fluoride

Hench and Spilman (1988) first incorporated fluoride into the original 45S5 Bioglass composition substituting CaF_2 for CaO and Na_2O. At first sight these substitutions appear logical and it is important to note that in the 1970s solid-state NMR was not readily available for either ^{29}Si, ^{31}P or ^{19}F. However as this would be seen later, if the F forms F—Ca/Na(n) complexes, these substitutions will result in an increase in network connectivity of the glass with a resulting reduction in the degradability of the glass and a consequent retardation of its ability to form apatite. Hench and Spilman also failed to consider that on adding fluoride, fluorapatite might form instead of hydroxyapatite. Since these two forms are almost impossible to distinguish from each other by XRD or FTIR and are only readily distinguishable by ^{19}F solid-state NMR this is not surprising. The group based in Modena in Italy published a number of studies (Lusvardi et al. 2009a, 2009b; Pedone et al. 2009; Cocchi et al. 2012) looking at the same glass compositions studied by Hench and Spilman but again failed to recognize that these compositions might form fluorapatite or a fluoridated apatite.

New Fluoride-Containing Bioactive Glasses

Brauer et al. (2009) also investigated fluoride-containing bioactive glasses and showed using ^{19}F Magic Angle Spinning Nuclear Magnetic Resonance (MAS-NMR) that the fluorine was complexed largely by calcium/sodium and formed F—M(n) species where M is Ca or Na and n is 3/4. In contrast to the previous studies, Brauer et al. (2009) added CaF_2, rather than substituting it for CaO. Substituting CaO with CaF_2 as seen Hench and Spilman's research would result in a reduction in the non-bridging oxygen content and a more cross-linked glass with a higher network connectivity that would dissolve and form apatite much more slowly or not at all. Brauer et al. confirmed that the silicon Q speciation in the glass structure and the NC did not change when CaF_2 was added. Brauer et al. (2010) subsequently investigated the dissolution behaviour and *in vitro* bioactivity of low phosphate content glasses on adding CaF_2. The glasses formed fluorapatite for CaF_2 contents <5 mol% and released fluoride in addition to Ca^{2+} and PO_4^{3-} ions. However above 5 mol%, the glasses formed fluorite at the expense of fluorapatite. These glasses with their low phosphate content were not commercially attractive because of the relatively small amounts of fluorapatite formed and the relatively long time to form apatite. Pedone et al. (2012) confirmed Brauer et al.'s fluorine speciation and the absence of Si—F bonds using more advanced solid-state NMR techniques including REDOR. Christie et al. (2011) carried out molecular dynamics simulations of fluoride-containing bioactive glass (BGs) and confirmed the fluorine speciation found by Brauer et al. (2009).

Brauer et al. (2011) also modelled the density of their fluoride-containing glasses successfully using a modified Doweidar model. However, density data on the original Spilman and Hench glasses from Modena was not successfully modelled suggesting loss of fluorine during melting. Fluorine analysis of the Brauer et al.'s (Brauer et al. 2009) composition indicated only small amounts of fluorine were being lost.

Attempts were made to produce high phosphate bioactive glasses with fluoride, but problems were encountered with crystallization of the compositions. However, Mneimne et al. (2011) subsequently investigated the role of fluoride in amorphous high phosphate content bioactive glasses of fixed network connectivity. The fluoride-containing glasses with <9 mol% CaF_2 formed fluorapatite within six hours. Lynch et al. (2012) showed a similar behaviour in more multicomponent glasses containing strontium.

The optimum CaF_2 concentration was found to be in the range 5–7 mol%, i.e. fluorite formation was suppressed slightly by a higher phosphate content in the glass (Liu et al. 2016b). Mneimne et al.'s studies were the foundation for the development of the BioMinF composition used in the toothpaste. Mneimne et al. also produced one sodium-free bioactive glass (QMMM7/CF9). This glass partially crystallized to fluorapatite during quenching and is the basis of the low or zero sodium-containing glasses for incorporating into resin matrices and for low sodium glasses that can be used for air abrasion cutting of enamel (Farooq et al. 2013). The lower sodium content results in a glass with a higher T_g and an increased hardness that is more efficient for cutting enamel. The glasses developed for this purpose had a reduced CaF_2 content (3 mol%) compared to the 9 mol% CaF_2 content in the QMMM9 composition to suppress the crystallization to fluorapatite on cooling in order to facilitate obtaining an amorphous glass. The QMMM7/H2 composition recoded as CF9 is also the glass composition used by Caluwe et al. (2016) in their studies that incorporating bioactive glass into GICs that they demonstrated was more bioactive than the 45S5 composition despite it crystallizes partially to fluorapatite.

Sol=Gel Fluoride-Containing Bioactive Glasses

Recently Mitchell and co-workers have investigated SiO_2—CaO—CaF_2—P_2O_5 bioactive sol-gel glasses incorporated into resin matrices (Dupree et al. 1989; Griffin and Hill 2000; Moshaverinia et al. 2008; Zainuddin et al. 2012; Orala et al. 2014; Vallittu et al. 2015; Zhao et al. 2017). They used tetraethyl orthosilane, calcium alkoxide and triethylphosphate as precursors for their sol-gel glasses. Tetraethyl orthosilane is an expensive precursor and calcium alkoxide and triethyl phosphate are not readily available and even more costly to synthesize. In their studies, it is not clear in what form the fluoride is incorporated into these sol-gel glasses. Table 8.2 gives some of the nominal compositions they produced. Unfortunately, there were no or very limited data on the dissolution rate, ion release kinetics and ability of these glasses to form apatite. Instead, this group largely bypassed these studies and directly incorporated the glasses into resin composites. Furthermore, there was no chemical analysis of the glass compositions post synthesis.

One of these glasses supplied by this group has been characterized by ^{19}F MAS-NMR and ^{31}P MAS-NMR at QMUL. No ^{19}F signal could be detected initially and the sample had to be run overnight for 20 hours to get a sufficiently low S/N and a reasonable quality spectrum. From the S/N it is reckoned the CaF_2 content is <<0.1 mol% compared to the original 3 mol%. The F in the glass reacts with silanol groups (Si—OH) in the sol-gel glass during processing to give volatile hydrofluoric acid (HF). As will be seen later, this explains the low fluoride release of the composite resins.

As a result of the large fluoride loss, the high cost of precursors and the long and complex synthesis process, these sol-gel glasses pose no competitive threat.

Marivalda and co-workers (2017) have put CaF_2 into sol-gel glasses; however, NMR shows the fluorine to be present after processing as a crystalline CaF_2 which is insoluble, consequently these glasses also do not release fluoride and do not form fluorapatite upon dissolution even though they have retained the fluoride.

Chloride-Containing Bioactive Glasses

Chloride-containing BGs are the most recently developed BGs (Chen et al. 2015, 2017; Swansbury et al. 2017). They are the basis of the fluoride-free BioMinC toothpaste sold by BioMin Technologies. The chloride in the glass expands the glass network and facilities glass dissolution. However, because of the high solubility of chlorides, these glasses offer no advantages for inclusion in resin or GIC matrices and will not be discussed further here.

Incorporating Bioactive Glasses into Resin Matrices

The strategy of putting bioactive glasses into composite resins is not new. Orthovita incorporated the 45S5 glass into a cold-cured BisGMA/TEGDMA resin system for use as a bioactive bone cement. However, problems were encountered with the high sodium content of the 45S5 glass, resulting in swelling and cracking of the resin matrix upon immersion. Consequently, the glass was heat treated to crystallize the glass to combeite (Erbe 1993); this solved the problem but crystallization reduces the reactivity and dissolution of the bioactive glass. The glass was also blended with a chemically inert barium alumino-silicate glass to confer radio-opacity.

Most studies for dental applications in the academic literature involve the use of the 45S5 glass without crystallizing it. The exception is the patent filed by Rusin from 3M that specifies a partially crystalline glass.

Yang et al. (2016a) investigated the ability of 45S5 glass with a particle size <25 μm into a BisGMA/TEGDMA (50//50) composite with inert glass filler with up to a 50% loading of the BG. The intended application was as a fissure sealant. The pH of the lactic acid solution to mimic caries-like conditions was measured over 180 minutes after immersion of a disc type specimen of the composites. They showed the pH rose to above 8 with the composite containing 50% BG. They measured flexural strength using three point beam specimens at 24 hours immersion in distilled water. The flexural strength decreased from 76.1 MPa with 0% BG to about 45 MPa for 50%. The short immersion time is too short to see the influence of the high sodium content glass on the flexural strength. The water sorption and solubility were measured according to ISO 4049 (2009), which is not appropriate for a composite with a reactive filler. The key finding from this study is that BGs can neutralize the type of acid produced in bacterial plaque.

Yang et al. (2016b) in a subsequent study also looked at three types of BG, 45S5, 53P4 and 45S5F, the latter one is a 45S5 glass with 12% CaO replaced by CaF_2 based on Spilman and Hench's composition. They again measure the lactic acid neutralizing ability and also measure the shear bond strength of orthodontic brackets bonded to teeth with these composites. Transbond XT is used as a reference material. They recognize the potential for BGs incorporated into orthodontic adhesives to prevent white spot lesion formation, which is a common problem after fixed orthodontic bracket treatment. The higher the loading of the BG the faster the neutralizing ability. The 45S5 and 53P4 with their lower NC and higher basicity not surprisingly neutralized the lactic acid more quickly. The shear bond strength for the 0% BG was about 15 MPa. Inclusion of the 45S5 or 53P4 reduced the shear bond strength to less than 5 MPa after 24 hours immersion in water. The least reactive 45S5F BG-based adhesive exhibited much higher shear bond strengths but still significantly reduced. Immersion for 24 hours is the standard test condition for shear bond tests, but given orthodontic brackets are applied for typically 18 months (28 × 18 days); 1 day is too short and the shear bond strength with BG-filled orthodontic adhesives may decline further with increased immersion time as the BG particles react further.

Morrel (2015) in a final-year project from the University of Birmingham titled Matching the Refractive Index Between Dimethacrylate Polymers and Bioactive Glass primarily looked at cure kinetics, so it will not be discussed further here.

Brown et al. (2011) measured the ion release and pH changes of four sol-gel BG composite adhesives at pH 4, two of which were fluoride-containing sol-gel glasses into SBF. The nominal glass compositions are given in Table 8.3.

It is worth noting that these four glasses contain no alkali metal. SBF is saturated with regard to calcium and phosphate. The phosphate concentration in SBF was found to reduce almost certainly as a result of these glasses forming apatite; however, the authors fail to

Table 8.3 Sol-gel bioactive glass compositions.

	mol% SiO_2	mol% CaO	mol% P_2O_5	mol% B_2O_3	mol% F
62BAG	62	31	4	1	3
65BAG	65	31	4	0	0
81BAG	81	11	4	0	4
85BAG	85	11	4	0	0

Source: Brown et al. (2011)/The EH Angle Education and Research Foundation, Inc.

look for apatite formation. All the glasses released Ca^{2+} ions under both immersion conditions. At pH 4 much greater concentrations of Ca^{2+} were detected. The authors attribute the higher Ca^{2+} concentrations to much greater ion exchange occurring at pH 4 due to the higher hydrogen ion concentration. All the glasses increased the pH significantly at pH 4, but changes were minimal at pH 7. However, no significant fluoride was detected at any condition or time point. It is possible the fluoride is being consumed in the formation of fluorapatite, resulting in no free fluoride being available. However, as we will see later the fluorine is probably almost entirely being lost during the synthesis of the two fluorine-containing glasses. The amount of glass in the composite is not given and the loading of glass was varied to give a viscosity matched to that of the reference adhesive Transbond XT which hinders analysis.

Manfred et al. (2013) looked at the microhardness adjacent to orthodontic brackets bonded to premolars using the same four BGs studied by Brown et al. These authors used a pH cycling regime to mimic the formation of white spot lesions. There was a significant reduction in hardness loss at 25 and 50 µm from the edge of the orthodontic bracket, but there was no significant further reduction in hardness. This would suggest a rather limited effectiveness of the BG adhesives.

Davis et al. (2014) looked at ion release and fluoride recharge of two fluoride-containing BG composites into distilled water. The composite resins were prepared by mixing the sol-gel BGs with inert glass to give a total filler loading by 72% of weight. The BG loading was 15% low. The fluoride released was less than 1 ppm and even recharging with 5,000 ppm NaF did not result in fluoride concentrations above 1 ppm. The composites released calcium in low amounts. The authors did not measure phosphate or look for apatite formation. They do state that the glasses formed hydroxyapatite in SBF, though no data were provided to support this. It is possible that these glasses could be forming fluorapatite or a fluoridated apatite not considered by the authors effectively repeating the mistakes of Hench and Spilman (1988) and the group from Modena (Lusvardi et al. 2009a, 2009b; Pedone et al. 2009; Cocchi et al. 2012). It should be noted that these glasses have probably lost nearly all their fluorine content and also possibly a significant amount of the phosphate content.

Hyun and Ferracane (2016) looked at biofilm formation and optical properties of BG composites including colour and translucency. The composites showed increased roughness and decreased translucency when a biofilm of *Streptococcus mutans* was grown on their surface. The changes in translucency observed could be due to increased acidity and increased BG degradation and consequent refractive index changes.

Miyaji et al. (1998) assessed the BG composite resins by incorporating an alkali-free bioactive glass $35.6SiO_2$ $46.7CaO$ $17P_2O_5$ and $0.5CaF_2$ in weight % into a cold-cured bisGMA/ TEGDMA resins and PMMA at a 70% loading by weight, and they also reported that PMMA inhibited the formation of an apatite layer whilst the bisGMA/TEGDMA resin failed to form a layer.

Miyaji et al. (1998) also investigated the influence of coupling agent on BisGMA/ TEGDMA composites filled with AW Glass-ceramic. Treating the glass-ceramic with coupling agents did not influence release but did influence their mechanical properties. Silylating agents that enabled the chemical bonding of the glass-ceramic particles to the resin gave improved strength.

Heid et al. (2016) reported the incorporation of particulate bioactive glasses into a dental root canal sealer. The BG used in this study was a flame-sprayed nano particulate BG. Since these glasses are not really true glasses and are extremely heterogeneous, these would not be discussed further.

Khvostenko et al. (2013) studied the mechanical performance of novel bioactive glass containing dental restorative composites. The objective of this study was to develop BG-containing dental restorative composites with adequate mechanical properties comparable to successful commercially available composites and to confirm the stability of these materials when exposed to a biologically challenging environment. The BG used was a sol-gel glass with 65% SiO_2, 31% CaO and 4% P_2O_5 (mol%); 15% BG was used and the total glass content was 72% by weight in a BisGMA/TEGDMA resin. Flexural strength, fracture toughness and fatigue crack growth resistance for the BAG-containing composites were unaffected by increasing BAG content up to 15% and were superior to Heliomolar after all post-cure treatments. The flexural strength of the BAG composites was unaffected by a two-month exposure to aqueous media and a bacterial challenge, whilst some decreases in fracture toughness and fatigue resistance were observed. The favourable mechanical properties compared to Heliomolar were attributed to higher filler content and a microstructure morphology that better promoted the toughening mechanisms of crack deflection and bridging.

Korkut et al. (2016) investigated the antimicrobial and mechanical properties of dental resin composite containing bioactive glass. These authors used the 53P4 BG composition that has a higher alkali metal content than 45S5 BG. Compressive and flexural strengths of the composites were measured after 24 hours immersion in distilled water and decreased significantly with an addition of 30% BAG. It was demonstrated that there was antibacterial activity against *S. Mutans*.

Chatzistavrou et al. (2014) assessed multicomponent sol gel synthesized BGs incorporating silver as a bacteriocide. It was shown an increased bacteriocidal effect against *S. Mutans* with silver incorporation. As this is a sol-gel-derived glass which would be expensive to produce it has limited applicability and will not be discussed further.

Brauer et al. (2017) reported a multicomponent resin composite system containing 45S5 and a fluoride with BG BAG-F with the following composition 42.7 mol% SiO_2, 26.2 mol% CaO, 26.1 mol% Na_2O, 4.0 mol% P_2O_5 and 1 mol% CaF_2. This composition falls just outside the boundary of the BioMin patents. The aim of this study was to evaluate the degradation of completely demineralized dentin specimens in contact with a filler-free or two ion-releasing resins containing micrometer-sized particles of bioglass 45S5 (BAG) or the fluoride-containing phosphate-rich bioactive glass (BAG-F). The fluoride-containing phosphate-rich bioactive glass incorporated into a resin-based material (BAG-F) showed greater ability in reducing the solubilization of C-terminal cross-linked telopeptide (ICTP) and C-terminal telopeptide (CTX) after prolonged AS storage. After 30 days of AS storage, BAG-F showed the greatest remineralizing effect on the stiffness of the completely demineralized dentin matrices. They claim the fluoride-containing phosphate-rich bioactive glass incorporated as micrometer-sized filler in dental composites may offer greater beneficial effects than bioglass 45S5 in reducing the enzyme-mediated degradation and promoting remineralization of demineralized dentin.

It is worth noting that if they had used a higher phosphate-containing glass with a higher fluoride content, their results would have been expected to have been even better.

Summary

Fluoride-containing bioactive glasses are a useful additive for developing dental restoratives for minimally invasive dentistry. These glasses can be added to dental cements and dental composites to provide remineralizing properties. The research on dental use of fluoride bioactive glasses has demonstrated the following:

1) BGs can neutralize the acids produced by cariogenic bacteria.
2) They degrade faster at acidic pH than neutral pH.
3) They inhibit cariogenic bacteria that prefer an acid environment.
4) High sodium-containing BGs result in a loss of composite mechanical properties upon immersion.
5) Fluoride release is negligible with sol-gel-derived glasses.
6) BGs have a capacity to remineralize dentine.

Further Reading

Brauer, D., Karpukhina, N., Law, R.V., and R.G. (2009). Hill Structural investigations of fluoride containing bioactive glass. *J. Mater. Chem.* 19: 5629–5636.

Hill, R., Calver, A., Skinner, S., Stamboulis, A., and Law, R. (2006). A MAS-NMR and combined Rietveldt study of mixed calcium/strontium fluorapatite glass-ceramics. *Key Eng. Mater.* 305–308.

Hill, R.G., and Wilson, A.D. (1988). Some structural aspects of glasses used in ionomer cements. *Glass Technol.* 29: 150–158.

Hill, R.G., Da Costa, N., and Law, R.V. (2005). Characterisation of a mould flux glass. *J. Non-Cryst. Solids* 351: 69–74.

Hill, R.G., Law, R.V., O'Donnell, M.D., Hawes, J., Bubb, N.L., Wood, D.J., Miller, C.A., Mirsaneh, M., and Reaney, I. (2009). Characterisation of fluorine containing glasses and glass-ceramics by 19F magic angle spinning nuclear magnetic resonance spectroscopy. *J. Eur. Ceram. Soc.* 29 (11): 2185–2219.

Hill, R.G., Stamboulis, A., Henry, R.V.L., and Hawes, J. (2004). A MAS-NMR study of the crystallisation process of barium fluorphlogopite glass-ceramics. *Glass Technol.* 45: 121–126.

Khvostenko, T.J., Hilton, J.L., Ferracane, J.C., and Mitchell, J.J. (2015). Kruzic Bioactive glass fillers reduce bacterial penetration into marginal gaps for composite restorations. *Dent. Mater.* 31: 701–710.

Matsuya, S., Robert, A.S., Spil, G., and Law, R.V. (2007). Structural characterization of Ionomer glasses by multinuclear solid state MAS-NMR spectroscopy. *J. Non-Cryst. Solids* 353: 237.

Salehi, S., Gwinner, F., Mitchell, J.C., Pfeifer, C., and Ferracane, J.L. (2015). Cytotoxicity of resin composites containing bioactive glass fillers. *Dent. Mater.* 31 (2): 195–203.

Stamboulis, A., Hill, R.G., and Law, R.V. (2005). Structural characterization of fluorine containing glasses by 19F, 27Al, 29Si and 31P MAS–NMR spectroscopy. *J. Non Cryst. Solids.* 351: 3289–3295.

Stamboulis, A., Law, R.V., and Hill, R.G. (2004). Characterisation of commercial ionomer glasses using magic angle nuclear magnetic resonance (MAS-NMR). *Biomaterials* 25: 3907–3913.

Yang, S.-Y., Piao, Y.-Z., Kim, S.-M., Lee, Y.-K., Kim, K.-N., and Kim, K.-M. (2013). Acid neutralizing, mechanical and physical properties of pit and fissure sealants containing melt-derived 45S5 bioactive glass. *Dent. Mater.* 29: 1228–1235.

References

Ana, I.D., Matsuya, S., Ohta, M., and Ishikawa, K. (2003). Effects of added bioactive glass on the setting and mechanical properties of resin-modified glass ionomer cement. *Biomaterials* 24 (18): 3061–3067. https://doi.org/10.1016/s0142-9612(03)00151-0.

Brauer, D.S., Karpukhina, N., Law, R.V., and Hill, R.G. (2009). Structure of fluoride-containing bioactive glasses. *J. Mater. Chem.* 19: 5629–5636.

Brauer, D.S., Karpukhina, N., O'Donnell, M., Law, R.V., and Hill, R.G. (2010). Fluoride containing bioactive glasses: effect of glass design and structure on degradation, pH and apatite formation in simulated body fluid. *Acta Biomater.* 6: 3275–3282.

Brauer, D.S., Al-Noaman, A., Hill, R.G., and Doweidar, H. (2011). Density–structure correlations in fluoride-containing bioactive glasses. *Mater Chem Phys* 130 (1–2): 121–125.

Brown, W., Eidelman, N., and Tomazic, B. (1987). Octacalcium phosphate as a precursor in biomineral formation. *Adv. Dent. Res.* 1 (2): 306–313.

Brown, M.L., Davis, H.B., Tufekci, E., Crowe, J.J., Covell, D.A., and Mitchell, J.C. (2011). Ion release from a novel orthodontic resin bonding agent for the reduction and/or prevention of white spot lesions an in vitro study. *Angle Orthod.* 81 (6): 1014–1020.

Chatzistavrou, X., Fenno, J.C., and Faulk, D. (2014). Fabrication and characterization of bioactive and antibacterial composites for dental applications. *Acta Biomater.* 10 (8): 3723–3732.

Chen, X., Karpukhina, N., Brauer, D.S., and Hill, R.G. (2015). Novel highly degradable chloride containing bioactive glasses. *Biomed. Glasses* 1: 108–118.

Chen, X., Karpukhina, N., Brauer, D.S., and Hill, R.G. (2017). High chloride content calcium silicate glasses. *Phys. Chem. Chem. Phys.* 19: 7078–7085.

Choi, J.Y., Lee, H.H., and Kim, H.W. (2008). Bioactive sol-gel glass added ionomer cement for the regeneration of tooth structure. *J. Mater. Sci. Mater. Med.* 19 (10): 3287–3294. doi: 10.1007/s10856-008-3464-8.

Chow, L.C., and Eanes, E. (2001). *Octacalcium Phosphate*, 18e. Basel: Karger.

Christie, J.K., Pedone, A., Menziani, M.C., and Tilocca, A. (2011). Fluorine environment in bioactive glasses: *ab Initio* molecular dynamics simulations. *J. Phys. Chem. B* 115: 2038–2049.

Cocchi, M., Durante, C., Lusvardi, G., Malavasi, G., and Menabue, L. (2012). Evaluation of the behaviour of fluorine-containing bioactive glasses: Reactivity in a simulated body fluid solution assisted by multivariate data analysis. *J. Mater. Sci. Mater. Med.* 23 (3): 639–648.

Curzon, M.E.J., Spector, P.C., and Iker, H.P. (1978). Association between strontium in drinking-water supplies and low caries Caries prevalence in man. *Arch. Oral Biol.* 23 (4): 317–321.

Davis, H.B., Gwinner, F., Mitchell, J.C., and Ferracane, J.L. (2014). Ion release from, and fluoride recharge of a composite with a fluoride-containing bioactive glass. *Dent. Mater.* 30: 1187–1194.

De Caluwe, T., Vercruysse, C.W.J., Declercq, H.A., Schaubroeckc, D., Verbeecka, R.M.H., and Martens, L.C. (2016). Bioactivity and biocompatibility of two fluoride containing bioactive glasses for dental applications. *Dent. Mater.* 32 (11): 1414–1428. https://doi.org/10.1016/j.dental.2016.09.014.

Dupree, R., Holland, D., Mortuza, M., Collins, J., and Lockyer, M. (1989). Magic angle spinning NMR of alkali phospho alumino silicate-glasses. *J. Non-Cryst. Solids* 112 (1–3): 111–119.

Earl, J.S., Ward, M.B., and Langford, R.M. (2010). Investigation of dentinal tubule occlusio using FIB-SEM milling and EDX. *J. Clin. Dent.* 21 (2): 37–41.

Earl, J.S., Topping, N., Elle, J., Langford, R.M., and Greenspan, D.C. (2011a). Physical and chemical characterization of the surface layers formed on dentin following treatment with a fluoridated toothpaste containing NovaMin. *J. Clin. Dent.* 22 (3): 68–73.

Earl, J.S., Leary, R.K., Muller, K.H., Langford, R.M., and Greenspan, D.C. (2011b). Physical and chemical characterization of dentin surface following treatment with NovaMin technology. *J. Clin. Dent.* 22 (3): 62.

Edén, M. (2011). The split network analysis for exploring composition–structure correlations in multi-component glasses: I. Rationalizing bioactivity-composition trends of bioglasses. *J. Non-Cryst. Solids* 357: 1595.

Erbe, J. Bioactive load bearing bone graft compositions WO 93/16738 9/1993.

Farooq, I., Tylkowski, M., Muller, S., Janicki, T., Brauer, D.S., and Hill, R.G. (2013). Influence of sodium content on the properties of bioactive glasses for use in air abrasion. *Biomed. Mater.* 8: 065008.

Fredholm, Y.C., Karpukhina, N., Law, R.V., and Robert, G. (2010). Hill Strontium containing bioactive glasses: glass structure and physical properties. *J. Non Cryst. Solids.* 356: 2546–2551.

Fredholm, F.C., Karpukhina, N., Brauer, D.S., Jones, J.R., Law, R.V., and Hill, R.G. (2012). Influence of Strontium for calcium substitution in bioactive glasses on degradation ion release and apatite formation. *J. R. Soc. Interface* 9: 880–889.

Gentlemen, E., Fredholm, Y., Jell, G., ODonnell, M.D., Lotibakhshaiesh, N., Stevens, M.M., and Hill, R.G. (2010). The effects of strontium substituted bioactive glasses on osteoblasts and osteoclasts in vitro. *Biomaterials* 31: 3949–3956.

Gillam, D.G., Tang, J.Y., Mordan, N.J., and Newman, H.N. (2002). The effects of a novel Bioglass dentifrice on dentine sensitivity: a scanning electron microscopy investigation. *J. Oral Rehabil.* 29: 305–313.

Greenspan, D.C. (2010). NovaMin and tooth sensitivity-an overview. *J. Clin. Dent.* 21 (special issue): 61–65.

Griffin, S.G. and Hill, R.G. (2000). Influence of glass composition on the properties of glass polyalkenoate cements. Part II: influence of phosphate content. *Biomaterials* 21 (4): 399–403.

Heid, S., Stoessel, P.R., Tauböck, T.T., Stark, W.J., Zehnder, M., and Mohn, D. (2016). Incorporation of particulate bioactive glasses into a dental root canal sealer. *Biomed. Glasses* 2 (1): https://doi.org/10.1515/bglass-2016-0004.

Hench, L.L. (2006). The story of Bioglass. *J. Mater. Sci. Mater. Med.* 17: 967–978.

Hench, L.L., Spilman, D.B., and Hench, J.W., inventors (1988). University of Florida, assignee. Fluoride-modified bioactive glass (Bioglass) and its use as implant material. US Patent 4,775,646.

Hench, L.L., Hench, J.W., and Greenspan, D. (2004). Bioglass: a short history and bibliography. *J. Aust. Ceram. Soc.* 40: 1–42. https://doi.org/10.1007/978-94-011-0541-5_1.

Hill, R. (1996). An alternative explanation of the bioactivity of bioglasses. *J. Mater. Sci. Lett.* 15: 1122–1125.

Hill, R.G. and Brauer, D.S. (2011). Predicting the bioactivity of glasses using the network connectivity or split network models. *J. Non-Cryst. Solids* 357: 3884–3887.

Hill, R.G., Stamboulis, A., Law, R.V., Clifford, A., Towler, M., and Crowley, C. (2004). The influence of strontium substitution in fluorapatite glasses and glass-ceramics. *J. Non-Cryst. Solids* 336 (3): 223–229.

Huang, M., Hill, R.G., and Simon, C.F. (2016). Rawlinson Strontium (Sr) elicits odontogenic differentiation of human dental pulp stem cells (hDPSCs): a therapeutic role for Sr in dentine repair? *Acta Biomater.* 1: 201–211.

Hyun, H.K. and Ferracane, J.L. (2016). Influence of biofilm formation on the optical properties of novel bioactive glass-containing composites. *Dent. Mater.* 32: 1144–1151.

Jones, J.R. (2013). Review of bioactive glass: from Hench to hybrids. *Acta Biomater* 9 (1): 4457–4486.

Khvostenko, D., Mitchell, J.C., Hilton, T.J., Ferracane, J.L., and Kruzic, J.J. (2013). Mechanical performance of novel bioactive glass containing dental restorative composites. *Dent. Mater.* 29: 1139–1148.

Korkut, E., Torlak, E., and Altunsoy, M. (2016). Antimicrobial and mechanical properties of dental resin composite containing bioactive glass. *J. Appl. Biomater. Funct. Mater.* 14 (3): e296–e301.

Lins, C.E.C., Oliveira, A.A.R., Gonzalez, I., Macedo, W.A.A., and Periera, M. (2017). Structural analysis of fluorine-containing bioactive glass nanoparticles synthesized by sol–gel route assisted by ultrasound energy. *J. Biomed. Mater. Res. Part B* 106: 360–366.

Liu, J., Rawlinson, S.C.F., Hill, R.G., and Fortune, F. (2016a). Strontium-substituted bioactive glasses in vitro osteogenic and antibacterial effects. *Dent. Mater.* 32: 416–422.

Liu, J., Rawlinson, S.C.F., Hill, R.G., and Fortune, F. (2016b). Fluoride incorporation in high phosphate containing bioactive glasses and *in vitro* osteogenic, angiogenic and antibacterial effects. *Dent. Mater.* 32: e221–e237.

Lotfibakhshaiesh, N., Gentleman, E., Hill, R., and Stevens, M. (2011). Strontium-substituted bioactive glass coatings for bone tissue engineering. *Clin. Biochem.* 44 (13): S36–S36.

Lucas, M., Arita, K., and Nishino, M. (2001). Strengthening a conventional glass ionomer cement using hydroxyapatite. *J. Dent. Res.* 80 (Special issue): 711.

Lusvardi, G., Malavesi, G., Menabue, L., Aina, V., and Monterra, C. (2009a). Fluoride-containing bioactive glasses: surface reactivity in simulated body fluids solutions. *Acta Biomater.* 53548–53562.

Lusvardi, G., Malavasi, G., Tarsitano, F., Menabue, L., Menziani, M.C., and Pedone, A. (2009b). Quantitative structure–property relationships of potentially bioactive fluoro phospho-silicate glasses. *J. Phys. Chem. B* 113: 10331–10338.

Lynch, E., Brauer, D.S., Karpukhina, N., Gillam, D.G., and Hill, R.G. (2012). Multicomponent bioactive glasses of varying fluoride content for treating dentin hypersensitivity. *Dent. Mater.* 18: 168–178.

Manfred, L., Covell, D.A., Crowe, J.J., Tufekci, E., and Mitchell, J.C. (2013). A novel biomimetic orthodontic bonding agent helps prevent white spot lesions adjacent to brackets. *Angle Orthod.* 83 (1): 97–103.

Martin, R.A., Twyman, H.L., Rees, G.J., Barny, E.R., Moss, R.M., Smith, M., Hill, R.G., Cibin, G., Charpentier, T., Smith, M.E., Hanna, J.V., and Newport, R.J. (2012). An examination of calcium and strontium site distribution in bioactive glasses through isomorphic neutron diffraction, X-ray diffraction EXAFS and multinuclear solid state NMR. *J. Mater. Chem.* 22: 22212.

Miyaji, F., Morita, Y., and Kokubo, T. (1998). Surface structural change of bioactive inorganic filler-resin composite cement in simulated body fluid: effect of resin. *J. Biomed. Mater. Res.* 42: 604–610.

Mneimne, M., Hill, R.G., Bushby, A., and Brauer, D.S. (2011). High phosphate contents significantly increase apatite formation of fluoride-containing bioactive glasses. *Acta Biomater.* 7: 1827–1834.

Morrel, A. (2015). *Matching the RFI between Dimethacrylate Polymers and Bioactive Glass Final Year Project*. University of Birmingham.

Moshaverinia, A., Ansari, S., Moshaverinia, M., Roohpour, N., Darr, J.A., and Rehman, I. (2008). Effects of incorporation of hydroxyapatite and fluoroapatite nanobioceramics into conventional glass ionomer cements (GIC). *Acta Biomater.* 4 (2): 432–440.

O'Donnell, M.D., Watts, S.J., Law, R.V., and Hill, R.G. (2008a). Effect of P2O5 content in two series of soda lime phosphosilicate glasses on structure and properties – Part I: NMR. *J. Non Cryst. Solids.* 354: 3554–3560.

O'Donnell, M.D., Watts, S.J., Law, R.V., and Hill, R.G. (2008b). Effect of P2O5 content in two series of soda lime phosphosilicate glasses on structure and properties – Part II: physical properties. *J. Non Cryst. Solids.* 354: 3561–3566.

O'Donnell, M.D., Fredholm, Y., de Rouffignac, A., and Hill, R.G. (2008c). Structural analysis of a series of strontium-substituted apatites. *Acta Biomater.* 4: 1455–1464.

O'Donnell, M.D., Watts, S.J., Law, R.V., and Hill, R.G. (2009). The effect of phosphate content on the bioactivity of soda-lime-phosphosilicate glasses. *J. Mater. Sci. Mater. Med.* 1611–1618.

Orala, O., Lassilaa, L.V., Kumbuloglu, O., and Vallittu, P.K. (2014). Bioactive glass particulate filler composite: effect of coupling of fillers and filler loading on some physical properties. *Dent. Mater.* 30: 570–577.

Pedone, A., Malavesi, G., and Menziani, M.C. (2009). Role of magnesium in soda-lime glasses: insight into structural, transport, and mechanical properties through computer simulations. *J. Phys. Chem. C* 113: 15723–15730.

Pedone, A., Charpentier, T., and Menziani, M.C. (2012). The structure of fluoride containing bioactive glasses: new insights from firs-principle calculations and solid state NMR spectroscopy. *J. Mater. Chem.* 22: 12599.

Sriranganathan, D., Kanwal, N., Hing, K.A., and Hill, R.G. (2016). Strontium substituted bioactive glasses for tissue engineered scaffolds: the importance of octacalcium phosphate. *J. Mater. Sci. Mater. Med.* 27: 39.

Sriranganathan, D., Chen, X., Hing, K.A., Kanwal, N., and Hill, R.G. (2017). The effect of the incorporation of fluoride into strontium containing bioactive glasses. *J. Non-Cryst. Solids* 457: 25–30.

Swansbury, L.A., Mountjoy, G., Chen, X., Karpukhina, N., and Hill, R. (2017). Modelling the onset of phase separation in CaO-SiO_2-$CaCl_2$ chlorine-containing silicate glasses. *J. Phys. Chem. B* 121: 5647–5653.

Tezvergil-Mutluay, A., Seseogullari-Dirihan, R., Feitosa, V.P., Cama, G., Brauer, D.S., and Sauro, S. (2017). Effects of composites containing bioactive glasses on demineralized dentin. *J. Dent. Res.* 96: 999–1005.

Thuy, T.T., Nakagaki, H., Kato, K., Phan, A.H., Inukai, J., and Tsuboi, S. (2008). Effect of strontium in combination with fluoride on enamel remineralization in vitro. *Arch. Oral Biol.* 53 (11): 1017–1022.

Tiskaya, M., Al-Eesa, N.A., Wong, F.S.L., and Hill, R.G. (2019). Characterization of the bioactivity of two commercial composites. *Dent. Mater.* 35 (12): 1757–1768.

Vallittu, P.K., Närhi, T.O., and Hupa, L. (2015). Fiber glass-bioactive glass composite for bone replacing and bone anchoring implants. *Dent. Mater.* 31 (4): 371–381.

Xiang, Y. and Du, J. (2011). Effect of strontium substitution on the structure of 45S5 bioglasses. *Chem. Mater.* 23 (11): 2703–2717.

Yang, S.-Y., Kim, S.-H., Choi, S.-Y., and Kim, K.-M. (2016a). Acid neutralizing ability and shear bond strength using orthodontic adhesives containing three different types of bioactive glass. *Materials* 9 (125): 1–12.

Yang, S.-Y., Kwon, J.-S., Kim, K.-N., and Kim, K.-M. (2016b). Enamel surface with pit and fissure sealant containing 45S5 bioactive glass. *J. Dent. Res.* 95 (5): 550–557.

Zainuddin, N., Karpukhina, N., Law, R.V., and Hill, R.G. (2012). Characterisation of a remineralising Glass Carbomer® ionomer cement by MAS-NMR spectroscopy. *Dent. Mater.* 28 (10): 1051–1058.

Zhao, I.S., Mei, M.L., Zhou, Z.L., Burrow, M.F., Lo, E.C.-M., and Chu, C.-H. (2017). Shear bond strength and remineralisation effect of a casein phosphopeptide-amorphous calcium phosphate-modified glass ionomer cement on artificial "caries-affected" dentine. *Int. J. Mol. Sci.* 18 (8): 1723.

9

Where Are We with a Minimally Invasive Approach in Periodontology?

David Gillam, Nik Pandya, and Wendy Turner

Key Topics

- Changing concepts: Dynamic paradigm shifts in dentistry and in periodontology
- History of minimally invasive periodontal surgery
- Concept of minimally invasive periodontal surgery
- Principles of minimally invasive periodontal surgery with advantages and disadvantages

Learning Objectives

- Be able to appreciate the dynamic paradigm shifts in clinical dentistry and in periodontology
- Be able to understand the history of the development of minimally invasive periodontal surgery procedures in clinical dentistry
- Be able to define the concept of minimally invasive periodontal procedures
- Be able to understand the principles with advantages and disadvantages of minimally invasive periodontal surgery

Introduction

> What do you think are the main reasons for this changes in the treatment of these diseases?

The traditional understanding of how to treat both dental caries and periodontal disease has been challenged over the last 30 years and there has undoubtedly been a seismic shift in how to treat both conditions. For example, in the treatment of dental caries there has been a greater emphasis in early detection and prevention (involving both the

Minimally Invasive Dentistry: Interdisciplinary Clinical and Scientific Approaches, First Edition.
Edited by Aylin Baysan and Paul Anderson.
© 2026 John Wiley & Sons Ltd. Published 2026 by John Wiley & Sons Ltd.
Companion website: www.wiley.com/go/baysan/minimally_invasive_dentistry

clinician and patient) and a move away from the 'extension for prevention' philosophy to a more conservative approach (MID). The advancement of adhesive materials has undoubtedly helped conserve tooth tissue with the use of sealants, glass ionomer cements, sealants and re-mineralising fluoride therapies. In a similar manner, the treatment of periodontal disease has also seen a paradigm shift in how to treat the condition. For example, the traditional methods of treating periodontal disease was either by non-surgical or surgical procedures depending on the severity of the condition with the emphasis on removing hard tissue (e.g., cementum) to render the root surface hard and smooth. This procedure also included the intentional removal of calculus. It is now recognised that the removal of diseased cementum is unnecessary and more minimally-invasive strategies have been implemented (Ower 2013). According to Ower (2013), the successful management of periodontal disease, by both non-surgical and surgical procedures is the establishment of optimal self-performed biofilm control by the patient prior to treatment. In other words, it is the disruption of the plaque biofilm by the patient and clinician that is clearly essential for the successful treatment and management of periodontal disease. The implementation of minimally invasive procedures such as MIS, MIST, M-MIST have also been developed to minimise the surgical trauma experienced by the patient and to reduce the duration of the surgical procedures. These procedures included minimal incisions and flap reflection and careful handling of the hard and soft tissues as well as the use of instruments such as operating microscopes, magnifying lenses, microsurgical instruments, and materials (Cortellini and Tonetti 2007, 2009; Harrel and Nunn 2001; Harrel and Rees 1995). Although minimally invasive therapeutic approaches have become the standard of care for numerous medical procedures, the use of minimally invasive techniques in both non-surgical and surgical periodontal therapy has not progressed at the same rate (Rethman and Harrell 2010).

> What are the reasons for the lack of progression in dentistry compared to medicine?

The aim of this chapter is to provide an overview of the current use of minimally invasive techniques and procedures in both non-surgical and surgical management of periodontal disease(s).

Changing Concepts: Dynamic Paradigm Shifts in Dentistry and in Periodontology

One of the more interesting aspects of innovative dentistry over the last two to three decades is the fundamental change in the understanding of basic concepts and the implementation into clinical practice. For example, in restorative dentistry the shift from the so-called 'extension for prevention' in cavity design to eliminate dental caries to a more minimally invasive approach which reduced the need to remove excessive amounts of hard tissue. Undoubtedly the advancement of dental materials has enabled the clinician to use adhesive materials that relied on chemical rather than mechanical retention. In a similar manner, there has been a major shift in the understanding in the treatment of periodontal disease from the misconception of the role of calculus and the unnecessary removal of hard tissue (e.g., cementum) to eliminate the pathogenic bacteria thought to be resident within the cementum to the current concept of easy removal of the plaque biofilm loosely adherent on the surface of the cementum (Checchi and Pelliccioni 1988; Moore et al. 1986; Smart et al. 1990). Our understanding of dental plaque has also changed, previously dental plaque was removed with a view that by reducing the amount of plaque containing bacteria this would reduce the risk of further progression of periodontal disease. A number of theories were introduced to support the non-specific plaque hypothesis, but it was evident that certain bacteria were associated with specific dental conditions e.g., Acute Ulcerative Gingivitis (AUG) (Currently classified as Necrotizing Ulcerative Gingivitis [NUG]). Further modifications were also proposed ranging from an environmental model to the keystone pathogen(s) hypothesis which identified key pathogens such as *Porphyromonas gingivalis* (P.g), *Treponema denticola*, and *Tannerella forsythia* that had a profound effect on the initiating and subsequent development of the disease process (Hajishengallis et al. 2012). There was also a realisation within the scientific community that dental plaque and its association with the oral microbiotia was not as simple as initially considered. For example, plaque bacteria were previously considered to be planktonic in nature but currently as indicated above, plaque can be considered as a dental biofilm with a highly organism interactive microbial community which interacts both with the host and other bacteria within the oral cavity. More recently the concept of the oral microbiome has been introduced which has wide ranging implications for the host in term of health (symbiosis) and disease (dysbiosis) (Killen et al. 2016). It therefore follows that key pathogens such as Porphyromonas gingivalis (P.g) can orchestrate inflammatory disease (e.g., periodontal disease) by 'remodelling a normally benign microbiota into a dysbiotic one' (Hajishengallis et al. 2012). Furthermore, it is evident from this research that there needs to be an adjustment on how the clinician managed a patient who is healthy, showing initial signs and symptoms of the disease and one who has established disease. For a practical day-to-day approach the clinician may be able to successfully manage this by both non-surgical and surgical procedures (supplemented with good oral hygiene instruction) provided the patient is complaint in terms of optimal self-performed biofilm control (Ower 2013). However, it is also apparent with the advances in the identification of key pathogens that treatment choices may benefit from adjunctive therapies that have a minimal effect on the oral tissues and commensal bacteria but have a profound effect on the humeral response of the host to maintain health (symbiosis).

Non-surgical and Surgical Procedures in Periodontology

The clinician has several techniques and procedures that are available to treat periodontal disease successfully ranging from non-surgical to surgical procedures which may be supplemented by adjunctive anti-microbial therapy, surgical material, etc. to either maintain or enhance both hard (bone) and soft (gingivae, connective) tissue. Using minimally invasive procedures to fulfil these aims has increased in popularity over the last two decades due in part to an improvement in dental material, equipment e.g., improvement in ultrasonic scaling tips) and improvement in surgical techniques designed to minimise the trauma to both hard and soft tissues. An important aspect that is often overlooked by clinician when treating patients with periodontal disease is the impact of providing oral hygiene instruction before the treatment phase. Several studies have reported on the importance of oral hygiene instruction prior to the treatment phase or during the treatment phase. For example, Axelsson and Lindhe (1981a, 1981b) reported on the beneficial effect of oral hygiene measures in children and adults on caries and periodontal disease. The high levels of oral hygiene and improvements in both caries and periodontal status reported in the Axelsson studies have been difficult to replicate in other studies. A study by Turner et al. (1994) in patients with chronic periodontitis reported that there were improvements in their periodontal condition by oral hygiene measures alone even in the deeper periodontal pockets. Although this study had a relatively small sample size ($n = 10$) nevertheless it suggested that oral hygiene measures alone could have an impact on the periodontium prior to treatment. This effect may be observed in the two photographs provided by Ower (2013) where he clearly demonstrated the importance and effect of good oral hygiene measures in a highly compliant patient prior to treatment (Figures 9.1 and 9.2). The importance of teaching aids in the form of video, charts and oral instruction in tooth brushing studies have also been shown to be beneficial in reducing plaque levels (Ashruff 2016; Pareek et al. 2015).

What evidence are you aware of to support this statement?

Non-surgical Procedures

According to Ower (2013) a very persuasive case can be made for non-surgical disease management, in terms of better treatment outcomes, compared to surgical procedures particularly in pockets up to 6 mm in depth. Surgical treatment has been shown in short-term studies to be of benefit in deeper pockets (≥ 6 mm) and while this would suggest that deeper pockets should be treated surgically, Ower argues that the evidence from long-term studies would suggest that non-surgical treatment may be as effective as surgical treatment in the deeper pocket.

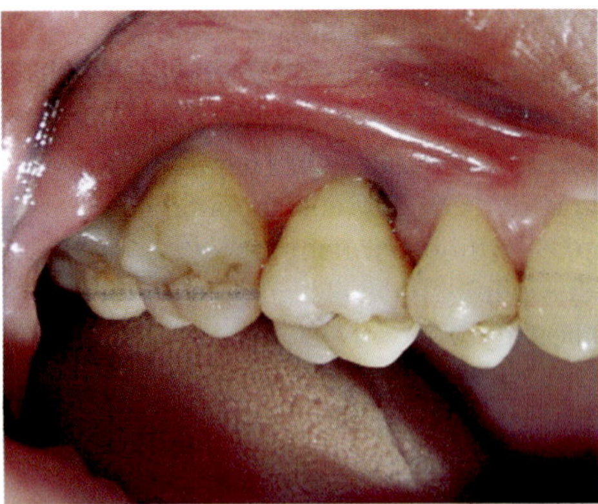

Figure 9.1 Patient with subgingival calculus prior to any periodontal treatment. Source: P. Ower (2013).

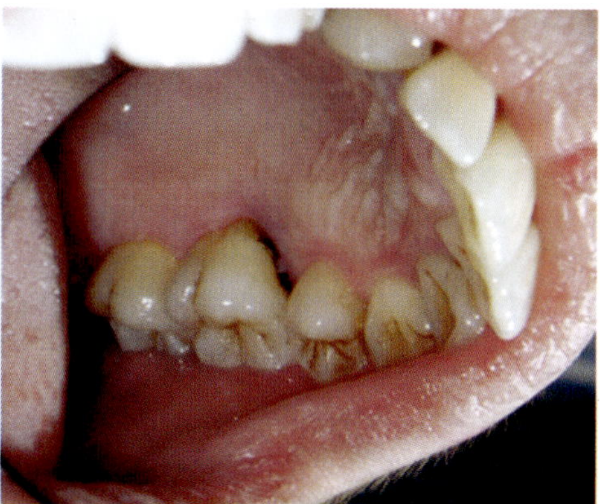

Figure 9.2 Results of meticulous oral hygiene in a compliant and motivated patient exposing the previously diagnosed subgingival calculus which is now easier to remove by debridement procedures. Source: P. Ower (2013).

A key component in the treatment of periodontal diseases is the disruption of the dental biofilm rather than the historical 'deliberate removal of the so-called disease cementum'. Evidence from the *in vitro* studies of the Kieser group (Cheechi et al. 1988; Moore et al. 1986; Smart et al. 1990) clearly indicated that the cementum and dentine was not permeated by calculus or contaminated with toxins or micro-organisms. This key finding subsequently changed the philosophical approach to periodontal treatment in that the removal of the cementum and underlying dentine was not required to remove the pathogenic bacteria. The question that may be posed, is what would be required to disrupt the dental biofilm in terms of educating the patient to be effective in their oral hygiene regime and what measures would the clinician need to take to help the patient reach this objective without initiating any damaging changes to either the soft or hard tissues? Several suggestions have been made that may minimise these effects for example, the use of a diode laser (e.g., Zingale et al. 2012), full mouth disinfectant procedures, sub gingival air polishing and the use of desensitising pastes to alleviate any discomfort from these procedures.

A recent review by Nibali et al. (2015) assessed the efficacy of minimally invasive non-surgical therapy (MINST) in the treatment of periodontal infrabony defects based on a retrospective analysis of 35 infrabony defects in 23 subjects. The authors concluded that MINST procedures led to both clinical and radiographic improvements in the infrabony defects. In summary, there is a recognition of the importance of non-surgical procedures in the treatment of periodontal disease not simply as a precursor to subsequent surgical intervention but as an alternative treatment within the minimally invasive philosophy. For example, the introduction of MINST procedures for the treatment of infra bony defects may not only have minimal effects on both the soft and hard tissues but have comparable results in terms of clinical relevance compared to more invasive surgical (MIST) interventions with negligible morbidity and acceptable patient satisfaction (Ribeiro et al. 2011). MINST procedures may also have an added advantage over MIST in terms of reduced surgical time.

Surgical Procedures in Minimally Invasive Periodontal Surgery (MIPS/MIST)

As previously indicated the implementation of minimally invasive procedures were developed to minimise the surgical trauma experienced by the patient and to reduce the duration of the surgical procedures such as conventional flap procedures (Guided Tissue Regeneration [GTR] with or without adjunctive therapy). These procedures included minimal incisions and flap reflection and careful handling of the hard and soft tissues as well as the use of innovative instruments, such as operating microscopes, magnifying lenses, microsurgical instruments, and materials.

A number of post-operative healing complications, such as pain and swelling have been associated with the traditionally used surgical procedures and this may have been related to flap design, duration of the procedures, extent of visualisation of the depth of the defect, and materials used during the procedures. For example, the wide extensive nature of the incisions within the flap design in order to visualise the extent of the periodontal problem may have an impact on post-operative healing. Several investigators have modified surgical periodontal procedures to preserve the periodontal tissues wherever possible for example in the papilla preservation technique and its subsequent modifications (modified and simplified papilla preservation techniques).

The application of microsurgical concepts recognised in medicine would therefore appear to be very appealing in periodontal surgery and it is evident from reviewing the periodontal literature that these concepts have gradually been implemented in dentistry. The development and modification of various techniques and procedures such as MIS, MIST, M-MIST, and Videoscope MIS (VMIS). These techniques have also been used in conjunction with regenerative materials in GTR, augmentation procedures, gingival recession defects using resorbable barrier membranes, connective tissue grafts, enamel matrix derivatives.

According to Dannan (2011), the main objectives of MIPS/MIST are as follows:

1) reduce surgical trauma,
2) increase flap/wound stability,
3) allow stable primary closure of the wound,
4) reduce surgical chair time, and
5) minimise patient discomfort and side effects.

Advantages of Minimally Invasive Periodontal Surgery

The concept of MIPS/MIST procedures would suggest that it is a method of gaining surgical access without the disadvantages associated with more traditional surgical procedures, such as minimising the flap design and tissue trauma, smaller incisions etc. (see Table 9.1). There are a number of relevant outcomes arising from this type of less invasive procedure, such as the maintenance of the blood supply to the surgical area and the stabilisation of the blood clot during the initial stages of the wound healing process. It has also been reported that there is less post-operative recession with MIPS/MIST procedures.

Table 9.1 Advantages of selected minimally invasive periodontal procedures and techniques.

Procedure	Authors	Comments
Minimally Invasive Periodontal Surgery (MIPS)		Allows for minimisation of soft tissue trauma and the removal of granulation tissue from periodontal defects using smaller less invasive procedures than in standard bone grafting techniques
Minimally Invasive Surgery (MIS)	Harrel and Rees (1995), Harrel and Nunn (2001), Cortellini and Tonetti (2001, 2005), Harrel et al. (2005)	The aim was to produce minimal (less extensive) wounds, minimal flap reflection and careful handling of the hard and soft tissues. Requires the application of very precise and delicate surgical procedures including the use of visualisation instruments such as operating microscopes, magnifying lenses, microsurgical instruments, and materials
Minimally Invasive Surgical Technique (MIST)	Cortellini and Tonetti (2007)	Stressed the importance of wound and blood clot stability and primary wound closure for blood clot protection
Modified Minimally Invasive Surgical Technique (M-MIST)	Cortellini and Tonetti (2009)	To enable sufficient space provision for periodontal regeneration
Periodontal Microsurgery (PS)	Tibbetts and Shanelec (1998)	Concentrates on soft tissue regeneration and augmentation procedures where visualisation of the defect is improved using a surgical operating microscope. Evidence from case reports would suggest that there are clinical improvements in clinical parameters such as pocket depth, attachment level gain, and minimal recession following MIPS
Videoscope Minimally Invasive Surgery (VMIS)	Tunnell and Harrell (2017)	Improved visual access to surgical sites, facilitated improved defect debridement and root planning. VMIS resulted in a gain in soft tissue height up to 3 years postoperatively

Source: Acknowledgement modified from Dannan (2011).

Disadvantages of Minimally Invasive Periodontal Surgery

One of the problems in using these minimally invasive techniques is that by minimising the extent of flap design, this may in turn restrict the field of vision for the operator. Another problem may relate to the development of MIPS/MIST procedures as clinicians have continually modified the original technique to improve the procedure, for example, using elements of a papilla preservation techniques with less invasive incision designs (Tunnel and Harrel 2017). There are, however, disadvantages associated with these procedures such as:

- Requires specialist training in MIPS/MIST procedures
- Specialist equipment may be required (e.g., microscopic visualisation [surgical microscopes and videoscopes], magnification loupes, fibre optics)

- Additional equipment may add considerable expense to the practice
- Some procedures may take longer compared to conventional procedures
- Precision and accuracy of microscopic visualisation may be limited in terms of the depth of field/access in periodontal defects, e.g., limitations within the fibre system (Jaffray cited by Dannan 2011 [modified]).

> Do you think there is sufficient evidence from clinical studies to justify the claims supporting the efficacy of MIPS/MIST procedures over conventional periodontal surgical techniques?

Although, there a number of studies in the published literature that have reported on the effectiveness of MIPS/MIST procedures in improving the clinical parameters and reducing patient morbidity they are generally confined to specific research teams or specialist clinical investigators. There is, therefore, a requirement to compare the effectiveness of these techniques with traditional techniques in randomised clinical studies.

One of the disadvantages of MIPS/MIST procedures as outlined above is the cost of specialised equipment. For example, in the Allen technique described in the case report, the cost of the specialised equipment may be prohibitive to most practitioners however, in order to achieve the required outcomes implicit in MIPS/MIST philosophy it may be considered essential to have this type of specialist instrumentation.

Example of Applying the Principles of Minimal Invasive Periodontal Surgery in a Periodontal Practice

This is a case report describing the procedures in a patient who was referred for the assessment and treatment of gingival recession and associated aesthetic concerns

A 53-year-old female who attended her dentist every 6 months and attended for dental hygienist treatment every 3 months was referred to a periodontal specialist concerned about the aesthetics relating to the UL1-UL5 area.

Relevant Medical and Dental History

There was no relevant medical history, she was a non-smoker and did not drink any alcohol.

Her oral hygiene was good, she brushed her teeth twice daily using an Oral B powered toothbrush and a fluoride toothpaste, she also used a mouthrinse on a daily basis and flossed very occasionally.

Clinical Examination

On examination there was minimal pocketing, plaque, and calculus but there was gingival recession on UL1, UL3, and UL4 ranging from 1 to 4 mm (Figure 9.3).

> How would you have treated the patient's gingival recession?

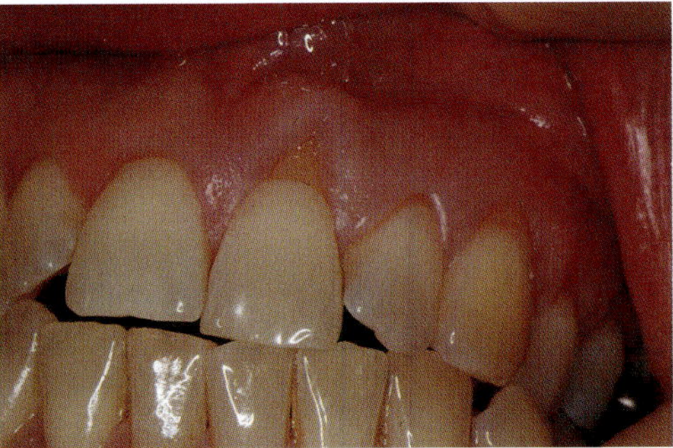

Figure 9.3 Clinical photograph of gingival recession on the anterior teeth.

Main Complaint

Her presenting complaint was related to concerns about UL1, which she was aware of for several years but thought that the recession was worsening. There was no sensitivity associated with the exposed root surface.

Surgical Procedure

Following inform consent, an appointment was made for periodontal surgery. The site (UR1-UL5) was anaesthetised with 2.2 mL Septanest 1;1000,000 (articaine hydrochloride with adrenaline) with buccal and palatal infiltrations. A buccal flap was raised using crevicular incisions but no relieving incision, root surface debridement to remove any plaque or calculus and conditioning with citric acid on the root surface of UL1 and UL3 was completed using an ultrasonic scaler and ethylenediaminetetraacetic acid (EDTA) conditioning of the exposed root surface. The Allen technique was utilised in this surgical procedure which involved preparation for a buccal pouch with two pieces of AlloDerm (BioHorizons IPH, inc.) placed in the pouch. A coronally advanced flap procedure was used and the flap secured using a modified continuous sling suture technique (6/0 monofilament [molypen]) (Figure 9.4). An extra suture was place buccal to UL1 and a cyanoacrylate tissue glue (PeriAcryl®90) was used to secure the flap, haemostasis was achieved. The surgical procedure was uneventful.

> What are the advantages of using a tissue glue during surgery?

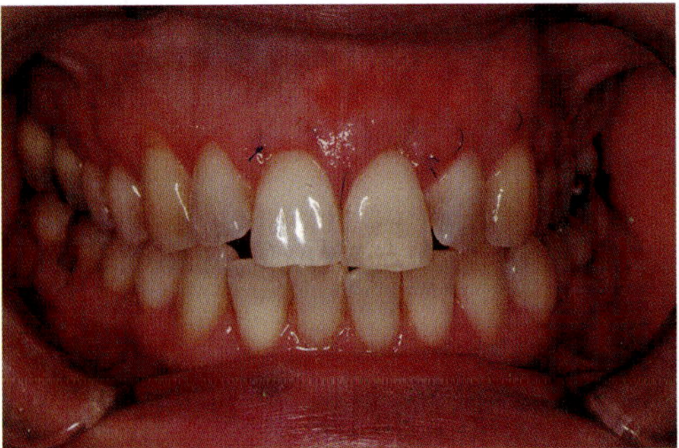

Figure 9.4 Clinical photograph immediately following the periodontal surgery, note the sutures in place with an additional interrupted suture securing the flap (UR1).

Post-operative Instructions

> What is the rationale for providing antibiotics following surgery? Is it justified?

> What is the rationale for using a mouthrinse following surgery? Is a chlorhexidine mouthrinse the most suitable choice following surgery?

Post-operative instructions were provided which included advice not to brush the upper arch. The patient was advised to rinse her mouth using a 0.2% chlorhexidine gluconate mouth rinse twice daily for two weeks. She was also given two ice packs to relieve any subsequent swelling and ibuprofen (400 mg–16 tablets [4 times a day for 4 days]) for pain relief. Antibiotics were also provided following the surgery (amoxycillin 500 mg for 5 days). The patient was reappointed 2 weeks later for a review and subsequently every 2 weeks for 6–8 weeks. No problems occurred during this period (Figure 9.5).

The sutures were removed 8 weeks post-op and the patient was advised to brush normally with a soft brush (TePe soft surgical brush) for 4–6 weeks (Figure 9.6).

The patient was monitored for every 2 weeks for next 1–2 months. At a subsequent review, clinical photographs were taken (Figure 9.7a, b).

> Do you know of any other evaluation method that could be used to assess patient outcomes?

Healing of the surgical site was uneventful and the patient maintain good oral hygiene during this period. The exposed root surface was successfully covered.

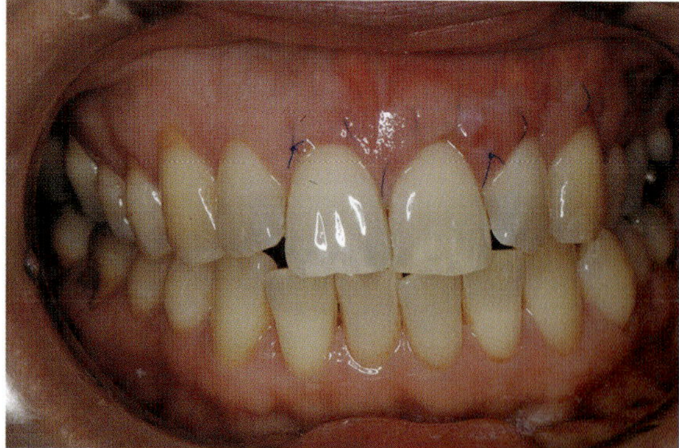

Figure 9.5 Clinical photograph two weeks post-op.

Patient Outcomes

The patient was very pleased with the outcome from this procedure and was very happy with her appearance (Figure 9.8).

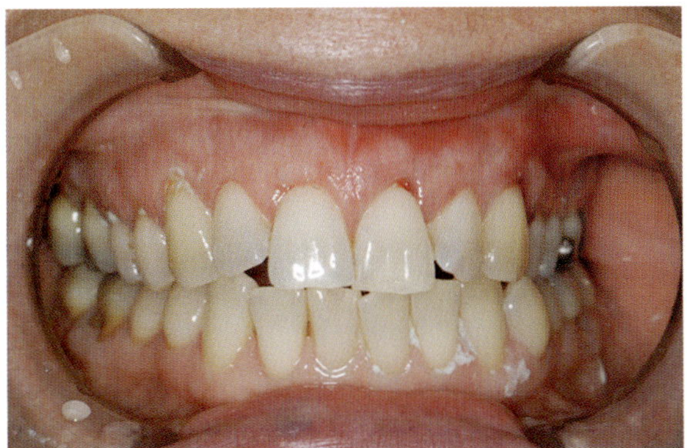

Figure 9.6 Clinical photograph of the surgical site at 8 weeks post-op following suture removal.

(a)   (b)

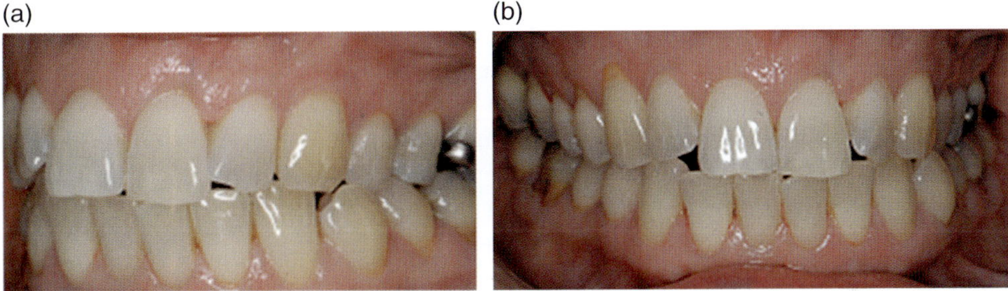

Figure 9.7 (a, b) Clinical photographs taken at a review appointment 2–3 months post-op.

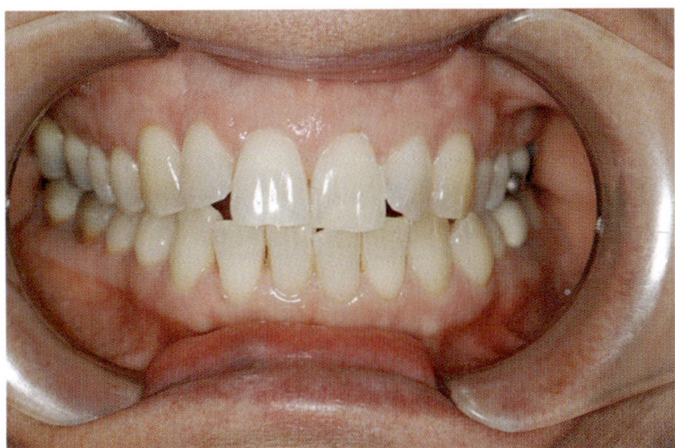

Figure 9.8 Clinical photograph 5 months post-op.

Post Script

It is important to acknowledge the role of non-surgical procedures in minimally invasive procedures in periodontal therapy and not solely focus on surgical procedures. Currently there is evidence that non-surgical debridement provided comparably results to surgical procedure in infra bony defects. The study by Zingale et al. (2012) using a diode laser compared a number of procedures such as 1) scaling/root planing using a closed approach, 2) a closed approach with laser-curettage, 3) a closed approach with laser-curettage/laser-sealing, and 4) an open approach (papilla reflection/flap closure). They reported that the closed approach therapies: SRP, laser-curettage/SRP, and laser-curettage/SRP/laser-sealing resulted in less gingival recession than the open approach (papilla reflection/flap closure). The implications from this study, if replicated in larger randomised clinical studies, would suggest there where aesthetics are a concern to the patient, the use of a diode laser maybe a less invasive option. Other non-invasive options may also be relevant in the treatment of exposed root surfaces, for example the use of desensitising toothpastes, mouthrinses, varnishes, or sealants in gingival recession rather than involving surgical procedures to cover the root surface. Depending on the extent and severity of the recession, this may be an alternative option for treatment of gingival recession and associated root sensitivity and avoid the necessity of invasive surgery.

The improvement in both surgical techniques and innovative materials over the last 20 years has also had a major impact in surgical procedures in periodontal therapy. For example, the use of Alloderm and Enamel Matrix Derivatives as well as resorbable barriers in GTR procedures in association with a less extensive flap design has also had a major impact in the subsequent outcomes. The advancement in visualisation techniques, magnification loupes, surgical microscopes, and improvements in surgical materials such as sutures etc. has also had an impact on post-operative outcomes. There are, however, some drawbacks to minimally invasive procedures in that the procedures are technique sensitive and the cost of the materials and instrumentation.

Concluding Remarks

The question proposed in the title of this chapter was 'Where Are we with a Minimally Invasive Approach in Periodontology?' Perhaps the question should have been rephrased 'Are we there yet?' since it appears to be a work in progress. There has undoubtedly been tremendous progress over the last two to three decades, nevertheless there appears to be limited data (in terms of evidence from randomised clinical trials and systematic reviews comparing both conventional and innovative MIPS. Although the introduction of MIPS into periodontal practice has made an impact on both clinical parameters and patient outcomes it was evident that most of the published studies was provided by clinicians with experience in MIPS/MIST procedures. The procedures are very technique sensitive and require considerable expenditure for the clinician in terms of specialised equipment and surgical instruments and this perhaps may be a barrier for the techniques to be transferred into clinical practices outside the hospital and specialist environment. Currently there is emphasis on observing patient outcomes in clinical research rather than just focussing on collecting clinical data looking at relatively small gains in pocket depth and attachment levels. Perhaps in future, focussing on the outcomes of the clinical procedures from the patient's point of view in terms of their quality of life such as reduced trauma during the surgery, the resultant aesthetics, minimising post-operative pain may be more meaningful.

Glossary

Term	Description
MIS	The definition of minimally invasive surgery separates the description of the surgical procedure from the technology used for visualising the surgical area using surgical operating microscopes or videoscopes. Minimally invasive surgery is a term that describes the application of very precise and delicate surgical procedures that require the use of magnifying devices, such as operating microscopes or magnifying lenses, and microsurgical instruments and materials.
MIPS	The MIPS technique allows for the minimisation of soft tissue trauma and the removal of granulation tissue from periodontal defects using a much smaller surgical incision than that used in standard bone graft techniques.
MIST	Cortellini and Tonetti (2007) proposed the Minimally Invasive Surgical Technique (MIST) to stress the aspects of wound and blood clot stability and primary wound closure for blood-clot protection. These concepts were further enforced with the Modified Minimally Invasive Surgical Technique (M-MIST, Cortellini and Tonetti 2009) that, additionally, incorporated the concept of space provision for regeneration. Two different minimally invasive techniques have been proposed: 1) procedures that include the elevation of a tiny buccal flap as well as the elevation of the interdental papilla and of the palatal flap and 2) techniques that are limited to the elevation of the buccal flap. These procedures can be applied for the treatment of shallow and deep intrabony defects (up to the apical third of the root surface).
M-MIST	Cortellini and Tonetti described a modified surgical approach of the minimally invasive surgical technique (modified minimally invasive surgical technique, M-MIST) to evaluate its applicability and clinical performances in the treatment of isolated deep intrabony defects in combination with amelogenins. The M-MIST consisted of a buccal incision of the defect-associated papilla, according to the principles of the papilla preservation techniques. Only a buccal flap was raised while the interdental papilla was left in situ. The granulation tissue filling the defect was dissected and removed, leaving the interdental and palatal tissues untouched. Root instrumentation and application of the regenerative material were performed before suturing. Primary closure of the flaps was attained with a single internal modified mattress suture. Surgery was performed with the aid of an operating microscope and microsurgical instruments. In summary, M-MIST associated with EMD resulted in improved clinical outcomes with no or minimal patient morbidity. It was easily applicable to isolated interproximal intrabony defects with a prevalent interdental component with no or minimal involvement of the lingual/palatal side. It appears to be that MIPS significantly enhances the clinical outcomes of periodontal treatment. More recently, a M-MIST has been proposed (Cortellini and Tonetti 2009). The overall idea of the M-MIST is to provide a very small interdental access to the defect only from the buccal side. The triangular buccal flap is minimally elevated in order to expose the residual buccal bone crest. According to the width of the interproximal space, the incision of the buccal aspect of the papilla follows the same principles described in the MIST approach. Once the buccal flap has been elevated, the supracrestal interdental tissue is dissected from the granulation tissue by means of a mini-blade. The interdental papilla is not detached from the residual interdental bone crest and supracrestal fibres, and the palatal flap is not elevated. The granulation tissue is further dissected from the bone with the mini-blade and then removed by means of mini-curettes. Then, the root surface is thoroughly scaled and planed by the combined action of mini-curettes and sonic/ultrasonic instruments. Special care has to be paid in order to avoid any trauma to the supracrestal fibres of the defect-associated papilla.

(Continued)

Glossary (Continued)

Term	Description
PS	Periodontal microsurgery concentrates on the soft tissue regeneration and augmentation procedures where visualisation of the area is essential. This can be improved by the use of a surgical operating microscope.
MINST	Minimally-invasive non-surgical periodontal therapy (MINST). More recently, MINST has been introduced as a concept aiming to obtain extensive subgingival debridement with minimal tissue trauma.
MIS (V-MIS)	The use of a videoscope has allowed for smaller surgical access openings when performing MIS, and the procedure is described as Videoscope-Assisted Minimally Invasive Surgery (V-MIS). With V-MIS, smaller access incisions and less flap reflection can be used than with traditional MIS surgical approaches. V-MIS/MIS is usually indicated for isolated defects.
GTR	Guided Tissue Regeneration. Of the techniques used in periodontics to reconstruct lost or diseased periodontal tissue in those with gingival recession. GTR often involves the use of absorbable barrier membranes or collagen. Regeneration of tissue directed by the physical presence or chemical activities of a biomaterial; often involves placement of barriers to exclude one or more cell types during healing or regeneration of tissue.
EMD	EMD is an extract of enamel matrix and contains amelogenins of various molecular weights. Amelogenins are involved in the formation of enamel and periodontal attachment formation during tooth development. Several surgical techniques have been developed to regenerate periodontal tissues including guided tissue regeneration (GTR), bone grafting (BG), and the use of enamel matrix derivative (EMD).
Papillary Preservation Technique	The objective of this procedure is to preserve papillary height. According to Dannan (2011) the buccal aspect of the flap is designed with a sulcular incision around each tooth, with no incisions made through the interdental papilla. The lingual/palatal flap design consists of a sulcular incision along the lingual or palatal aspect of each tooth, with a semi-lunar incision across each interdental papilla. This incision dips apically from the line angles of the tooth so that the papillary incision line is at least 5 mm from the gingival margin. This allows the interdental tissue to be dissected from the lingual/palatal aspect so that it can be elevated intact with the facial flap. After treatment of the bony defect, the buccal flap, including the palatal/lingual aspect of the papilla, is repositioned. The palatal/lingual papilla is sutured with the palatal/lingual flap.
Modified Papilla Preservation Techniques	This is a modification of the papillary preservation techniques. A horizontal incision is performed on the buccal papillary tissue at the base of the papilla. A full-thickness palatal flap, which includes the interdental papilla, is elevated. A buccal full-thickness flap is elevated with vertical releasing incisions and/or periosteal incisions, when needed. A barrier membrane is positioned to cover the defect. The interdental tissues are repositioned and sutured to completely cover the membrane. A horizontal internal crossed mattress suture is placed beneath the mucoperiosteal flaps between the base of the palatal papilla and the buccal flap. This suture relieves all the tension of the flaps. A second suture (vertical internal mattress suture) is placed between the buccal aspect of the interproximal papilla and the most coronal portion of the buccal flap to ensure primary closure. This technique is applicable in wide interdental spaces (>2 mm), especially in the anterior dentition. This technique allows for achieving primary closure of the tissue and preserving the papilla in 75% of cases.

Glossary (Continued)

Term	Description
Simplified Papilla Preservation Technique	This is a simplification of the modified papilla preservation technique. It is initiated with an oblique incision across the defect-associated papilla, from the gingival margin at the buccal line angle of the involved tooth to the mid interproximal portion of the papilla under the contact point of the adjacent tooth. A full-thickness palatal flap, including the papilla, and a split-thickness buccal flap are then elevated. The interdental tissues are positioned and sutured to obtain primary closure of the interdental space. The SPPT is applicable in narrow interdental spaces (<2 mm).

Further Reading

Cortellini P., Prato, G.P., and Tonetti, M.S. (1999). The simplified papilla preservation flap: A novel surgical approach for the management of soft tissues in regenerative procedures. *Int. J. Periodontics Restorative Dent.* 19: 589–599.

Cortellini, P., and Tonetti, M.S. (2009). Improved wound stability with a modified minimally invasive surgical technique in the regenerative treatment of isolated interdental intrabony defects. *J. Clin. Periodontol.* 36: 157–163.

Cortellini, P., Prato, G.P., and Tonetti M.S. (1995). The modified papilla preservation technique. A new surgical approach for interproximal regenerative procedures. *J. Periodontol.* 66: 261–266.

Harrel, S.K., and Wilson, T.G. (2015). *Minimally Invasive Periodontal Therapy: Clinical Techniques and Visualization Technology*, 1e (eds. S.K. Harrel and T.G. Wilson, Jr.). Iowa, USA: John Wiley & Sons Inc.

Harrel, S.K. (2015b). Ch 2. Visualization for minimally invasive periodontal therapy: An overview. In: *Minimally Invasive Periodontal Therapy: Clinical Techniques and Visualization Technology*, 1e (eds. S.K. Harrel and T.G. Wilson, Jr.), 3–12. Iowa, USA: John Wiley & Sons Inc.

Jaffray, B. (2005). Minimally invasive surgery. *Arch. Dis. Child.* 90: 537–542.

Tunnell, J.C., and Harrel, S.K. (2017). Minimally invasive surgery in periodontal regeneration: A review of the literature. *Compend. Contin. Educ. Dent.* 38 (4): e13–e16.

Wang, S.-Y., Yang, Y.-H., and Chang, H.-P. (2007). The effect of an oral hygiene instruction intervention on plaque control by orthodontic patients *J. Dent. Sci.* 2 (1): 45–51.

References

Ashruff, F. (2016). Impact of oral hygiene instructions in the maintenance of periodontal health of patients. *Int. J. Pharm. Sci. Res.* 8 (10): 1212–1214.

Axelsson, P., and Lindhe, J. (1981a). Effect of controlled oral hygiene procedures on caries and periodontal disease in adults. Results after 6 years. *J. Clin. Periodontol.* 8 (3): 239–248.

Axelsson, P., and Lindhe, J. (Dec 1981b). Effect of oral hygiene instruction and professional tooth cleaning on caries and gingivitis in schoolchildren. *Community Dent. Oral Epidemiol.* 9 (6): 251–255.

Checchi, L., and Pelliccioni, G.A. (1988). Hand verses ultrasonic instrumentation in the removal of endotoxins from root surfaces in vitro. *J Periodontol.* 59(6): 398–402. doi: 10.1902/jop.1988.59.6.398. PMID: 3292754.

Cortellini, P. and Tonetti, M.S. (2001). Microsurgical Approach to Periodontal Regeneration. Initial Evaluation in a Case Cohort. *J Periodontol.* 72: 559–569. doi: 10.1902/jop. 2001.72.4.559.

Cortellini P. and Tonetti M.S. (2005). Clinical performance of a regenerative strategy for intrabony defects: scientific evidence and clinical experience. *J Periodontol.* 76(3): 341–350. doi: 10.1902/jop.2005.76.3.341.

Cortellini, P., and Tonetti, M.S. (2007). A minimally invasive surgical technique with an enamel matrix derivative in the regenerative treatment of intra-bony defects: A novel approach to limit morbidity. *J. Clin. Periodontol.* 34 (1): 87–93.

Cortellini, P., and Tonetti, M.S. (2009). Improved wound stability with a modified minimally invasive surgical technique in the regenerative treatment of isolated interdental intrabony defects. *J. Clin. Periodontol.* 36 (2): 157–163.

Dannan, A. (Oct–Dec 2011). Minimally invasive periodontal therapy, *J. Indian Soc. Periodontol.* 15 (4): 338–343.

Harrel, T.K., and Nunn, M.E. (2001). Longitudinal comparison of the periodontal status of patients with moderate to severe periodontal disease receiving no treatment, non-surgical treatment, and surgical treatment utilizing individual sites for analysis. *J. Periodontol.* 72: 1509–1519.

Harrel, S.K., and Rees, T.D. (1995). Granulation tissue removal in routine and minimally invasive procedures. *Compend. Contin. Educ. Dent.* 16 (9): 960–964.

Harrel, S.K. (2015a). Ch 7. The MIS and V-MIS surgical procedure. In: *Minimally Invasive Periodontal Therapy: Clinical Techniques and Visualization Technology*, 1e (eds. S.K. Harrel and T.G. Wilson, Jr.), 81–116. Iowa, USA: John Wiley & Sons Inc.

Harrel, S.K., Wilson, T.G., Nunn, M.E. (2005). Prospective assessment of the use of enamel matrix proteins with minimally invasive surgery. *J Periodontol.* 76(3): 380–384. doi: 10.1902/jop.2005.76.3.380.

Hajishengallis, G., Darveau, R.P., and Curtis, M.A. (October 2012). The keystone pathogen hypothesis *Nat. Rev. Microbiol.* 10 (10): 717–725.

Killen, M., Chapple, I.L.C., Hannig, M., Marsh, P.D., Meuric, V., Pedersen, A.M., Tonetti, M.S., Wade, W.G., and Zaura, E. (2016). The oral microbiome – an update for oral healthcare professionals. *Br. Dent. J.* 221: 657–666.

Moore, J., Wilson, M., and Kieser, J.B. (1986). The distribution of bacterial lipopolysaccharide (endotoxin) in relation to periodontally involved root surfaces. *J. Clin. Periodontol.* 13: 748–751

Nibali, L., Pometti, D., Chen T.T., Tu, Y.K. (2015). Minimally invasive non-surgical approach for the treatment of periodontal intrabony defects: A retrospective analysis. *J Clin Periodontol.* 42(9): 853–859.

Ower, P. (May 2013). Minimally-invasive non-surgical periodontal therapy. *Dent. Update.* 40 (4): 289–290.

Pareek, S., Nagaraj, A., Yousuf, A., Ganta, S., Mansi Atri, M., and Singh, K. (May–Jun 2015). Effectiveness of supervised oral health maintenance in hearing impaired and mute children- A parallel randomized controlled trial. *J. Int. Soc. Prev. Community Dent.* 5 (3): 176–182.

Rethman, M.P., and Harrell, S.K. (2010). Minimally invasive periodontal therapy: Will periodontal therapy remain a technologic laggard? *J. Periodontol.* 81: 1390–1395.

Ribeiro, F.V., Casarin, R.C., Palma, M.A., Júnior, F.H., Sallum, E.A., and Casati, M.Z. (Sep 2011). Clinical and patient-centered outcomes after minimally invasive non-surgical or surgical approaches for the treatment of intrabony defects: a randomized clinical trial. *J. Periodontol.* 82 (9): 1256–1266.

Smart, G.J., Wilson, M., Davies, E.H., and Kieser, J.B. (1990). Assessment of ultrasonic root surface debridement by determination of residual endotoxin levels. *J Cin Periodontol.* 17: 174–178.

Tibbetts, L.S., and Shanelec, D. (1998). Periodontal microsurgery. *Dent. Clin. North Am.* 42 (2): 339–359.

Tunnell, J.C., and Harrel, S.K. (Apr 2017). Minimally invasive surgery in periodontal regeneration: A review of the literature. *Compend. Contin. Educ. Dent.* 38 (4): e13–e16.

Turner, Y., Ashley, F.P., and Wilson, R.F. (1994). Effectiveness of oral hygiene with and without root planing in treating subjects with chronic periodontitis. *Br. Dent. J.* 177 (10): 367–7.

Zingale, J., Harpenau, L., Chambers, D., and Lundergan, W. (Oct 2012). Effectiveness of root planing with diode laser curettage for the treatment of periodontitis. *J. Calif. Dent. Assoc.* 40 (10): 786–793.

10

Pulp and Endodonic Regeneration

Alastair J. Sloan

Key Topics

- Dentin/pulp complex structure
- Vital Pulp Therapies
- Dental Pulp Stem Cells
- Non-vital Pulp Therapies

Learning Objectives

- Be able to understand the relationship between the pulp and dentin and bioactive nature of dentin
- Be able to recognize biological responses within the pulp can be harnessed to facilitate tissue repair
- Understand the biological basis of current research with respect to pulp regeneration

Introduction

Over the past 20 years there have been numerous developments in tissue engineering that have been led by development, synthesis and manufacture of novel materials acting as scaffolds to support cell attachment, growth, and differentiation. This work has been enhanced, in parallel by the identification of novel stem cell sources (Nakashima and Iohara 2011) and bioactive molecules (Lu and Atala 2014). These approaches in tissue engineering have targeted the regeneration of tissues and organs lost due to trauma or disease (Langer and Vacanti 1993). As such tissue engineering has been seen as being key to the development and translational impact of regenerative dentistry and specifically endodontic tissue regeneration. The goal of any regenerative approach to dentistry is to direct or mediate biological activity leading to the replacement of dental tissues and their supporting structures with

Minimally Invasive Dentistry: Interdisciplinary Clinical and Scientific Approaches, First Edition.
Edited by Aylin Baysan and Paul Anderson.
© 2026 John Wiley & Sons Ltd. Published 2026 by John Wiley & Sons Ltd.
Companion website: www.wiley.com/go/baysan/minimally_invasive_dentistry

natural tissue. The potential for a clinical application of regenerative therapies in dentistry is possible to some degree due to significant advances in our understanding of the dentine/pulp complex, its innate biological ability to respond to infection, inflammation and trauma and repair compromised tissues and the increasing understanding of the role dental stem cells play in the regenerative processes. By applying the underlying principles of tissue engineering with these biological processes (spatial assembly of stem cells, growth factors, matrix and scaffolds) it may be possible to achieve the functional regeneration required for successful clinical translation of regenerative dentistry.

The Dentin-Pulp Complex

Dentin is the most abundant tissue of the tooth and is a thick, tubular mineralized tissue found beneath the enamel in the crown of the tooth and beneath the cementum in the root of the tooth. It serves as a barrier to infectious agents that threaten the pulp tissue. Dentin is synthesized and secreted by the odontoblast cell, a post-mitotic mesenchymal-derived cell that is found on the periphery of the dental pulp in contact with the dentin. They maintain this position throughout dentinogenesis and for the life of the healthy tooth. It is because of this anatomical structure of the dentin and underlying pulp and odontoblast layer that we consider the dentin and pulp as one complex. It is cells on the periphery of the one tissue (the pulp) that secretes the other (dentin) and their biological activity, specifically in response to trauma, infection, inflammation and repair are exquisitely intertwined. The composition of dentin is approximately 70% inorganic mineral, 20% organic matrix and 10% water by weight. The inorganic material is crystalline hydroxyapatite whilst the organic matrix is similar to bone consisting of collagen fibrils embedded in a non-collagenous matrix. The principal collagen fibre is type I collagen and these fibres are closely packed in mineralised dentin. The collagen content contributes 90% of the organic matrix, with the remaining 10% being non-collagenous proteins, including the proteoglycans decorin and biglycan, with the glycosaminoglycan side chains of chondrotin-4-sulphate and chondroitin-6-sulphate. Also within this non-collagenous matrix are specific dentine phosphoproteins, acidic proteins, including osteopontin and osteonectin and a cocktail of bioactive growth factors. Dentin is not an inert tissue, more a bioactive extracellular matrix (ECM) whose molecular constituents may influence cellular behaviour in the dentin–pulp complex, mediating reparative responses of the tissue. Several ECM components have been identified with protein binding sites, allowing adherence and incorporation of growth factors within the ECM. Biglycan and decorin are the main proteoglycans found in dentine matrix, and studies have demonstrated that TGFβ is present in dentin matrix associated with its latency-associated protein (LAP), biglycan and decorin (Smith et al. 1998). Real time kinetic measurements to observe the interactions of the TGFβ with biglycan and decorin suggest that TGFβ-1 and β3 bind to both molecules, but that the association with TGFβ-1 is strongest (Baker et al. 2009). This concept of dentin as a bioactive matrix has allowed us to determine how dentin matrix components may be utilised for novel therapies to drive dental tissue repair and regeneration. Release of bioactive molecules from the dentin matrix occurs during carious demineralisation but local release may take place during various dental procedures such as cavity preparation and restoration (Sadaghiani et al. 2016). By understanding the biological activity of these bioactive molecules, both in isolation but more importantly as a synergistic combination of matrix molecules, on cells of the dentin–pulp complex provides opportunities to exploit them clinically.

The pulp is a dynamic matrix that has an important role in controlling the activity of the cells residing within it. The structural framework of collagen type I and III and associated proteoglycans and glycoproteins creates a porous scaffold to stabilise the pulp, however the nature of the organic molecules within it allow it to influence cell migration, proliferation, adhesion and differentiation. The pulp contains significant quantities of the glycosaminoglycans (GAGs) chondrotin sulphate, with dermatan sulphate being detected in much smaller amounts. These GAGs are hydrophilic and form biological gels that fill most of the extracellular space. When hydrated they will swell which may explain the high fluid pressure detected within the pulp. These GAGs are also thought to contribute to the broader mechanical support of the tissue. Hyaluronan is found unbound to protein and is thought to facilitate cell migration through the matrix. Thus, the proteoglycans found within the pulp not only contribute to the bulk and stability of the matrix, but also influence bioactivity by binding and conferring protection to growth factors whilst functioning as adhesion molecules to influence cell behaviour. The pulp is also highly vascularized and this extensive capillary network is confined by the surrounding dentin with the only access being through the apical foramen. Vascularization of the pulp occurs through the process of vasculogenesis during tooth development. The presence of such an extensive capillary network also provides a potential second progenitor cell niche within the pulp, with pervascular cells being present around capillaries. Due to the presence of large neural plexuses in the pulp and their extensive innervations, the presence of variety of neuropeptides found in the dental pulp is considerable. The most significant is calcitonin gene-related peptide (CRGP), a potent vasodilator and the major agent controlling blood flow locally in the periphery of the pulp. CRGP may also have role to play in initiating and controlling mineralized tissue secretion. Nerve growth factor (NGF) has also been identified in the peripheral pulp tissue and the expression of NGF and its receptor is increased during pulpal injury, where it may act as a chemoattractant for leukocytes. A range of other neuropeptides and transmitters have also been identified within the pulp however their roles are still fully not understood and are something of conjecture.

Histologically, the pulp consists of four distinct regions. There is, at its periphery the odontoblast layer followed by a cell-free zone which contains extensive nerve and capillary networks. Beneath this is a cell-rich zone, characterized by high cellular density consisting of spindle-shaped pulpal fibroblasts and a population of undifferentiated mesenchymal cells that are polyhedral in shape with large nuclei. The central core of the pulp sits beneath this cell-rich layer containing predominately fibroblasts. Dendritic cells are present beneath the odontoblast layer and these cells increase in number following trauma/infection to identify and present foreign antigens to immune cells. Transient immune cell populations including macrophages, neutrophils, antigen-presenting cells and T-lymphocytes are also found within the pulp and essential for tissue homeostasis. In addition, they are key to the host defense during tissue injury, including caries and may facilitate or negate.

Dental Pulp Stem Cells and Regeneration of the Dentine-Pulp Complex

Mesenchymal stem cells (MSCs) are now recognized as the cell population ultimately responsible for the synthesis of the collagenous connective tissue of the dentin-pulp complex. Within the dental pulp these MSCs have been reported to represent between 1% and 9% of the total cell population (Gronthos et al. 2002; Lizier et al. 2012). This is higher than estimates of MSCs in bone marrow which have been estimated to represent 0.001–0.001% of the total bone marrow mononuclear cells (Jones et al. 2002). These MSCs derived from the pulp also exhibit significant heterogeneity due in part to the fact that they fall into a hierarchical order of cell types observed in many other connective tissues. Multiple niches of MSCs are also likely, suggesting that multiple distinct progenitors may reside in the pulp. As mentioned previously, the presence of an extensive capillary network in the pulp and mesenchymal stem cells are normally closely associated with blood vessels. Such progenitor cells associated with the vasculature are termed peri-vascular cells or pericytes. It is also now thought that cells of the dental pulp also contain neural crest stem cells (NCCs) that derive from the external ectoderm (Chai et al. 2000). During early embryogenesis, these NCCs migrate from their original positon and, in relation of craniofacial development, undergo an epithelial to mesenchymal transition and contribute to the formation of the presumptive dentin-pulp complex. NCCs thus contribute to the formation of mesenchymal tissues, including the dentine and dental papilla. The population of NCCs decreases as tooth development progresses and they become progressively restricted in terms of their differentiation ability (Tucker and Sharpe 1999). However, a population of NCCs is retained within the post-natal dental pulp and presence of these cells, along with pulpal MSCs and pericytes further reflect the significant heterogeneity of progenitor cells isolated from this tissue.

The so-called dental pulp stem cells (DPSCs) were first isolated by Gronthos and colleagues (Gronthos et al. 2000, 2002; Shi and Gronthos 2003) and these DSPSs and selected clonal cell lines derived from isolated DPSCs have successfully been differentiated through adipogenic, chondrogenic, myogenic, neurogenic and osteogenic lineages (d'Aquino et al. 2007; Gronthos et al. 2002; Laino et al. 2005; Song et al. 2016; Young et al. 2016; Zhang et al. 2006). It has been suggested that DPSCs are more lineage restricted compared to BMSCs. BMSCs, transplanted into the dorsal surface of immuno-compromised mice resulted in synthesis of a bone-like tissue but transplantation of DPSCs produced a dentin-like tissue (Gronthos et al. 2000).

The dental pulp of teeth from the primary dentition also contains a population of progenitor cells. Isolation of a population of Stem cells from Human Exfoliated teeth (SHEDs) suggest that these teeth contain a more immature progenitor cell population compared with DPSCs. SHEDs are highly proliferative (and clonogenic) and have demonstrated a greater potentiality in differentiating into a multiple cell types compared with DPSCs (Miura et al. 2003). Progenitor cells have also been isolated from the apical papilla of developing teeth. These cell have been referred to as SCAPs (stem cells from apical papilla) (Sonoyama et al. 2008) It is likely that these cells are responsible for the formation of root dentin and the radicular dentin-pulp complex as well as cementum and alveolar bone.

The odontoblasts of the post-natal dental pulp remain viable throughout the life of the tooth and protect the it by localised up-regulation of dentin synthesis, called reactionary dentine, in response of mild caries or trauma (Lesot et al. 1993). Significant injury to the pulp leads to odontoblast cell death and in this scenario, the population of DPSCs resident within the pulpal tissue (from the multiple niches within the pulp) are recruited to the site of tissue injury where they proliferate and subsequently differentiate into odontoblast-like cells, synthesizing an atubular, dysplastic reparative dentin matrix. Reparative dentinogenesis is regulated by the numerous growth factors sequestered in the dentin matrix and known to play a role in recruitment and functional control of DPSCs. This cocktail of growth factors is extensive and it is thought that they function synergistically to to lead to cell differentiation and upregulation of matrix synthesis (Smith et al. 2012). Several studies have demonstrated TGF-β1, TGF-β3 and BMP-7 may mediate dentin matrix secretion in a 3D organotypic culture system (Sloan et al. 2000; Sloan and Smith 1999) and release of these (and other growth factors) from the dentin matrix through carious demineralization has been postulated as one of the key promoters of dentin-pulp complex repair. How we can exploit this growth factor release with clinically acceptable agents and materials provides a key challenge in regenerative dentistry. It has been shown that acidic, basic and neutral chelating agents are capable of releasing bioactive molecules and other ECM components from dentin (Graham et al. 2006; Sadaghiani et al. 2016).

The extensive vasculature of the dental pulp is fundamental to the supply of nutrients during active dentinogenesis in development and to maintain a vital post-natal pulp. During tissue repair, there is a need to maintain that blood supply to facilitate repair and at sites of repair neo-angiogenesis is observed. Pulp tissue bioengineering has highlighted the potential role of release of pro-angiogenic factors from dentin matrix in signalling angiogenic events during dentin–pulp regeneration (Cordeiro et al. 2008). Pro-angiogenic growth factors are sequestered in the dentin matrix (Roberts-Clark and Smith 2000) and if released will provide a possible mechanism for signaling angiogenesis during regeneration of the dentin–pulp complex. In support of this hypothesis, it is worth noting that lyophilized dentin matrix components have been demonstrated to exhibit potent pro-angiogenic properties *in vitro* (Zhang et al. 2011).

Greater understanding is now required of the response of DPSCs to pro-inflammatory cytokines and the role inflammation may play in dentin-pulp complex repair. It is clear that repair of the pulp and dentin-pulp complex best occurs when infection and subsequent inflammation are controlled or mediated. Chronic inflammation in the pulp will negate tissue repair (Rutherford and Gu 2000). Such inhibition has been observed during rapidly progressing caries (Bjorndal et al. 1999) and high levels of pro-inflammatory cytokines such as TNF-α as well as dentin matrix components released by bacterial acids during caries can lead to pulpal cell death and inhibition of progenitor cell proliferation and differentiation (Silva et al. 2005; Smith et al. 2005). Significantly lower levels of such pro-inflammatory cytokines present during early caries or following treatment may modulate the reparative processes including progenitor cell differentiation (Goldberg et al. 2008; Saito et al. 2011). Clearly, inflammation is required to initiate cellular repair and cellular responses for tissue repair. If prolonged or inappropriate inflammatory responses can adversely modulate the function of dentin sequestered growth factors reducing progenitor cell recruitment, differentiation and dentin synthesis, there is a fine line dividing required and positive inflammatory which is required and longer lasting chronic inflammation that whilst promoting immune cell recruitment in response to infective agents significantly hinders repair.

Utilizing the DPSCs *in situ* for clinically controlled tissue regeneration is one possible therapeutic avenue to explore, however exogenous use of DPSCs is another possible therapeutic route for both dental tissue regeneration and regeneration of other tissues using tissue engineering approaches. An important requirement for the tissue engineering exploitation of progenitor cells is the requirement for *in vitro* cell expansion to obtain sufficient cell numbers for subsequent use. Here however, lies a significant limitation in that extensive expansion *in vitro* leads to alterations in cell behavior including a decline in cell proliferation, cellular senescence and impaired regenerative potential. For many cell types, *in vitro* expansion and associated cellular senescence is a consequence of replicative senescence which is telomere dependent and is characterised by progressive telomere shortening due to repeated cell divisions. Such differences in the expansion limitations of individual DPSC populations has been recognized and a recent study examining differences in telomere lengths and associated susceptibilities to cellular senescence between individual DPSC populations demonstrated significant variability in the proliferative and differentiation capabilities for individual DPSC populations expanded from individual human teeth from donors within a similar age range and differences between DPSC populations derived from the same patient (Alraies et al. 2017). Such information may allow the optimization of population selection by selectively screening and isolating better quality DPSCs from whole dental pulp tissues for *in vitro* expansion and assessment and is something commercial tissue banks may want to consider. Isolating and storing the best 'quality' DPSCs will facilitate translational development of effective and further evidenced DPSC-based therapies for clinical evaluation.

Vital Pulp Therapy

As discussed in the previous section, it is known that a highly proliferative population of progenitor/stem cells reside within the dental pulp and can differentiate into cells of a mineralizing phenotype when appropriately stimulated. As such, odontoblasts compromised by infection or trauma may be replaced by newly differentiated populations of odontoblast-like cells derived from the DPSC populations(s) in the healthy portion of the pulp (Huang et al. 2009, 2010; Nakashima and Akamine 2005). Vital pulp therapy works with these physiological process to induce dentinal bridge formation to maintain pulp vitality and function after reversible pulpal injury. However, pulp capping in carious teeth has been considered unpredictable and are usually limited to well-selected clinical cases. Successful outcomes for vital pulp therapy are also highly dependent on the type and location of the dentin-pulp injury, the age of the tooth, the treatment modality (capping material to be used) and the integrity of the cavity restoration (Tziafas 2004).

Several clinical materials, such as calcium hydroxide and mineral trioxide aggregate (MTA), are believed to promote the reparative dentinogenesis (Graham et al. 2006; Huang et al. 2009).

These materials seal off the exposed pulp or dentinal tubules from external environment and mediate release of growth factors sequestered in the dentin ECM. *In vivo* studies have demonstrated that MTA capping may lead to mild necrotic changes followed by new dentin matrix formation and a calcified bridge. Pulpal responses to MTA capping involve proliferation and migration of progenitor cells followed by differentiation into odontoblast-like cells, a mechanism very similar to that found in the response of the dentin-pulp complex to calcium hydroxide. Here, osteopontin is thought to play a triggering role in initiation of the pulpal reparative process (Kuratate et al. 2008). Calcium hydroxide has been considered the gold standard for direct pulp capping procedures for over sixty years, however the newer clinical materials designed to have better biocompatibility and inductive effects on progenitor cells, including MTA and tricalcium silicate cements (e.g. Biodentine), have increased the success and, more importantly, the clinical predictability of pulp capping treatments. As mentioned above, the desired clinical outcomes of pulp capping procedures rely heavily on the effects these materials have on the local environment and extent of tissue injury. They have the ability to modulate inflammation whilst promoting the recruitment, proliferation and differentiation of DPSCs. It has been demonstrated using *ex vivo* models that both MTA and Biodentine when used as direct capping materials induces greater reparative tertiary dentinogenesis compared with calcium hydroxide through both direct and indirect mechanisms. The direct mechanism concerns calcium mediated increase in proliferation and recruitment of progenitor cells whilst indirect effects are through the release of transforming growth factor β-1 from dentin (Laurent et al. 2012; Tecles et al. 2008). Together, these materials have demonstrated the ability to reproducibly promote significant regeneration of the infected and injured dental pulp and have quickly translated to clinical practice.

Robust clinical studies are required if we are to deduce which pulp capping materials may elicit the best, and most reproducible, biological response to lead to a desired clinical outcome. Randomized control trials are increasing to provide key data to provide this clinical and biological evidence. One such trial recently demonstrated that the use of MTA as a direct pulp capping agent resulted in significantly greater clinical success (81.3%) compared those patients where patients were treated with calcium hydroxide (68.5%) (Hilton et al. 2013). These results concur with another clinical study that reported a 80.5% success with the use of MTA as compare to 59% when calcium hydroxide was used (Mente et al. 2014). It is worth noting that desirable clinical outcomes including resolution of disease and loss of symptoms is directly influenced by the biocompatibility of these materials and their effects on pulpal progenitor cells and sequestered growth factors. The histological evaluation of human dental pulp capped with MTA or calcium hydroxide following extraction of treated teeth (for orthodontic reasons) has led to the opportunity to evaluate what effects these materials elicit on the tissue (Accorinte Mde et al. 2008). Similar histological findings were found in study by Nowicka and colleagues (Nowicka et al. 2013). These findings included the presence of a dentinal bridge lined with odontoblast-like cells and minimal inflammation. It is now possible to hypothesize that the greater clinical success rates achieved with contemporary biomaterials in pulp capping procedures could be directly related to the ability of these materials to facilitate DPSC-mediated pulp regeneration with the differentiation of new odontoblast-like cells and synthesis of tertiary dentin leading to the restoration of normal pulp physiology.

Current endodontic practice, therapies and materials have led to successful clinical outcomes for vital pulp therapy in mature teeth diagnosed with reversible pulpitis (Simon et al. 2013). A problem, which must be overcome for vital pulp therapy to be a routine primary choice of treatment for these cases, is the ability to determine the extent of pulpal inflammation and an understanding of how this negates pulpal repair (naturally and mediated by application of clinical materials). It is also important to understand to what extent pulpal progenitor cells may operate in these compromised conditions, thus providing the clinician with knowledge that regenerative treatments on significantly inflamed teeth (pulpitis) would be successful. Currently clinicians use highly subjective measures to determine if pulpal inflammation is reversible or irreversible. A clinical case recently reported that a pulpotomy was capable of reversing the irreversible pulpitis status of a secondary mandibular molar in a 19 year-old patient (Chueh and Chiang 2010). Extraction of this tooth (for orthodontic reasons) was undertaken 10 months post procedure allowing the histological evaluation of the tissue. In this case, a vital pulp was observed with normal appearance with presence of a mineralized barrier in intimate contact with the MTA capping material.

Despite such significant advances reported in the literature, and isolated cases with promising results reported clinically, vital pulp therapy is still not the routine treatment alternative for teeth with vital pulps requiring endodontic treatment. We require a better understanding of the inherent regenerative potential of the dental pulp if we are to tap into it to mediate tissue repair clinically. As we understand better the ability of the pulpal progenitor cells to function in highly inflamed tissues, the molecular mechanisms regulating dentinogenesis and pathogenesis of pulpal infection we will create new opportunities to design innovative regenerative methods of treatment including materials which exert antimicrobial properties, but also treatments where partial pulpotomies result in regeneration of healthy pulp tissue.

Regenerative Endodontics

A situation where there is pulpal necrosis presents a different clinical challenge. Apexification procedures allow for healing of apical periodontitis, but do not promote continued root development or repair/regeneration of a physiological pulp. This presents a particular challenge with immature permanent teeth. Regenerative endodontic procedures include, but not restricted to, procedures described in the literature as revascularization procedures (Banchs and Trope 2004). Revascularization refers to the reestablishment of the vasculature of an ischemic tissue, such as the dental pulp of an avulsed tooth. Initially it was thought that the blood clot created during invoked bleeding promoted the wound healing but recent evidence has suggested that revascularization procedures promotes the influx of a significant number of undifferentiated mesenchymal stem cells into the root canals (Lovelace et al. 2011). Clinical success observed with regenerative endodontic procedures has been observed in a patient with a necrotic pulp. Here, there was a complete resolution of pre-operative sinus tract and symptoms alongside thickening and elongation of the root and apical closure (Diogenes et al. 2013). Additionally these treated teeth were vital to testing. Numerous cases demonstrating successful clinical outcomes using regenerative endodontic procedures have also been reported (Diogenes et al. 2013). It is worth mentioning that the patient is the greatest variable in predicting success with regenerative endodontics. The patient's age and the stage of root development may play a key role in predicting clinical outcomes. Most clinical cases have been undertaken on young patients with an age range of 6–20 years (Kontakiotis et al. 2015). This success is likely to be due to the number, differentiation state and cellular properties of progenitor cells present in young patients as opposed to adult patients. It is now accepted that there is a decrease in the number as well as a decrease in the proliferative and differentiation capacity of progenitor cells in older patients (Yu et al. 2011). This is related to changes in cell-cycle regulation, signaling mechanisms, cell damage over time (Piccin and Morshead 2010) and significantly reduces the regenerative potential of the tissue and thus unpredictability of clinical outcome and success.

Angiogenesis is thus clearly a requirement for tissue regeneration, however this needs to be taken together alongside the role of the progenitor cells, local bioactive molecules (e.g. growth factors, cytokines) and tissue engineering scaffolds. If bleeding into the root canal is invoked a blood clot will form and it was initially thought that this clot mediated healing by inducing angiogenesis. However, bleeding also results in not only vascular components entering the canal but also, as mentioned above, the influx of progenitor cells that naturally circulate in the blood. The fibrin clot may also act as a suitable scaffold for these cells. The source of progenitor cells for regenerative endodontics is also varied, and includes those located in the periapical region (Diogenes et al. 2013). SCAPs, and bone marrow stromal cells (BMSCs) appear to be the most likely of sources. SCAPs have been demonstrated to exhibit a high proliferation rate, telomerase activity, and cell migration ability (Sonoyama et al. 2008). It is likely then that regeneration of pulp tissue is mediated, if not controlled, by progenitor cell function and determined by the plasticity of these cells to differentiate into numerous connective tissue phenotypes including collagenous connective tissue, endothelium and dentin. To this end, the environment into which these cells migrate is critical to mediating their final phenotype.

The ability of stem cells to proliferate and differentiate into the desired phenotypes is dependent on signaling from bioactive molecules such as growth factors and their 3 dimensional carrier, a biodegradable scaffold. Tissue engineering for endodontics should be designed to use biological materials to replace damaged tissues including dentin, root and cells of the dentin-pulp complex. To achieve this, there is a need to optimize differentiation of DPSCs or SCAPs if they are to be utilized, to their final phenotype. The environment in which these cells will be carried and biologically manipulated is critical to mediating cell differentiation. Increasing the bioavailability of growth factors already sequestered in root dentin will facilitate this. It is this combination of requisite numbers of progenitor cells, appropriate growth factors and a suitable scaffold that form the basis of this tissue engineering (Murray et al. 2007). As mentioned earlier, dentin contains a cocktail of growth factors including transforming growth factor beta (TGF-β), basic fibroblast growth factor (bFGF), vascular endothelial growth factor (VEGF), bone morphogenetic proteins (BMPs), platelet derived growth factor (PDGF) alongside numerous others (Smith et al. 2012). *In vitro* studies have demonstrated the potency of demineralized dentin matrix in driving progenitor cell differentiation to a mineralizing cell phenotype (Avery et al. 2017). It has also been shown *in vitro* that dentin conditioning with either calcium hydroxide, MTA or 17%

ethylenediamine tetraacetic acid (EDTA) solubilizes dentin-matrix components (Casagrande et al. 2010; Graham et al. 2006; Tomson et al. 2007) and influences DPSC behvaviour (Sadaghiani et al. 2016). Additionally, platelet-rich plasma (PRP) from patient's own blood has been used to act as an autologous scaffold as well as being a rich source of growth factors (Sachdeva et al. 2014; Torabinejad and Turman 2011). Other options include delivery of exogenous growth factors to drive cell differentiation and and this has been demonstrated *in vitro* (Melling et al. 2018) and *in vivo* (Huang et al. 2010; Iohara et al. 2011; Kodonas et al. 2012). As mentioned above, the environment is key to regeneration of the pulp. It is not desirable for all progenitor cells to differentiate into a mineralizing phenotype. New blood vessels, neurons and a collagenous matrix are also required for a fully engineered pulpal tissue. Hypoxia is a major regulator of angiogenesis, stimulating paracrine angiogenic activity of pulp cells (Rombouts et al. 2017) and DPSCs have been shown to have the potential to differentiate though a neuronal and glial lineage (Young et al. 2016). Ideally, exploiting the endogenous progenitor cells and growth factors to regenerate the dentin-pulp complex *in situ* would be the better approach. All the ingredients required for this tissue engineering approach, cells (DPSCs or SCAPs), growth factors (sequestered in dentin) and appropriate scaffold (pulp tissue) are present.

If delivery of cells or bioactive molecules is required then there will be a need for a scaffold that can carry or deliver progenitor cells and growth factors and act as a structural template for tissue regeneration. Ideal characteristics of a such a scaffold include biocompatibility, biodegradablity, defined mechanical properties to mimic the pulp and consistent porosity to allow for adequate loading of cells and penetration of nutrients and growth factors to facilitate cell proliferation, adhesion and migration (Galler et al. 2011). Ideal scaffolding materials include natural polymers, synthetic polymers, hydrogels and bioceramics (Galler et al. 2011) but decellularised pulp tissue (Matoug-Elwerfelli et al. 2018) has also recently been explored as an alternative scaffold. Given the anatomy of a root canal system, injectable scaffolds may provide an attractive alternative and *in vitro* and *in vivo* models have demonstrated that providing the necessary scaffold such as poly(lactic) acid (PLA) and poly(glycolic) acid (PGA) in combination with growth factors may provide a suitable environment for progenitor cells and may lead to desirable outcomes clinically and biologically (Huang et al. 2010; Iohara et al. 2004).

Summary

If we are to realize the potential for true regenerative endodontics we first need to agree what it is we are willing accept. Are we wanting to recapitulate tooth development and regenerate the perfect dentin-pulp complex? This complete tissue regeneration sounds ideal but is it more idealistic. Should we look to encourage routine clinical treatments based on biological evidence and look at regenerative endodontics as tissue repair? It is now well established that the dentin matrix contains a broad cocktail of bioactive molecules, which if released appropriately can act to modulate a significant majority of the cellular and molecular events underpinning regeneration of the dentin-pulp complex. The heterogenous population of progenitor cells which reside in the pulp are able to respond appropriately to released dentin matrix components and when bleeding into a root canal is invoked, SCAPs and circulating MSCs from the blood can enter the canal and respond in a similar manner. All the ingredients required for endogenous repair or regeneration of the dentin-pulp complex exist and it may be prudent to pursue this innate repair mechanism as a route to novel clinical treatments. Delivery of cells for regenerative endodontics proves a different tissue engineering challenge. Design of appropriate scaffolds is required along with isolation of patient cells. How growth factors are delivered in such exogenous approaches also provides another challenge. Whilst several of these hurdles have been overcome in *in vitro* studies, translation into patient treatments remains some distance away. However, our increasing knowledge of the biology of dentin-pulp complex regenerative processes and our better understanding of the cellular behavior and function of pulpal progenitor cells allows us to modify existing clinical treatments based on biological evidence. Thus, techniques which result in sporadic success at present are becoming more reliable and this offers exciting opportunities to exploit biological processes for new clinical therapies.

References

Accorinte Mde, L., Holland, R., Reis, A., Bortoluzzi, M.C., Murata, S.S., Dezan, J.E., Souza, V., and Alessandro, L.D. (2008). Evaluation of mineral trioxide aggregate and calcium hydroxide cement as pulp-capping agents in human teeth. *J. Endod.* 34 (1): 1–6.

Alraies, A., Alaidaroos, N.Y., Waddington, R.J., Moseley, R., and Sloan, A.J. (2017). Variation in human dental pulp stem cell ageing profiles reflect contrasting proliferative and regenerative capabilities. *BMC Cell Biol.* 18 (1): 12. Feb 2.

Avery, S.J., Sadaghiani, L., Sloan, A.J., and Waddington, R.J. (2017). Analysing the bioactive makeup of demineralised dentine matrix on bone marrow mesenchymal stem cells for enhanced bone repair. *Eur. Cell Mater.* 34: 1–14.

Baker, S.M., Sugars, R.V., Wendel, M., Smith, A.J., Waddington, R.J., Cooper, P.R., and Sloan, A.J. (2009). TGF-beta/extracellular matrix interactions in dentin matrix: A role in regulating sequestration and protection of bioactivity. *Calcif. Tissue Int.* 85 (1): 66–74.

Banchs, F., and Trope, M. (2004). Revascularization of immature permanent teeth with apical periodontitis: New treatment protocol? *J. Endod.* 30 (4): 196–200.

Bjørndal, L., Simon, S., Tomson, P.L., and Duncan, H.F. (2019). Management of deep caries and the exposed pulp. *Int. Endod. J.* 52 (7): 949–973.

Casagrande, L.F., Demarco, F., Zhang, Z., Araujo, F.B., Shi, S., and Nor, J.E. (2010). Dentin-derived BMP-2 and odontoblast differentiation. *J. Dent. Res.* 89 (6): 603–608.

Chai, Y., Jiang, X., Ito, Y., Bringas, P. Jr, Han, J., Rowitch, D.H., Soriano, P., McMahon, A.P., and Sucov, H.M. (2000). Fate of the mammalian cranial neural crest during tooth and mandibular morphogenesis. *Development* 127 (8): 1671–1679.

Chueh, L.H., and Chiang, C.P. (2010). Histology of Irreversible pulpitis premolars treated with mineral trioxide aggregate pulpotomy. *Oper. Dent.* 35 (3): 370–374.

Cordeiro, M.M., Dong, Z., Kaneko, T., Zhang, Z., Miyazawa, M., Shi, S., Smith, A.J., and Nor, J.E. (2008). Dental pulp tissue engineering with stem cells from exfoliated deciduous teeth. *J. Endod.* 34: 962–969.

d'Aquino, R., Graziano, A., Sampaolesi, M., Laino, G., Pirozzi, G., De Rosa, A., and Papaccio, G. (2007). Human postnatal dental pulp cells co-differentiate into osteoblasts and endotheliocytes: A pivotal synergy leading to adult bone tissue formation. *Cell Death Differ.* 14: 1162–1171.

Diogenes, A.M., Henry, A., Teixeira, F.B., and Hargreaves, K.M. (2013). An update on clinical regenerative endodontics. *Endod. Topics* 28 (1): 2–23.

Galler, K.M., D'Souza, R.N., Hartgerink, J.D., and Schmalz, G. (2011). Scaffolds for dental pulp tissue engineering. *Adv. Dent. Res.* 23 (3): 333–339.

Goldberg, M.1., Farges, J.C., Lacerda-Pinheiro, S., Six, N., Jegat, N., Decup, F., Septier, D., Carrouel, F., Durand, S., Chaussain-Miller, C., Denbesten, P., Veis, A., and Poliard, A. (2008). Inflammatory and immunological aspects of dental pulp repair. *Pharmacol. Res.* 58 (2): 137–147.

Graham, L., Cooper, P.R., Cassidy, N., Nor, J.E., Sloan, A.J., and Smith, A.J. (2006). The effect of calcium hydroxide on solubilisation of bio-active dentine matrix components. *Biomaterials* 27 (14): 2865–2873.

Gronthos, S., Mankani, M., Brahim, J., Robey, P.G., and Shi, S. (2000). Postnatal human dental pulp stem cells (DPSCs) in vitro and in vivo. *Proc. Natl. Acad. Sci. U. S. A.* 97: 13625–13630.

Gronthos, S., Brahim, J., Li, W., Fisher, L.W., Cherman, N., Boyde, A., DenBesten, P., Robey, P.G., and Shi, S. (2002). Stem cell properties of human dental pulp stem cells. *J. Dent. Res.* 81: 531–535.

Hilton, T.J., Ferracane, J.L., and Mancl, L. (2013). Northwest Practice-based Research Collaborative in Evidence-based Dentistry (NWP). Comparison of CaOH with MTA for direct pulp capping: A PBRN randomized clinical trial. *J Dent Res.* 92 (7 Suppl): 16S–22S.

Huang, G.T., Gronthos, S., and Shi, S. (2009). Mesenchymal stem cells derived from dental tissues vs. those from other sources: Their biology and role in regenerative medicine. *J. Dent. Res.* 88: 792–806.

Huang, G.T., Yamaza, T., Shea, L.D., Djouad, F., Kuhn, N.Z., Tuan, R.S., and Shi, S. (2010). Stem/progenitor cell-mediated de novo regeneration of dental pulp with newly deposited continuous layer of dentin in an *in vivo* model. *Tissue Eng. Part A* 16 (2): 605–615.

Iohara, K., Imabayashi, K., Ishizaka, R., Watanabe, A., Nabekura, J., Ito, M., Matsushita, K., Nakamura, H., and Nakashima, M. (2011). Complete pulp regeneration after pulpectomy by transplantation of CD105+ stem cells with stromal cell-derived factor-1. *Tissue Eng. Part A* 17 (15-16): 1911–1920.

Iohara, K., Nakashima, M., Ito, M., Ishikawa, M., Nakasima, A., and Akamine, A. (2004). Dentin regeneration by dental pulp stem cell therapy with recombinant human bone morphogenetic protein 2. *J. Dent. Res.* 83: 590–595.

Jones, E.A., Kinsey, S.E., English, A., Jones, R.A., Straszynski, L., Meredith, D.M., Markham, A.F., Jack, A., Emery, P., and McGonagle, D. (2002). Isolation and characterization of bone marrow multipotential mesenchymal progenitor cells. *Arthritis Rheum.* 46: 3349–3360.

Kodonas, K., Gogos, C., Papadimitriou, S., Kouzi-Koliakou, K., and Tziafas, D. (2012). Experimental formation of dentin-like structure in the root canal implant model using cryopreserved swine dental pulp progenitor cells. *J. Endod.* 38 (7): 913–919.

Kontakiotis, E.G., Filippatos, C.G., Tzanetakis, G.N., and Agrafioti, A. (2015). Regenerative endodontic therapy: A data analysis of clinical protocols. *J. Endod.* 41 (2): 146–154.

Kuratate, M., Yoshiba, K., Shigetani, Y., Yoshiba, N., Ohshima, H., and Okiji, T. (2008). Immunohistochemical analysis of nestin, osteopontin, and proliferating cells in the reparative process of exposed dental pulp capped with mineral trioxide aggregate. *J Endod.* 34 (8): 970–974.

Laino, G., d'Aquino, R., Graziano, A., Lanza, V., Carinci, F., Naro, F., Pirozzi, G., and Papaccio, G. (2005). A new population of human adult dental pulp stem cells: A useful source of living autologous fibrous bone tissue (LAB). *J. Bone Miner. Res.* 20: 1394–1402.

Langer, R. and Vacanti, J.P. (1993). Tissue engineering. *Science* 260 (5110): 920–926.

Laurent, P., Camps, J., and About, I. (2012). Biodentine(TM) induces TGF-beta1 release from human pulp cells and early dental pulp mineralization. *Int. Endod. J.* 45 (5): 439–448.

Lesot, H., Beguekirn, C., Kubler, M.D., Meyer, J.M., Smith, A.J., Cassidy, N., Ruch, J.V., Aubin, J.E., Goldberg, M., and Magloire, H. (1993). Experimental induction of odontoblast differentiation and stimulation during reparative processes. *Cells Mater.* 3: 201–217.

Lizier, N.F., Kerkis, A., Gomes, C.M., Hebling, J., Oliveira, C.F., Caplan, A.I., and Kerkis, I. (2012). Scaling-up of dental pulp stem cells isolated from multiple niches. *PLoS One* 7: e39885.

Lovelace, T.W., Henry, M.A., Hargreaves, K.M., and Diogenes, A. (2011). Evaluation of the delivery of mesenchymal stem cells into the root canal space of necrotic immature teeth after clinical regenerative endodontic procedure. *J. Endod.* 37 (2): 133–138.

Lu, B., and Atala, A. (2014). Small molecules and small molecule drugs in regenerative medicine. *Drug Discov. Today* 19 (6): 801–808.

Matoug-Elwerfelli, M., Duggal, M.S., Nazzal, H., Esteves, F., and Raïf, E. (2018). A biocompatible decellularized pulp scaffold for regenerative endodontics. *Int. Endod. J.* 51 (6): 663–673.

Melling, G.E., Colombo, J.S., Avery, S.J., Ayre, W.N., Evans, S.L., Waddington, R.J., and Sloan, A.J. (2018). Liposomal delivery of demineralized dentin matrix for dental tissue regeneration. *Tissue Eng. Part A. Feb* 21.

Mente, J., Hufnagel, S., Leo, M., Michel, A., Gehrig, H., Panagidis, D., Saure, D., and Pfefferle, T. (2014). Treatment outcome of mineral trioxide aggregate or calcium hydroxide direct pulp capping: Long-term results. *J. Endod.* 40 (11): 1746–1751.

Miura, M., Gronthos, S., Zhao, M., Lu, B., Fisher, L.W., Robey, P.G., and Shi, S. (2003). SHED: Stem cells from human exfoliated deciduous teeth. *Proc. Natl. Acad. Sci. U. S. A.* 100: 5807–5812.

Murray, P.E., Garcia-Godoy, F., and Hargreaves, K.M. (2007). Regenerative endodontics: A review of current status and a call for action. *J. Endod.* 33 (4): 377–390.

Nakashima, M. and Akamine, A. (2005). The application of tissue engineering to regeneration of pulp and dentin in endodontics. *J. Endod.* 31 (10): 711-.

Nakashima, M. and Iohara, K. (2011). Regeneration of dental pulp by stem cells. *Adv. Dent. Res.* 23: 313–319.

Nowicka, A., Lipski, M., Parafiniuk, M., Sporniak-Tutak, K., Lichota, D., Kosierkiewicz, A., Kaczmarek, W., and Buczkowska-Radlinska, J. (2013). Response of human dental pulp capped with biodentine and mineral trioxide aggregate. *J. Endod.* 39 (6): 743–747.

Piccin, D. and Morshead, C.M. (2010). Potential and pitfalls of stem cell therapy in old age. *Dis. Model Mech.* 3 (7-8): 421–425.

Roberts-Clark, D.J. and Smith, A.J. (2000). Angiogenic growth factors in human dentine matrix. *Arch. Oral Biol.* 45: 1013–1016.

Rombouts, C., Giraud, T., Jeanneau, C., and About, I. (2017). Pulp vascularization during tooth development, regeneration and therapy. *J. Dent. Res.* 96 (2): 137–144.

Rutherford, R.B., and Gu, K. (2000). Treatment of inflamed ferret dental pulps with recombinant bone morphogenetic protein-7. *Eur. J. Oral Sci.* 108 (3): 202–206.

Sachdeva, G.S., Sachdeva, L.T., Goel, M., and Bala, S. (2014). Regenerative endodontic treatment of an immature tooth with a necrotic pulp and apical periodontitis using platelet-rich plasma (PRP) and mineral trioxide aggregate (MTA): A case report. *Int. Endod. J.* 48 (9): 902–910.

Sadaghiani, L., Gleeson, H.B., Youde, S., Waddington, R.J., Lynch, C.D., and Sloan, A.J. (2016). Growth factor liberation and DPSC response following dentine conditioning. *J. Dent. Res.* 95 (11): 1298–1307.

Saito, A., Saito, E., Yoshimura, Y., Takahashi, D., Handa, R., Honma, Y., and Ohata, N. (2011). Attachment formation after transplantation of teeth cultured with enamel matrix derivative in dogs. *Journal of Periodontology*, 82: 1462–1468. doi: 10.1902/jop.2011.100596.

Shi, S., and Gronthos, S. (2003). Perivascular niche of postnatal mesenchymal stem cells in human bone marrow and dental pulp. *J. Bone Miner. Res.* 18: 696–704.

Silva, T.A., Lara, V.S., Silva, J.S., Oliveira, S.H., Butler, W.T., and Cunha, F.Q. (2005). Macrophages and mast cells control the neutrophil migration induced by dentin proteins. *J. Dent. Res.* 84: 79–83.

Simon, S., Perard, M., Zanini, M., Smith, A.J., Charpentier, E., Djole, S.X., and Lumley, P.J. (2013). Should pulp chamber pulpotomy be seen as a permanent treatment? Some preliminary thoughts. *Int. Endod. J.* 46 (1): 79–87.

Sloan, A.J., and Smith, A.J. (1999). Stimulation of the dentine–pulp complex of rat incisor teeth by transforming growth factor-β isoforms 1–3. *Arch. Oral Biol.* 44: 149–156.

Sloan, A.J., Rutherford, R.B., and Smith, A.J. (2000). Stimulation of the rat dentine-pulp complex by bone morphogenetic protein-7 *in vitro*. *Arch. Oral Biol.* 45: 173–177.

Smith, A.J., Matthews, J.B., and Hall, R.C. (1998). Transforming growth factor-beta 1 (TGF-beta 1) in dentine matrix – ligand activation and receptor expression. *Eur. J. Oral Sci.* 106: 179–84.

Smith, A.J., Patel, M., Graham, L., Sloan, A.J., and Cooper, P.R. (2005). Dentine regeneration: Key roles for stem cells and molecular signaling. *Oral Biosic. Med.* 2: 127–132.

Smith, A.J., Scheven, B.A., Takahashi, Y., Ferracane, J.L., Shelton, R.M., and Cooper, P.R. (2012). Dentine as a bioactive extracellular matrix. *Arch. Oral Biol.* 57 (2): 109–121.

Song, B., Jiang, W., Alraies, A., Liu, Q., Gudla, V., Oni, J., Wei, X., Sloan, A., Ni, L., and Agarwal, M. (2016). Bladder smooth muscle cells differentiation from dental pulp stem cells: Future potential for bladder tissue engineering. *Stem Cells Int.* 6979368. doi: 10.1155/2016/6979368.

Sonoyama, W., Liu, Y., Yamaza, T., Tuan, R.S., Wang, S., Shi, S., and Huang, G.T. (2008). Characterization of the apical papilla and its residing stem cells from human immature permanent teeth: A pilot study. *J. Endod.* 34 (2): 166–171.

Tecles, O., Laurent, P., Aubut, V., and About, I. (2008). Human tooth culture: A study model for reparative dentinogenesis and direct pulp capping materials biocompatibility. *J. Biomed. Mater. Res. B Appl. Biomater.* 85 (1): 180–187.

Tomson, P., Grover, L.M., Lumley, P.J., Sloan, A.J., Smith, A.J., and Cooper, P.R. (2007). Dissolution of bio-active dentine matrix components by mineral trioxide aggregate. *J. Dent.* 35 (8): 636–642.

Torabinejad, M., and Turman, M. (2011). Revitalization of tooth with necrotic pulp and open apex by using platelet-rich plasma: A case report. *J. Endod.* 37 (2): 265–268.

Tucker, A.S., and Sharpe, P.T. (1999). Molecular genetics of tooth morphogenesis and patterning: The right shape in the right place. *J. Dent. Res.* 78 (4): 826–834.

Tziafas, D. (2004). The future role of a molecular approach to pulp-dentinal regeneration. *Caries Res.* 38 (3): 314–320.

Young, F.I., Telezhkin, V., Youde, S.J., Langley, M.S., Stack, M., Kemp, P.J., Waddington, R.J., Sloan, A.J., and Song, B. (2016). Clonal heterogeneity in the neuronal and glial differentiation of dental pulp stem/progenitor cells. *Stem Cells Int.* 2016: 1290561.

Yu, J.M., Wu, X., Gimble, J.M., Guan, X., Freitas, M.A., and Bunnell, B.A. (2011). Age-related changes in mesenchymal stem cells derived from rhesus macaque bone marrow. *Aging Cell* 10 (1): 66–79.

Zhang, W., Walboomers, X.F., Shi, S., Fan, M., and Jansen, J.A. (2006). Multilineage differentiation potential of stem cells derived from human dental pulp after cryopreservation. *Tissue Eng.* 12: 2813–2823.

Zhang, R., Cooper, P.R., Smith, G., and Nor, J.E. (2011). Angiogenic activity of dentin matrix components. *J. Endod.* 37: 26–30.

11

Minimally Invasive Dentistry in Paediatric Dentistry

Paul Ashley and Ferranti Wong

Key Topics

- Introduction to dental decay
- IM approaches to primary and permanent teeth
- IM approaches when treating children and adults

Learning Objectives

- Understand how the MI approach can be applied to children
- Understand the differences between primary and permanent teeth
- Understand the differences between caries management and the MI approach in children vs adults

Introduction

Dental decay is one of the most common human diseases and affects almost 100% of adults and 60–90% of school children across the world (World Health Organisation 2012). Dental caries and related treatment are the main contributors to the healthcare cost of dental disease, which is estimated at US $442 billion (Listl et al. 2015), globally. Untreated teeth become infected, causing pain, loss of tooth vitality, and dental abscess formation. Ultimately this will lead to surgical extraction of the tooth.

In children, untreated carious teeth may affect sleeping, eating, general health, and well-being. Dental infections in primary teeth can damage the underlying adult teeth and early extraction of decayed primary teeth may lead to abnormalities in tooth alignment (Faculty of Dental Surgery 2015). Management of carious teeth in children is complicated by the difficulties of providing more complex treatment to this group (Figure 11.1).

Minimally Invasive Dentistry: Interdisciplinary Clinical and Scientific Approaches, First Edition.
Edited by Aylin Baysan and Paul Anderson.
© 2026 John Wiley & Sons Ltd. Published 2026 by John Wiley & Sons Ltd.
Companion website: www.wiley.com/go/baysan/minimally_invasive_dentistry

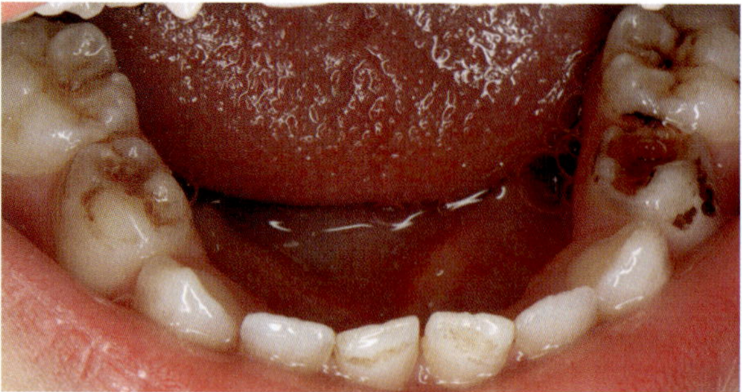

Figure 11.1   Image of a carious dentition in a child.

Children may be anxious or not have sufficient intellectual development to cope with local anaesthesia, caries removal, etc. As a result untreated dental decay can lead to emergency hospital admission for management. In England, dental decay is currently the most common reason for a young child to be admitted to hospital in order for the infected teeth to be surgically removed under general anaesthesia (Faculty of Dental Surgery 2015). In the United States, 50% of the 215,073 emergency room visits in children from dental causes were because of dental caries (Allareddy et al. 2014). The additional hidden cost of sleepless nights, days off school, etc. is unknown.

Maintaining tooth structure and preventing the development of caries is the new paradigm for caries management and is well described in this book and elsewhere. Much of the evidence and discussion concerns permanent teeth in adults. Evidence in children and for primary teeth is sometimes lacking. This group is important as they are very different to adults in terms of behaviour, management, and the structure of their dentition. Potentially they could benefit most from the MI approach as it will reduce or eliminate the need for difficult and complex dental treatment. Therefore in this chapter we will consider how the MI approach can be applied to children. We will do this first by thinking about some of the differences between primary and permanent teeth and how MI evidence from permanent teeth could be extrapolated to primary teeth. We will then consider some of the other differences between caries management and the MI approach in children vs. adults.

Differences between Primary and Permanent Teeth and How This Will Influence the MI Approach

Eruption and Exfoliation

Primary teeth start to develop in utero and erupt from 6 months onwards. Exfoliation happens from approximately 6 years of age, finishing at about 11 (Cleghorn et al. 2011). The early emergence of teeth in human developmen inevitably limits the range of possible treatments that can be provided, particularly technical approaches such as resin infiltration or fissure sealants that require good moisture control. As a consequence MI approaches that rely less on cooperation have greater benefit, *e.g.*, fluoride varnish application. The fact that primary teeth will eventually exfoliate also influences how we might think about MI.

As these teeth are ultimately temporary structures, it could be argued preservation of tooth structure is less significant. Whilst this is relevant, we should also consider the importance of maintaining primary teeth to allow normal development and eruption of the permanent successors, and the fact that many MI approaches are easier to provide for a young child than more complex restorative procedures.

The other factor to consider in this group is the risk of fluorosis. At the same time as the primary teeth are erupting the permanent teeth are also in development and prolonged exposure to fluoride can result in disturbance of enamel development. This is relevant for MI practitioners as use of topical fluoride is one of the most effective and commonly used methods for caries prevention. In order to minimise the risk of fluorosis, systemic methods of fluoride delivery (e.g., tablets) should be avoided and topical methods (e.g., fluoride varnish) promoted. Fluoride toothpaste use should be encouraged with the best combination for high caries risk children being higher concentration fluoride pastes in small quantities (Public Health England 2017).

Thinner Enamel and Dentine

Primary teeth are smaller than permanent teeth, so inevitably the enamel and dentine is thinner in primary teeth when compared to permanent teeth.

One of the implications of the decreased depth of enamel and dentine in primary teeth when compared to permanent teeth is the effect this has on caries progression rates. Caries progression rates have been shown to vary widely within permanent teeth, with progression being faster in the years immediately following eruption (Mejàre et al. 2004). Although laboratory investigation does not show any significantly different demineralisation rate between primary and permanent enamel (Hassanali 2018), there is some clinical evidence to suggest that overall progression of caries is more rapid in primary teeth when compared to permanent teeth (Vanderas et al. 2003). This possible increased rate of progression should not preclude use of an MI approach. However, it may be advisable to consider more frequent recalls to monitor any change in lesion depth.

Pulp Chamber and Canals

The pulp of primary teeth differs from permanent teeth in two important respects (Figure 11.2). The first is that the pulp chamber in primary molars is proportionally larger relative to the whole tooth when compared to the permanent dentition. As the enamel and dentine are thinner and the caries progression is higher, the pulp is often involved when removing caries. Taking an MI approach of selective or minimal caries removal is therefore beneficial in primary teeth as it further minimises the risk of inadvertent pulp involvement.

The other difference between the pulpal anatomy of primary and permanent teeth is that in primary teeth, root canal systems are complex and variable (Cleghorn et al. 2011). Conventional concepts of endodontic therapy in primary teeth do not apply, and the fundamentals of endodontic treatment (such as isolation with rubber dam) are difficult for young children to tolerate. Procedures to manage and maintain endodontically involved primary teeth exist, but clearly avoidance of this is preferable. Currently, best evidence is that in primary molars with deep caries, an MI approach of selective caries removal and sealing

Primary tooth has:

- Thinner enamel than permanent tooth
- Pulp horns that are closer to amelo-dentinal junction
- Larger pulp relative to overall size of tooth when compared to permanent tooth

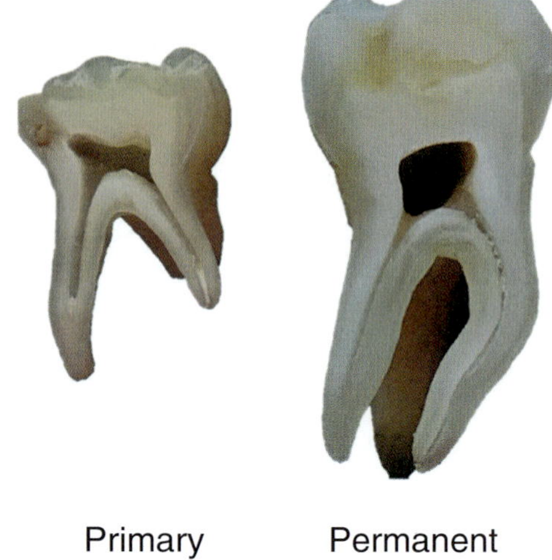

Figure 11.2 Differences between primary and permanent teeth.

caries in (sometimes referred to as indirect pulp therapy) is preferable to approaches such as an elective pulpotomy (Coll et al. 2017). At present there is no clear consensus on whether any particular liners or filling materials should be used in this situation, clearly maintenance of an adequate seal around the restoration will be important.

Dental Materials for Primary Teeth

Dental materials used in primary teeth are usually identical to those used in permanent teeth with little thought as to the different structure and composition of primary teeth vs. permanent teeth. Evidence for use of materials in primary teeth is sparse and much of what we know is inevitably extrapolated from data in permanent teeth. This may not be ideal, for instance there is some evidence to suggest that bond strengths in primary teeth with a range of different systems are not as strong as those in permanent teeth (Burrow et al. 2002).

How will these possible differences in material properties influence MI management of caries in primary teeth? It's important to note first that whilst differences almost certainly exist they are unlikely to result in an enormous impact on bonding and other desirable properties. However they should be considered particularly if prescribing MI approaches that rely on bonding alone, e.g. sealing in of caries following selective removal. One example of this is the atraumatic restorative technique in primary molars (ART). Conventionally, ART is minimal removal of caries followed by placement of a glass ionomer cement to seal caries in. There is some evidence to suggest that in children with high caries levels and poor oral hygiene that this may not be effective (Melgar et al. 2017). Also, due to the physical property of the restorative materials, the marginal ridge is not often maintained, resulting in a loss of arch length and potential crowding in the posterior region. This does not mean that the ART approach should be abandoned, but perhaps with primary molars the definitive restoration might be better being a preformed metal crown (hall crown) where reliance on the bond to enamel and dentine is less critical.

Differences between Treating Children and Adults and How This Will Influence the MI Approach

The other element to consider when thinking about the MI approach in paediatric dentistry are some of the implications when considering treatment provision in children vs. adults. Children, particularly young children will be cognitively and emotionally unable to cope with complex treatment. They will also be unable to understand or interact on complex health messages. This will of course justify the MI approach, particularly those MI approaches that do not require much cooperation from the patient, as early intervention with a simple therapy may well prevent later intervention with a more complex therapy. However this will also throw up additional complications.

Managing Behaviour

Managing anxious or pre-cooperative children will often result in diagnostic and treatment compromises, it will also influence treatment planning. Early and accurate diagnosis in young children can be complicated—examination may be difficult in an anxious child and standard diagnostic tools such as use of bitewing radiography may well be impossible. Therefore identifying caries lesions suitable for an MI approach, and monitoring subsequent progression cannot be carried out with the same accuracy as perhaps is possible in a more cooperative adult. This, coupled with the rapid progression of caries in primary teeth, requires a more cautious MI approach. Mode of treatment delivery and behaviour management will also influence MI treatment planning i.e., if treatment is provided under deep sedation or general anaesthesia (GA). In these situations, one of the aims is to eliminate the risk of the patient requiring deep sedation or GA again as these procedures carry their own risks of morbidity (and even mortality). It may be appropriate to consider more drastic approaches (i.e., to extract the affected tooth) for primary teeth where the success of an MI approach is less predictable.

Health Promotion for Children

When considering health promotion in adults it is important to appreciate that the evidence linking oral health promotion and clinically relevant outcomes such as a reduction in dental caries is weak ((B) Kay et al. 2016b). Delivering simple messages around diet advice, use of diet diaries, and other conventional techniques are part of the standard approaches used by oral health professionals, arguably though the evidence to support their effectiveness is not available. Part of the problem is that changing behaviour is a complex and challenging field, understanding the benefits of a particular behaviour often does not lead to the individual then acting on this.

Children (particularly very young children) are different as they are wholly dependent on their caregivers for nourishment. This potentially increases the efficacy of preventive advice. In most cases the caregivers will want to act in the child's best interest, the child has little or no autonomy with regards to their diet so changes may be straightforward to implement. Advice is particularly important in the early years of life when children are bottle fed or transitioning from a bottle to drinking from a cup, poor nutritional practices often include use of a bottle during night-time containing sweetened milks or other sugar containing beverages. Motivational interviewing techniques in this instance to influence the caregiver to make the right nutritional choices may lead to reductions in caries ((B) Kay et al. 2016b).

MI Therapies for Children

From what has been discussed above, the main aim in treating caries in primary teeth is to allow them to exfoliate at the normal time free of pain and infection. This will maintain the arch length and should be applied with minimal behavioural adjustment especial in pre-cooperative and anxious children. This next section concentrates on MI techniques that are particularly suitable for the management of existing carious lesions in children. The use of fluoride, sealants, and health promotion as an MI approach for managing caries can be found in other chapters in this book.

Silver Diamine Fluoride

Fluoride, whether it is delivered in the form of toothpaste, mouth rinse solution, gel or varnish, is known to be effective on preventing enamel caries. The most effective professionally delivery method is sodium fluoride (NaF, 5%) vanish containing 22,600 ppm F. However, its effectiveness in arresting dentinal caries might be limited (Chu et al. 2002). Silver diamine fluoride (SDF, 38% containing 44,800 ppm F) might be a more effective alternative for arresting and remineralising enamel and dentine lesions. This silver containing compound is thought to have an anticaries effect by utilising the combined effect of the antimicrobial properties of silver and the anticaries properties of fluoride. Rather than just preventing caries, it arrests any existing dentinal caries and leaves behind a mineral rich surface layer that prevents further degradation, thus it could be viewed as a permanent therapy, at least until the primary teeth are exfoliated. Evidence supports its use (Chibinski et al. 2017; Horst 2018), however it does come with a significant side effect—any treated areas are stained black (Burgess and Vaghela 2018). This side effect is less significant in primary teeth that will eventually exfoliate and be lost, it is also easy to place making it ideal for use in young children. Therefore this therapy is one that should be considered when reviewing the appropriate MI strategy in a young child.

Sealing in Caries

It is well established that fissure sealants are effective, not only in preventing fissure caries, but arresting progression in non-cavitated lesions (Wright et al. 2016). Use of sealants is well covered elsewhere in this book, they should be one of the techniques used by the MI practitioner when managing children. For this to be successful, the sealant has to be placed correctly and maintained subsequent to that. Sealants need regular monitoring, and defective areas need to be repaired and/or topped up (Scottish Dental Clinical Effectiveness Programme 2018). This requires a level of cooperation which might not be achievable in a child. They are also of little value when a lesion is cavitated.

Another approach commonly used in MI dentistry (and described elsewhere in this book) is resin infiltration. ICON® infiltrant (DMG, Hamburg, Germany) was developed for this particular purpose. Whilst there is strong evidence to support its use in permanent teeth, effectiveness in primary molars is unclear (Chatzimarkou et al. 2018). The other issue with these resins are that they can be time consuming and difficult to place. As these materials are hydrophobic, good moisture control, which may involve the placement of rubber dam and local anaesthetic, is required to achieve maximum effectiveness. As above, this makes use in a young child difficult.

One approach to sealing caries in that requires significantly less cooperation is the Hall crown (Figure 11.3).

Preformed metal crowns have been used for many years in paediatric dentistry with good success to restore primary molar teeth. Conventionally they were placed after crown preparation, however this usually required local anaesthetic and significant patient cooperation. The Hall technique developed in Scotland (Innes et al. 2017) is a method of placing the crown with little or no preparation, consequently no local anaesthetic is needed. Evidence shows that it is highly effective at arresting and preventing further caries and is generally acceptable by very young children. Covering the entire crown of a tooth with a metal cap may seem the opposite of a minimal intervention approach, however because there is no caries removal or crown preparation this approach embodies all the key features of the MI philosophy.

Use of Hall crowns is also indicated as an MI approach when managing children with enamel defects affecting the primary molars. There is evidence to suggest that a proportion of children will have second primary molars that are affected by enamel defects 2.7–21.8%, usually hypomineralisations (Owen et al. 2017). Reasons for these defects are not clear, however they do present a management problem as these teeth are more prone to become decayed and may present with pain or sensitivity. These defects are well suited for an MI approach.

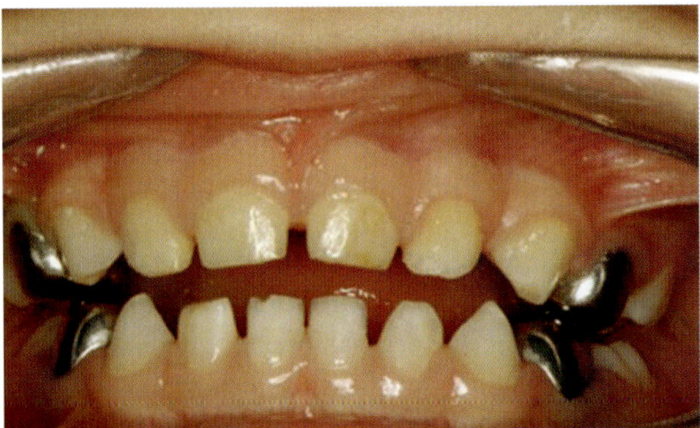

Figure 11.3　Hall crown in place.

Atraumatic Restorative Technique

The ART approach for caries management was first used in the developing world where there are limited resources such as electricity and dental equipment such as handpieces. The principal is that soft caries is removed using a simple excavator and then the cavity restored with a glass ionomer cement. As well as being a technique that can be used in resource scarce environments, it is also easier for children to accept as the use of drills and local anaesthetic are avoided. It could be considered as an MI approach as caries is only partially removed. However, current evidence suggests that in terms of clinical effectiveness it may not perform as well as conventional restorations (Dorri et al. 2017).

Summary

The MI approach applies equally to primary teeth and children as it does to permanent teeth and adults. Evidence for some of the MI therapies may not be from primary teeth directly and this should be kept in mind when planning treatment. Therapies such as use of silver diamine fluoride and the Hall crown have particular value in this group.

References

Allareddy, V., Nalliah, R.P., Hague, M., Johnson, H., Rampa, S.B., and Lee, M.K. (2014). Hospital-based emergency department visits with dental conditions among children in the United States: Nationwide epidemiological data. *Pediatr. Dent.* 36: 393–399.

Burgess, J.O., and Vaghela, P.M. (2018). Silver diamine fluoride: A successful anticarious solution with limits. *Adv. Dent. Res.* 29: 131–134.

Burrow, M.F., Nopnakeepong, U., and Phrukkanon, S. (2002). A comparison of microtensile bond strengths of several dentin bonding systems to primary and permanent dentin. *Dent. Mater.* 18: 239–245.

Chatzimarkou, S., Koletsi, D., and Kavvadia, K. (2018). The effect of resin infiltration on proximal caries lesions in primary and permanent teeth. A systematic review and meta-analysis of clinical trials. *J. Dent.* doi: 10.1016/j.jdent.2018.08.004.

Chibinski, A.C., Wambier, L.M., Feltrin, J., Loguercio, A.D., Wambier, D.S., and Reis, A. (2017). Silver diamine fluoride has efficacy in controlling caries progression in primary teeth: A systematic review and meta-analysis. *Caries Res.* 51: 527–541.

Cleghorn, B.M., Boorberg, N.B., and Christie, W.H. (2012). Primary human teeth and their root canal systems. *Endod. Topics* 23: 6–33.

Coll, J.A., Seale, N.S., Vargas, K., Marghalani, A.A., Al Shamali, S., and Graham, L. (2017). Primary tooth vital pulp therapy: A systematic review and meta-analysis. *Pediatr. Dent.* 39: 16–23.

Chu, C.H., Lo, E.C., and Lin, H.C. (2002). Effectiveness of silver diamine fluoride and sodium fluoride varnish in arresting dentin caries in Chinese pre-school children. *J. Dent. Res.* 81: 767–770.

Dorri, M., Martinez-Zapata, M., Walsh, T., Marinho, V.C.C., Sheiham (Deceased), A., and Zaror, C. (2017). Atraumatic restorative treatment versus conventional restorative treatment for managing dental caries. *Cochrane Database Syst. Rev.* 12. Art. No.: CD008072. doi: 10.1002/14651858.CD008072.pub2.

Faculty of Dental Surgery. (2015). The state of children's oral health in England. https://www.rcseng.ac.uk/fds/policy/documents/fds-report-on-the-state-of-childrens-oral-health (accessed March 2016).

Horst, J.A. (2018). Silver fluoride as a treatment for dental caries. *Adv. Dent. Res.* 29: 135–140.

Kay, E., Vascott, D., Hocking, A., Nield, H., Dorr, C., and Barrett, H. (2016b). A review of approaches for dental practice teams for promoting oral health. *Community Dent. Oral Epidemiol.* 44: 313–330.

Hassanali, L. (2018). Quantitative measurements of the demineralisation rates and mineral masses of deciduous and permanent enamel. PhD Thesis, Queen Mary University of London.

Innes, N.P., Evans, D.J., Bonifacio, C.C., Geneser, M., Hesse, D., Heimer, M., Kanellis, M., Machiulskiene, V., Narbutaité, J., Olegário, I.C., Owais, A., Araujo, M.P., Raggio, D.P., Splieth, C., van Amerongen, E., Weber-Gasparoni, K., and Santamaria, R.M. (2017). The hall technique 10 years on: Questions and answers. *Br. Dent. J.* 222 (6): 478–483.

Listl, S., Galloway, J., Mossey, P.A., and Marcenes, W. (2015). Global economic impact of dental diseases. *J. Dent. Res.* 94: 1355–1361.

Mejàre, I., Stenlund, H., and Zelezny-Holmlund, C. (2004). Caries incidence and lesion progression from adolescence to young adulthood: A prospective 15-year cohort study in Sweden. *Caries Res.* 38: 130–141.

Melgar, X.C., Opdam, N.J.M., Correa, M.B., Franzon, R., Demarco, F.F., Araujo, F.B., and Casagrande, L. (2017). Survival and associated risk factors of selective caries removal treatments in primary teeth: A retrospective study in a high caries risk population. *Caries Res.* 51: 466–474.

Owen, M., Ghanim, A., Elsby, D., and Manton, D. Hypomineralised second primary molars: Prevalence, defect characteristics and relationship with dental caries in Melbourne preschool children. *Aust. Dent. J.* Accepted Author Manuscript. doi: 10.1111/adj.12567.

Public Health England. Delivering better oral health: An evidence-based toolkit for prevention Third edition. https://www.gov.uk/government/uploads/system/uploads/attachment_data/file/605266/Delivering_better_oral_health.pdf. (accessed October 2017).

Scottish Dental Clinical Effectiveness Programme (SDCEP). (2018). Prevention and Management of Dental Caries in Children, 2e.

Vanderas, A.P., Manetas, C., Koulatzidou, M., and Papagiannoulis, L. (2003). Progression of proximal caries in the mixed dentition: A 4-year prospective study. *Pediatr. Dent.* 25: 229–234.

World Health Organisation. (2012). Oral health factsheet. http://www.who.int/mediacentre/factsheets/fs318/en (accessed March 2016).

Wright, J., Tampi, M., Graham, L., Estrich, C., Crall, J.J., Fontana, M., Gillette, E.J., Nový, B.B., Dhar, V., Donly, K., Hewlett, E.R., Quinonez, R.B., Chaffin, J., Crespin, M., Iafolla, T., Siegal, M.D., and Carrasco-Labra, A. (2016). Sealants for preventing and arresting pit-and-fissure occlusal caries in primary and permanent molars; a systematic review. *J. Am. Dent. Assoc.* 147: 631–645.

12

Minimally Invasive Dentistry in Orthodontics

Tarek EL-Bialy

Key Topics

- Traditional orthodontics (diagnosis and treatment planning)
- Side effects in orthodontics
- New technologies in orthodontics (diagnosis and treatment options)
- How new technologies in orthodontics help achieving minimally invasive orthodontics
- Summary and future of orthodontics

Learning Objectives

- Be able to aware of the evolution of orthodontics and to diagnose and manage someone malocclusion
- Be able to diagnosis and give advice on orthodontic treatment to someone with craniofacial disorders
- Be able to identify problems of retreatment and avoiding side effects
- Be able to identify patients for specific orthodontic treatment

Introduction

Orthodontics (Orthos = Straight, odous, odont = teeth in Greek language), also called orthodontia, is the dental specialty and practice of preventing and correcting irregularities of the teeth, as by the use of orthodontic appliances either removable or fixed orthodontic appliances (fixed braces). Orthodontics started as an independent specialty by Edward Hartley Angle who founded the Angle School of Orthodontia in St. Louis in 1899 and schools in other regions of the United States. The initial orthodontic appliances proposed by Angle included gold wires, headgears, and removable appliances (Figure 12.1) (Matasa and Graber 2000).

Minimally Invasive Dentistry: Interdisciplinary Clinical and Scientific Approaches, First Edition.
Edited by Aylin Baysan and Paul Anderson.
© 2026 John Wiley & Sons Ltd. Published 2026 by John Wiley & Sons Ltd.
Companion website: www.wiley.com/go/baysan/minimally_invasive_dentistry

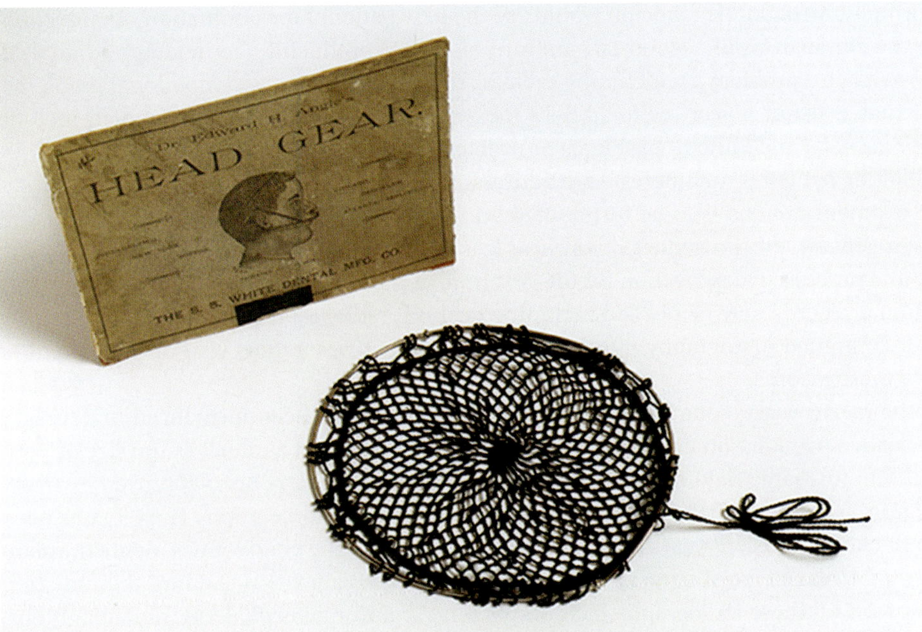

Figure 12.1 Headgear and head cap as proposed and used by Angle, in 1900s.

In 1930, Tweed introduced first bracket system with rectangular slot that can house rectangular wires for controlling tooth position in three dimensions of space. Since then many developments in the field of orthodontics from diagnostic tools including lateral cephalometric radiographs and many cephalometric analyses have been introduced in the field of orthodontics with the intention to provide a diagnostic set up for orthodontic treatment plan that cannot only improves teeth position and bite, but also to improve facial aesthetics of the teeth and face altogether.

New Technologies in Orthodontics (Diagnosis and Treatment Options)

Traditionally, orthodontic diagnosis and treatment planning included stone dental study casts and in difficult cases stone model diagnostic set up as well as lateral cephalometric radiograph/analysis, panoramic radiographs, full mouth periapical radiographs, and in cases with transverse problems, frontal or also known as postero-anterior cephalometric radiographs are to be taken and analyzed. Due to the known limitations of panoramic radiographs that include magnification distortions that is very sensitive to patient positioning in the radiographic machine and also ghost images, superimposition of different structures on top of each other makes the use of panoramic radiographs limited to be a screening not a diagnostic tool. Periapical radiographic films as well suffer from magnification distortion and being a two-dimensional radiograph, normally many information about tissues in the buccal and lingual sides to be missed or poorly diagnosed.

Normally, orthodontic clinician would see the new patient for examination, then records then the clinician would spend fair amount of time reproducing the models and analyse them to reach a problem list including skeletal, dental, soft tissue, and functional problems. After that, a list of objectives to address these problems to be formulated which include wither accept some difficult problems or problems that are seen or diagnosed by the clinician but the patient is not interested in addressing these problems. Then a list of an alternative treatment options is to be formulated and presented to the patient at a consultation visit. In general, this procedure involves at least three visits assuming that the records are done and processed to perfection for the first time, if the clinical find out that in some cases additional records may be needed including occlusal radiograph and regular tomography and or computed tomography may be needed. This involves a third visit of the patient to obtain these records.

In the recent years, cone beam computed tomography has been introduced in dentistry specifically low radiation dose and different fields of view from as small as the size of periapical film to a large field of view including the whole skull have been approved by many regulatory bodies in North America. Cone beam computed tomography (CBCT) has been the best choice in recent years in many dental fields including endodontics, dental implantology, oral/maxillofacial surgery, and orthodontics (El-Bialy 2013). Adding the radiation exposure of all these radiographs including lateral and frontal cephalometric radiographs, panoramic radiographs, and periapical radiographs are collectively higher radiation exposure than the available contemporary CBCT radiographic units.

The advantages of new CBCT machines in orthodontics include but not limited to the followings: 1) evaluation of alveolar bone widths in three dimensions (labio-lingual, mesio-distal, and occlusogingival) around each tooth, a feature that can be viewed by regular panoramic, cephalometric, occlusal, or periapical radiographs (Figure 12.2); 2) evaluation

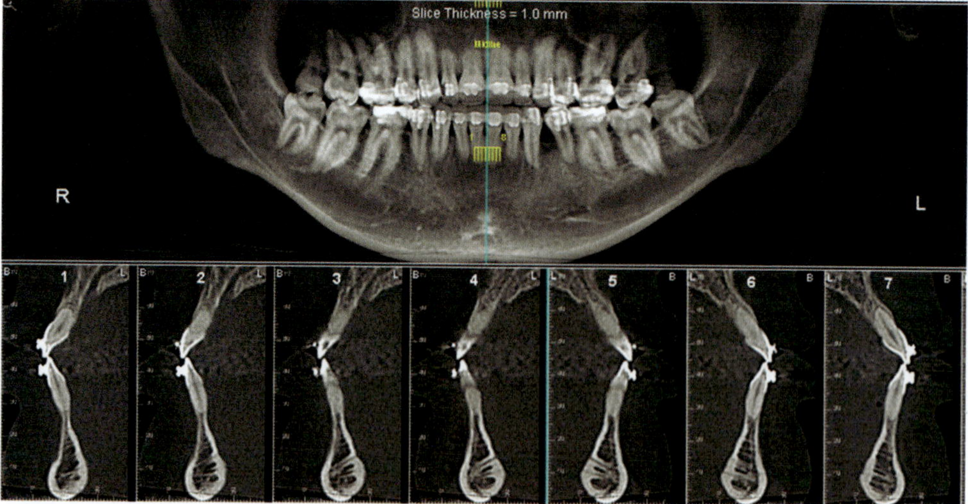

Figure 12.2 A panoramic X-ray for a patient (top) showing normal alveolar bone, while sagittal screenshots driven from CBCT (bottom) showing severe resorption of the alveolar bone labial and lingual that compromises the crown/root ratio.

of the temporomandibular joint (TMJ), which helps clinicians identifying if there is a shift between centric relation (CR) of the condyle within the TMJ and centric occlusion (CO) or not. Normally CO should be coincident with CR; and 3) airway evaluation. CBCT provide more information than regular X-rays about airway, especially when the patients have sleep disorder in combination with recessive upper and/or lower jaws; 4) better evaluation of root resorption and crown to root ratio (Alqerban et al. 2011); 5) evaluation of patients asymmetry better than regular postero-anterior or frontal cephalometric radiographs (Damstra et al. 2013); 6) possible measure changes of orthodontic and or orthognathic surgical treatment in three dimensions and possibly reproduce a 3D study models without the need to take impressions or scans to produce dental models (Luu et al. 2014).

Transitionally and still, many orthodontists still use dental stone study casts for treatment planning orthodontic cases. Issues with dental stone costs not only hard to produce (gagging induced impressions need to be taken in majority of cases) and requires a dirty lab to produce and afterwards require storage that many orthodontists suffer from its increasing cost of storing stone models over many years after finishing orthodontic treatment to cover any malpractice litigations that might appear after 15–25 years of finishing orthodontic cases. New and minimal invasive techniques to produce digital models including high speed digital scanners have been introduced in the last decade that has been improved to about one minute scan for both upper and lower arches to produce digital models that can be analysed with high accuracy like data obtained from stone models (Luu et al. 2014; Koretsi et al. 2017; Aragón et al. 2016). Digital impression is by far minimally invasive technique compared to traditional impression techniques using alginate or rubber base impression materials.

How New Technologies in Orthodontics Help Achieving Minimally Invasive Orthodontics

In the past few decades, changes in types of orthodontic bracket systems has increased exponentially. Literally, every year at the American Association of Orthodontists meeting and other large dental/orthodontic meetings, most companies have to come up with a new product to differentiate themselves from other competitors. Either there is a real need of the practitioners for newly introduced bracket system or materials or not, companies have been competing with each other by introducing new products. Most recent bracket systems that have been introduced are self-ligating brackets with aim to reduce treatment time, more hygienic, and may make orthodontic offices more profitable. However, a recent systematic review has shown that this is not true (Ehsani et al. 2009). In general, all fixed orthodontic appliances regardless of their being regular or self-ligating systems, directly bonded or indirectly bonded/delivered to teeth, suffer from common complications. These complications include but not limited to white spot lesions, decalcification, poor oral hygiene, and gingivitis/periodontitis, trauma from pocking wires or broken brackets and root resorption. Root resorption mainly happened due to the fact that orthodontic forces delivered through all fixed appliances are considered as undetermined system. This is simply because regardless of the ample evidence about force delivery by different archwires, the exact forces and moments applied to each tooth cannot be precisely determined due to variability of teeth dimensions (crowns, roots) as well as level of bone surrounding the involved roots. A new orthodontic appliance that can precisely control forces applied to each tooth is highly needed based on a comprehensive cone beam computed tomography evaluation and calculation of each tooth root volume as well as volume of invested bone. Another factor is the thickness and stiffness of the periodontal ligament which also affects the transmissibility of the forces to alveolar bone. The closest to this system nowadays is the Invisalign system. Using Invisalign, the amount of force can be determined, changing the rate of tooth movement for each individual tooth or restricting tooth movement is an option that can be performed using the Invisalign system. However, future development of the system to provide an individualised force system still yet to be available.

Anchorage

Anchorage in orthodontics is another challenge since the inception of orthodontics especially when considering space closure either after extraction of teeth or closing existing spaces. First reported appliances to control anchorage was headgear as introduced by Angle, 1990. Compliance with headgear wearing is not always the best and may have never reached 100% regardless of how the patient is compliant or committed to finish his/her treatment faster. Over the last few decades, many non-compliance appliances have been introduced for example for maxillary molar distalisation, pendulum appliance for example has been introduced and extensively studied. Recent review of the efficacy of this device has shown that loss of anchorage occurred which negates the purpose of its use (Kinzinger et al. 2008).

Temporary anchorage devices (TADs) has been introduced many years ago but in the last few decades has been re-introduced with different shapes, dimensions, with aim to provide non-compliance devices that can produce maximum anchorage to retract, protract teeth, or the whole jaw if needed. However, the efficiency of these TADs have been reported in addition to their invasive procedures that make them not immune from complications (Reynders et al. 2009).

Restricting tooth movement of some teeth is doable suing clear aligners like Invisalign system. It is doable to move one single tooth using the rest of the entire dental arch as an anchorage in three dimension. For example, it is doable to distalise one single tooth, upper second molar for example to achieve class I correction then continuous anchorage levels can be achieved by reprograming anchorage within or between both arches. Changing moment to force ratio for a tooth or group of teeth is doable using Invisalign system, hence providing maximum anchorage can be done without the need for TADs or other similar invasive orthodontic appliance or auxiliaries.

Dentofacial Orthopedics

Dentofacial orthopedics has been proposed long time ago and hence the American Journal of Orthodontics has changed its name to the American Journal of Orthodontics and Dentofacial Orthopedics because of the commonly believed that there are group of appliances that can or may change or modify the growth amount and/or direction or either or both jaws during the growth period of growing patients or in some cases even after the growth period (in adults). Some of these appliances are widely used in orthodontic practice these days like Herbst appliance, face mask, headgears, etc. (Von Bremen et al. 2014; Ruf and Pancherz 2004, 2006). As mentioned before, removable appliance including all functional appliances and or headgears suffer from major issue in achieving the proposed treatment, is patient compliance. Also, major removable functional orthopedic appliances are bulky and patients cannot speak while wearing these appliances. Fixed functional appliances on the other hand suffer from many other complications that have been documents in the literature (Wiechmann et al. 2015). A minimal invasive mandibular forward positioning or growth modification appliance or complication free appliance is yet to be available for both patients and clinicians.

New Invisalign modification feature has incorporated upper and lower inclined wings that can provide progressive mandibular advancement during growing patients to allow for mandibular advancement or commonly known as growth modification. Although this modified Invisalign aligner is still in experimental or trial stage, it seems promising but still has the disadvantage of being a removable appliance that requires patient's cooperation. Regardless, this device is less bulky compared to other available functional appliances like Twin Block, activator, bionator, or other similar devices.

Accelerated Tooth Movement

Over the last few decades, there have been many devices or techniques that have been introduced to accelerate tooth movement with the intention that orthodontic treatment time can be shortened so that patients can have minimum complications including white spot lesions, gingivitis/periodontitis, and or root resorption. Many of the reported techniques are invasive which include corticotomy, surgical flap, and or micro-osteoperofration (Alikhani et al. 2013; Tsai et al. 2016). Also, low frequency and high frequency devices have been introduced to accelerate tooth movement as minimal invasive techniques. A recent review has shown that low frequency vibration is not effective in accelerating tooth movement (Uribe et al. 2017).

Two new techniques have been introduced recently that are non-invasive and have shown effectiveness in accelerating tooth movement. These are light emitting diodes (LED) (Cruz et al. 2004) and low intensity pulsed ultrasound (LIPUS) (Al-Daghreer et al. 2014). LIPUS also has been reported to minimise orthodontically induced tooth root resorption, which is unavoidable side effect of orthodontic treatment (Al-Daghreer et al. 2014; Raza et al. 2016).

Summary

Minimally invasive techniques in orthodontics at this time include the following:

1. Digital scan of teeth to produce diagnostic orthodontic models;
2. Cone bean computed tomography that can provide better diagnosis and effective treatment planning;

3. The use of minimal invasive orthodontic appliances like clear aligners, especially the highly developed Invisalign aligners;
4. The use of auxiliary systems or techniques to minimise side effect and in the same time accelerate orthodontic tooth movement like low intensity pulsed ultrasound (LIPUS).

References

Al-Daghreer, S., Doschak, M.R., Sloane, A.J., Major, P.W., Heo, G., Scurtescu, C., Tsui, Y.Y., and El-Bialy, T. (2014). Effect of LIPUS on orthodontically induced root resorption in Beagle dogs. *Ultrasound Med. Biol.* 40: 1187–1196.

Alikhani, M., Raptis, M., Zoldan, B., Sangsuwon, C., Lee, Y.B., Alyami, B., Corpodian, C., Barrera, L.M., Alansari, S., Khoo, E., and Teixeira, C. (2013). Effect of microosteoperforations on the rate of tooth movement. *Am. J. Orthod. Dentofacial Orthop.* 144: 639–648.

Alqerban, A., Jacobs, R., Fieuws, S., Nackaerts, O., and Willems, G. (2011). Comparison of 6 cone-beam computed tomography systems for image quality and detection of simulated canine impaction-induced external root resorption in maxillary lateral incisors. *Am. J. Orthod. Dentofacial Orthop.* 140: e129–139.

Aragón, M.L., Pontes, L.F., Bichara, L.M., Flores-Mir, C., and Normando, D. (2016). Validity and reliability of intraoral scanners compared to conventional gypsum models measurements: A systematic review. *Eur. J. Orthod.* 38: 429–434.

Cruz, D.R., Kohara, E.K., Ribeiro, M.S., and Wetter, N.U. (2004). Effects of low-intensity laser therapy on the orthodontic movement velocity of human teeth: A preliminary study. *Lasers Surg. Med.* 35: 117–120.

Damstra, J., Fourie, Z., and Ren, Y. (2013). Evaluation and comparison of postero-anterior cephalograms and cone-beam computed tomography images for the detection of mandibular asymmetry. *Eur. J. Orthod.* 35: 45–50.

Ehsani, S., Mandich, M.A., El-Bialy, T.H., and Flores-Mir, C. (2009). Frictional resistance in self-ligating orthodontic brackets and conventionally ligated brackets. *Angle Orthod.* 79: 592–601.

El-Bialy, T. (2013). Cone-beam Computed Tomography (CBCT) an Essential for Proper Orthodontic Diagnosis and Treatment Planning, 241–254. *Hauppauge NY, USA: Computed Tomography: New Research Editor: Jae Hyun Park*; Nova Science Publishers, Inc.

Kinzinger, G.S., Eren, M., and Diedrich, P.R. (2008). Treatment effects of intraoral appliances with conventional anchorage designs for non-compliance maxillary molar distalization: A literature review. *Eur. J. Orthod.* 30: 558–571.

Koretsi, V., Tingelhoff, L., Proff, P., and Kirschneck, C. (2017). Intra-observer reliability and agreement of manual and digital orthodontic model analysis. *Eur. J. Orthod.* 22. doi: 10.1093/ejo/cjx040.

Luu, N.S., Mandich, M.-A., Flores-Mir, C., El-Bialy, T., Heo, G., Carey, J.P., and Major, P.W. (2014). The validity, reliability and time requirement of study model analysis using conebeam computed tomography generated virtual study models. *Orthod. Craniofac. Res.* 17: 14–26.

Matasa, C.G., and Graber, T.M. (2000). Angle, the innovator, mechanical genius, and clinician. *Am. J. Orthod. Dentofacial Orthop.* 117: 444–452.

Raza, H., Major, P.W., Dederich, D., and El-Bialy, T. (2016). Effect of low intensity pulsed ultrasound on orthodontically induced root resorption caused by torque: A prospective double blind controlled clinical trial. *Angle Orthod.* 35: 349–358.

Reynders, R., Ronchi, L., and Bipat, S. (2009). Mini-implants in orthodontics: A systematic review of the literature. *Am. J. Orthod. Dentofacial Orthop.* 135: 564.e1–19.

Ruf, S., and Pancherz, H. (2004). Orthognathic surgery and dentofacial orthopedics in adult Class II Division 1 treatment: Mandibular sagittal split osteotomy versus Herbst appliance. *Am. J. Orthod. Dentofacial. Orthop.* 126: 140–152.

Ruf, S., and Pancherz, H. (2006). Herbst/multibracket appliance treatment of Class II division 1 malocclusions in early and late adulthood. A prospective cephalometric study of consecutively treated subjects. *Eur. J. Orthod.* 28: 352–360.

Tsai, C.Y., Yang, T.K., Hsieh, H.Y., and Yang, L.Y. (2016). Comparison of the effects of microosteoperforation and corticision on the rate of orthodontic tooth movement in rats. *Angle Orthod.* 86: 558–564.

Uribe, F., Dutra, E., and Chandhoke, T. (2017). Effect of cyclical forces on orthodontic tooth movement, from animals to humans. *Orthod. Craniofac. Res.* 20 (Suppl 1): 68–71.

Von Bremen, J., Erbe, C., Pancherz, H., and Ruf, S. (2014). Facial-profile attractiveness changes in adult patients treated with the Herbst appliance. *J. Orofac. Orthop.* 75: 167–174.

Wiechmann, D., Vu, J., Schwestka-Polly, R., Helms, H.J., and Knösel, M. (2015). Clinical complications during treatment with a modified Herbst appliance in combination with a lingual appliance. *Head Face Med.* 11: 31. doi: 10.1186/s13005-015-0088-3.

Index

Note: Page numbers in "*italics*" represents figures and "**bold**" represents table in text.